AF780966

THE POLITICS OF SOCIAL, ECOLOGICAL, AND STRUCTURAL DETERMINANTS OF HEALTH IN CANADA

THE POLITICS OF SOCIAL, ECOLOGICAL, AND STRUCTURAL DETERMINANTS OF HEALTH IN CANADA

Elizabeth McGibbon

CANADIAN SCHOLARS
Toronto | Vancouver

The Politics of Social, Ecological, and Structural Determinants of Health in Canada
Elizabeth McGibbon

First published in 2024 by
Canadian Scholars, an imprint of CSP Books Inc.
180 Bloor Street West, Suite 1401
Toronto, Ontario
M5S 2V6

www.canadianscholars.ca

Library and Archives Canada Cataloguing in Publication

Title: The politics of social, ecological, and structural determinants of health in Canada / Elizabeth McGibbon.
Names: McGibbon, Elizabeth Anne, 1955- author.
Series: Politics of health series.
Description: Series statement: The politics of health series | Includes bibliographical references and index.
Identifiers: Canadiana (print) 20240414284 | Canadiana (ebook) 20240414322 | ISBN 9781773384443 (softcover) | ISBN 9781773384467 (EPUB) | ISBN 9781773384450 (PDF)
Subjects: LCSH: Public health—Social aspects—Canada. | LCSH: Public health—Political aspects—Canada. | LCSH: Public health—Environmental aspects—Canada. | LCSH: Equality—Health aspects—Canada.
Classification: LCC RA418.3.C3 M38 2024 | DDC 362.10971—dc23

Cover photo by Alexander Raphael
Cover design by Lizzie Di Giacomo
Page layout by S4Carlisle Publishing Services
Printed and bound by CPI Group (UK) Ltd, Croydon, CR0 4YY

EU Authorized Representative: Mare Nostrum Group B.V., Mauritskade 21D, 1091 GC Amsterdam, The Netherlands, gpsr@mare-nostrum.co.uk.

Canadä

CONTENTS

INTRODUCTION TO THE POLITICS OF HEALTH SERIES

It is becoming increasingly evident that the sources of health, as well as inequities in health—the unfair and avoidable differences in health outcomes—are primarily due to how resources are distributed among a society's members. These resources include economic resources, such as income and wealth, and social resources, such as access to social services, health care, employment, housing, and food, as well as the power and influence to shape the legislation and regulations that distribute these same resources.

Increasingly, attention is also being directed to economic and political systems and the transnational global capitalist system and how the making of public policy is embedded within these systems. This type of analysis looks at the societal structures and processes that determine how public policy enacted by governing authorities shapes the quality and distribution of these resources. Such an analysis is far more useful than discredited approaches that focus on so-called healthy behaviours and lifestyle choices as the determinants of health.

This structural analysis of society therefore draws attention to how public policy shapes the quality and distribution of the social determinants of health—the living and working conditions that are the primary determinants of people's health. But it goes deeper. A structural analysis also looks at the politics of health—how issues of power and influence skew the making of public policy either in the service of or to the detriment of health. The politics of health therefore focuses on political ideologies held by governing authorities as well as the public; political parties and their positions; and the politics of everyday life—that is, how these ideologies and political parties shape the living and working conditions that lead to health or illness.

In this third volume of this series, *The Politics of Social, Ecological, and Structural Determinants of Health in Canada*, Elizabeth McGibbon of St. Francis Xavier University takes a novel approach towards understanding these influences upon health by developing a three-pronged analysis of the factors that shape health. Social Determinants of Health include the now commonly accepted—though little acted upon by governing authorities—classic factors of housing, health care services, food security, living wage, and education; isms of ableism, ageism, classism, genderism, and racism; and geographies of built environments such as segregation, ghettoization, and toxic dump locations, among others.

Ecological Determinants of Health are clearly linked to their structural drivers. These determinants include pollution, ecotoxicity, and environmental racism; resource extraction and depletion; climate and atmospheric emergency; desertification and deforestation; ocean and soil acidification; biodiversity loss, species endangerment, and extinction.

Structural Determinants of Health are the less commonly considered factors associated with political-economic determinants of health such as neoliberal epidemics and neoliberal global capitalism; worker unionization rates; commercial and corporate determinants of health; digital determinants of health; colonialism, white supremacy, social murder, necropolitics, and slow violence.

Professor McGibbon's wide lens for understanding the determinants of health therefore offers a profoundly new way of understanding the forces that are shaping our health. It also suggests what needs to be done to respond to these forces by proving examples from across the globe of people, groups, and social and political movements mobilizing for health. The breadth of Professor McGibbon's work is sure to provoke reflection and discussion. Hopefully, it will also provoke action in the service of health.

Like the first two volumes in this series—*The Politics of Health in the Canadian Welfare State* by Toba Bryant of Ontario Tech University and Dennis Raphael of York University, and *The Politics of Dental Care in Canada*, by Carlos Quiñonez of the University of Toronto—this volume will be of special interest to practising and aspiring health care and social service professionals in a variety of fields—dentistry, health care, medicine, public health, social work, and nursing—and policymakers and policy analysts in governments, non-governmental organizations, and advocacy groups, as well as the public. The social, environmental, and structural forces adversely affecting our health must be identified and then responded to. Considering how these deteriorating social, ecological, and structural determinants of health are impacting our lives, governing authorities' continuing disregard of these developments is not acceptable.

We invite readers to contribute to the Politics of Health Series by submitting manuscripts exploring issues aligned with their interests and expertise but that are consistent with the series' aim of transforming the ways Canadians think about the health of Canadians. This series seeks to raise awareness of how broader societal forces—especially politics in Canada—promote as well as threaten health. By becoming aware of these issues, Canadians will gain the means of responding to them, thereby promoting health. The alternative is to continue ineffective and wasteful approaches to promoting health that not only divert attention from the important causes of ill health but also make the improvement of health more difficult.

Dennis Raphael, Series Editor
February 2024

PREFACE

The origins of this book are many and varied. I stand on the shoulders of my colleagues, in academia as well as in many other spaces, who, like me, are in a perpetual state of outrage about the entirely preventable unfairness of public policy–created poverty, unhappiness, and dwindling chances for achieving "the good life" that we all deserve and wish for ourselves, our families, and all our people. Howard Zinn (1922–2010), American historian, playwright, philosopher, socialist intellectual, World War II veteran, and civil rights activist in the Southern United States, championed an approach to history from the bottom up or from the perspective of "the people." His autobiography *You Can't Be Neutral on a Moving Train* has long been an inspiration for me. Most importantly, Zinn's explanation of the myth of neutrality gave me a way to reframe the constant presence of neoliberal global capitalism's assault on humans, all life on Earth, and planet Earth itself. If there is a debate about whether or not the train should be stopped to avoid an imminent crash, it is impossible to be "neutral" because silence is assent—the train will just keep going towards its crash. In the presence of this faux neutrality, opposing opinions very often sound "biased." Zinn told his students that he did not "pretend to an objectivity that was neither possible nor desirable. 'You can't be neutral on a moving train,' I would tell them. . . Events are already moving in certain deadly directions, and to be neutral means to accept that" (Taylor, 2018).

The goal of this book is to trace politics to the on-the-ground outcomes of inequities in the social, ecological, and structural determinants of health (DoH). The aim is to present a justice-minded critical perspective, not to provide an overview of all perspectives. There is already an abundance of "neutral" information about the benefits of neoliberal capitalism, if the reader should want to engage with it. Here, the stance of writing is intentionally from a critical perspective, one that focuses on societal, cultural, economic, and political power—who has it, how they "get it and keep it," and how power can be redistributed for a just world.

The chapters are stand-alone; however, there is consistent reference to other chapters throughout the book. This process is a necessary step in maintaining the logical flow of the complex topics that are explored in the book. The objectives at the beginning of each chapter closely match the chapter content. Critical thinking questions are broader and meant to stimulate discussion and debate. Each chapter has a glossary based on key words in the chapter. I have chosen the location of the bolded glossary terms to best fit the description of the terms, rather than sequentially as they first appear.

The book was a challenge to write due to the synergistic nature of the social, ecological, and structural DoH. The end result is an intentional and systematic integration of all three DoH areas in each chapter. Chapter 1 introduces the main ideas in the book, including a brief introduction to the usefulness of a complex adaptive systems (CAS) approach to framing the DoH. Complexity science is increasingly being used as a core application for disentangling the polycrisis of current inequities in the social, ecological, and structural DoH. The fields of environmental sciences are becoming especially known for their detailed complexity applications in the face of alarming (not too strong a word these days) climate emergency changes. Chapter 2 is the result of the first round of proposal reviews for the book. Reviewers correctly suggested that a policy analysis frame needed to be made clear early in the book. Public and other forms of policy are central root causes of inequities, so Chapter 2 policy knowledge is integrated throughout the book.

Chapter 3 is about the social DoH, again explained through the lens of criticality. The "social determinants of health" is now the academic and public policy version of "a household word." Yet, the term still proliferates amidst worsening health outcomes for the marginalized and the racialized. This disconnect is analyzed, along with persistent evidence of inequities in equitable access across intersections of the social DoH. Chapter 4 focuses on the ecological DoH. It layers critical lenses within the sciences and social sciences of the Anthropocene(s), demonstrating the breadth and depth of the current polycrisis. Chapter 5 analyzes the structural DoH, another contested area with variations ranging from micro (one's social environments) to macro, where the beneficiaries of increasing poverty and climate damage are exposed, as well as the problems caused by capitalism, especially inequality, exploitation, and alienation. The chapter emphasizes the structural violence of social murder, necropolitics, and slow violence.

Chapter 6 revisits complexity science with more detailed descriptions of CAS characteristics and two direct applications: the Alberta Tar Sands and the COVID-19 pandemic. Chapter 7 integrates the ideas throughout the book, with a focus on citizen mobilization and global alternatives to neoliberal capitalism, including alternative political economies. Explanatory, solution-focused approaches, such as Gene Sharpe's 198 Methods for nonviolent action and Gaventa's power cube, are detailed with the goal of providing concrete pathways to enact change for tacking the current global polycrisis.

REFERENCES

Taylor, K-Y. (2018). Foreword. In H. Zinn, *You can't be neutral on a moving train: A personal history*. Beacon Press.

ACKNOWLEDGEMENTS

I thank my loving family. Pat Gardner, partner in all things life, who has been unwaveringly along for the journey for almost 40 years. We have always been on the same page politically, sharing our outrage at the "way things are." Our children, the firstborn, Case Eugenie Gardner, has been on their own journey for justice since at least Grade 6, when they were told that they couldn't take a lead singing role in the school's holiday performance because they were "too short." "And what about the people in wheelchairs?" was their response—the beginning of a lifelong dedication to speaking out for justice. Sophie Margaret McGibbon, born in a big storm, has also carved a life of speaking out for justice, integrating union activism alongside all things personal and science-bound. These two beautiful humans make me ever hopeful that a just and compassionate world is at hand. They are a joyful outcome of "radicalizing the kid's table."

I thank Dr. Dennis Raphael for his ongoing support of my work, including the invitation to write this book for his Politics of Health series. I also thank Dr. Barry Lavallee (MD), a member of the Métis community of St. Laurent, Manitoba, and a descendent of Duck Bay and Lake Manitoba First Nations. He has quietly and steadfastly supported key pieces of my work since the first publication of the Oppression book in 2012 (*Oppression: A Social Determinant of Health*), and this support has meant a great deal to me.

Finally, I thank Caitlin Winter of Canadian Scholars for her steadfast support throughout the creation of this book, and Nikki Bell-Morrison for her first-rate copyediting. This book was largely written in Mi'kma'ki, the ancestral and unceded territory of the Mi'kmaq People. Per the IWK Foundation (n.d)., "This territory is covered by the 'Treaties of Peace and Friendship' which Mi'kmaq Wəlastəkwiyik (Maliseet), and Passamaquoddy Peoples first signed with the British Crown in 1726. The treaties did not deal with surrender of lands and resources but in fact recognized Mi'kmaq and Wəlastəkwiyik (Maliseet) title and established the rules for what was to be an ongoing relationship between nations."

REFERENCES

IWK Foundation. (n.d.). *Land acknowledgement.* https://iwkfoundation.org/land-acknowledgement

CHAPTER 1

How Politics are Determinants of Health

CHAPTER OBJECTIVES

Using as many examples as possible:

1. Explain what is meant by the overall term "determinants of health."
2. Describe the relationship between politics and health.
3. Describe at least three examples of the root determinants of health.
4. List and describe examples of the three areas of the Root Determinants of Health Framework: social determinants of health, ecological determinants of health, and structural determinants of health.
5. Explain why it is not possible to derive static, rigid definitions of the determinants of health.

CRITICAL THINKING QUESTIONS

1. What is meant by Stevens and Hall's (1992) claim that "All research, theory, policy, and practice are political because they are intimately affected by the social, economic, and political processes of the society"?
2. How would you explain the claim that "it is racism, not race, that socially determines health outcomes"?
3. How are the social DoH connected to the structural DoH?
4. How are the ecological DoH connected to the structural DoH?
5. How does this chapter help to explore Aesop's story about "belling the cat"?

INTRODUCTION

> Long ago, the mice had a general council to consider what measures they could take to outwit their common enemy, the Cat. Some said this, and some said that; but at last a young mouse got up and said she had a proposal to make, which she thought would meet the case. "You will all agree," said she, "that our chief danger consists in the sly and treacherous manner in which the enemy approaches us. Now, if we could receive some signal of their approach, we could easily escape from them. I venture, therefore, to propose that a small bell be procured, and attached by a ribbon round the neck of the Cat. By this means we should always know when the Cat was about and could easily retire while they were in the neighborhood." This proposal met with general applause, until an old mouse got up and said: "That is all very well, but who is to bell the cat?" (Blair, 2004)

Understanding how politics are determinants of health (DoH) is all about belling the cat—naming and analyzing the connections between public policy and governance choices and population health outcomes. Through case studies, and numerous other examples and applications, this book demonstrates how health-damaging public policies happen in a "sly and treacherous" manner through largely hidden processes. The overall aim of the book is to demonstrate how these DoH shape, and actually determine, health. This chapter begins with a discussion of foundational ideas about the DoH, emphasizing the limitations of individualistic and behavioural perspectives about health. Politics, power, and the DoH are explained in terms of how health outcomes are, for better or for worse, the results of structural, political choices.

These **structural DoH**, described further in the chapter, are referred to as root causes, often described as the "cause-of-the-causes" of worsening health outcomes for marginalized and racialized peoples across the globe as well as for planet Earth. A Root Determinants of Health Framework is introduced to explain the connections among the **social DoH**, **ecological DoH**, and structural DoH. Each of these areas is briefly described to set the groundwork for the following chapters. At the same time, readers will gain a better sense of who is benefiting from health and social inequities, and how power, privilege, dominance, and wealth are sustained over time. This knowledge will provide readers with effective tools to address and ultimately challenge and disrupt political choices that continue to create and sustain health-damaging inequities across the DoH. The chapter concludes with a brief explanation of how the social, ecological, and structural DoH form a **complex adaptive system** (CAS). Complexity science framings of the DoH are increasingly recognized as a necessary footing for understanding the multitude of changing contexts and variables that inform our comprehension of inequities across the DoH. Most importantly, a CAS approach provides clear entry points for tackling the polycrisis that is deepening inequities across the social, ecological, and structural DoH.

DETERMINANTS OF HEALTH: FOUNDATIONAL IDEAS

What are the Determinants of Health?

Health is most often seen as an overall descriptor for our sense of well-being, including physical, mental, and spiritual well-being. Furthermore, "health" often infers individual health, such as absence of disease. However, copious evidence demonstrates that health is much more than only the absence of individual ill health (World Health Organization [WHO], n.d., 2008). Health can also refer to collective aspects of health, such as a family's or community's overall health. More and more, these aspects of health are seen as also connected to planet health. The question then becomes, what shapes or determines health? There have been major advances in the ways that health is framed and understood and the focus is increasingly on what factors and influences actually determine health. This thinking rests on century-old insights, research, and theoretical developments about how, along with biological determinants, health is also powerfully determined by one's social, economic, and political contexts throughout the lifecourse. These contexts are often referred to as the **politics of health**.

However, there is still considerable resistance to the integration or synthesis of the two fields of politics and health. Researchers, practitioners, and policymakers in the health fields have generally not had the opportunity to learn about or explicitly integrate politics in their thinking or their work. The strong dominance of biomedical models of health continues to be a major barrier, due to its focus on the individual body, individual body parts, and related beliefs that introducing social and political contexts also introduces unacceptable bias in assessment, intervention, policymaking, education, and research. One of the main challenges in understanding the politics of health is that even the mention of politics is disconcerting for some, because discussions of politics necessarily infers an opinion about situations such as increasing, and some would say alarming, health and social inequities—and especially what causes these inequities in the first place. These opinions thus become tethered to the politics of what causes inequities—to talk about the politics of health means talking about root causes, such as the decisions made by particular governments and other governance structures. Root-cause discussions then lead us directly to politics and power so that we can name and change these unfair and unjust structures in the interest of equitable redistribution of resources to achieve health-for-all.

POLITICS, POWER, AND THE DETERMINANTS OF HEALTH

Politics and power are the foundations that determine health. Humans and all living things on Earth cannot stay healthy, or even become healthy, unless inequities in these determinants and their root causes are named and tackled. Individualistic, behavioural perspectives about health keep the analysis, and hence the solutions, at the micro level—for example, within individual, human, or micro-ecosystems levels (e.g., species endangerment). In contrast, moving forward for human and planet health equity requires a focus on how health is political, including a close examination and critique of worsening health inequities across the DoH.

Limitations of Individualistic, Behavioural Perspectives about Health

With some exceptions, individualistic, behavioural perspectives about health are by far the dominant approach in health and related fields and throughout public and institutional policymaking, further described in Chapter 2. A classic example is federally funded lifestyle campaigns, such as ParticipACTION ("Encouraging people living in Canada to get healthy by getting active since 1971"), where wellness and fitness largely involve the financial resources and the free time to engage in exercise and to be outdoors, as well as to buy the most expensive food options, such as fresh fruits and vegetables. Time is a largely hidden aspect of these approaches to achieving health and well-being. Many people recognize the financial constraints of not being able to join a gym or buy healthy exercising shoes; however, time is also a precious commodity for individuals and families who live in poverty, or near poverty. As Dutch artist Willem de Kooning famously said, "The trouble with being poor is that it takes up all of your time" (AZQuotes, n.d.). Time-related barriers include not having a predictable time schedule of work if one has a job, the time and the resources to even go for an exercise-related walk if you are a lone parent, and the sheer energy it takes to find the time to exercise after a long day at a stressful, low-paying job. These health and well-being contexts are pivotal on-the-ground examples of how micro solutions, such as ParticipACTION, are unlikely to change population health outcomes because they do not integrate the politics of why some people have persistently worse health than others.

Understanding mental health struggles is often similarly confined within the limitations of individualistic, behavioural thinking. For example, 2SLGBTQIA+ (two-spirit, lesbian, gay, bisexual, trans, queer, intersex, asexual) people have disproportionately high rates of suicide when compared to the general population (Gorse, 2022). If we, including policymakers, remain stuck at the individual area of analysis/understanding, then deeply embedded societal discrimination remains hidden (e.g., racism, genderism, homophobic hatred). We essentially silence these relentless, everyday experiences of oppression as if they are happening somewhere else, or more egregiously, do not even exist.

How is Health "Political"?

There is increasingly urgent attention to political processes that determine health. The meanings of politics and policy are complex and tend to differ along political and philosophical lines. But what does "political" mean in the everyday world of thinking about health? Power and politics are central DoH, especially when we consider whether health is viewed from dominant neoliberal and biomedical perspectives or from critical perspectives. As Kickbusch (2015) points out,

> Health is a political choice, and politics is a continuous struggle for power among competing interests. Looking at health through the lens of political determinants means analyzing how different power constellations, institutions, processes, interests, and ideological positions affect health within different political systems and cultures and at different levels of governance... The key political debates in public health revolve around the primacy of economic over social policies (often referred to as neoliberalism), charity versus entitlements, and concepts of liberty. (p. 1)

Analyzing policy and politics is all about analyzing power because, as the evidence throughout this book demonstrates, different forms of power (e.g., political, economic, cultural) literally determine who lives and who dies. Kickbusch (2015) describes these forms of power as the political DoH. The term *politics* has many meanings in everyday speech and in the context of political parties and in formal governance. Politics—the process of making and executing decisions—has many political structures, such as parliaments, governments, and government ministries (Mackenbach & McKee, 2015). According to Mackenbach and McKee, political processes can include elections, lobbying, and law-making and can be characterized by, for example, their levels of democracy. Policy is thus the result of interactions among many actors and organizations with particular ideas about what course of action should be taken.

These activities are known as the policy process (Luttrell et al., 2007). Policy processes, in turn, determine public policies that have direct and indirect impacts on the health of nations, including their environmental health. As described throughout the book, the worldview or political compass of dominant political structures most potently determines health outcomes across generations. Knowledge about these political determinants, described further in Chapter 5, and the policy analysis process, described in Chapter 2, are foundations for taking action to bell the cat.

Stevens and Hall's (1992) germinal work describes the relationship between politics and health:

1. "All research, theory, policy, and practice are political because they are intimately affected by the social, economic, and political processes of the society.
2. Oppressive power relations are common in society; usually they operate without much notice and are taken for granted.
3. Scientific and practical ways of thinking and getting things done are open to systematic questioning and criticism.
4. Social, economic, and political conditions have a history.
5. One can better understand the changing conditions of society's health by studying the historical development of unsafe physical surroundings, oppressive social arrangements, economic inequities, and political disenfranchisement.
6. Liberation from oppressive environmental constraints is an indispensable part of any group's pursuit of wellbeing and integrity." (p. 203)

As Stevens and Hall (1992) point out, understanding the relationships among politics, policy, and health involves systematic questioning about "the ways things are." These political aspects of the policy environment are pivotal entry points for tackling inequities in the DoH. They include the distribution of power, the range of organizations involved and their interests, and the formal and informal rules that govern interactions among the players (Luttrell et al., 2007). Naming and understanding political conditions can expose the root causes of inequity and thus promote and provoke action for health and environmental justice.

Root Causes, Root Determinants of Health

Root cause analyses bring us directly into the realm of politics and power because they open up discussion about why some groups of people have persistently worse health across the lifecourse than others, and why some people persistently have much better health outcomes. **Root causes** refer to the social, political, economic, and cultural origins of health and social inequities, where health refers to the health of all life on Earth, including all aspects of planet Earth itself. Consideration of concepts of inequality, equality, equity, and justice (depicted in Figure 1.1) are paramount. These terms support an understanding of how disadvantage may be framed in terms of supporting, or not supporting, a root cause approach.

Inequality refers to the assumption that everyone has the opportunity to benefit from the same supports. This assumption results in public policy that supports a "one-size-fits-all" approach. For example, prenatal community care may be designed so that prenatal classes are advertised as available to everyone. This approach produces unequal access to care because it requires transportation and perhaps the money to pay for a babysitter so that parents can attend the classes. *Equality* is the related assumption that everyone is equal. Public transportation, babysitters, and so on are assumed to be available to everyone. *Equity* involves creating custom tools and mechanisms so that everyone has access to prenatal classes. An example is engaging in the important and complex planning involved in creating a fully accessible, low-cost transportation system. *Justice* is "fixing" the system (the systemic structures) to ensure equal access to the tools and mechanisms to ensure universally accessible transportation, often involving lobbying/advocating for municipal and provincial/territorial changes to existing transportation infrastructures.

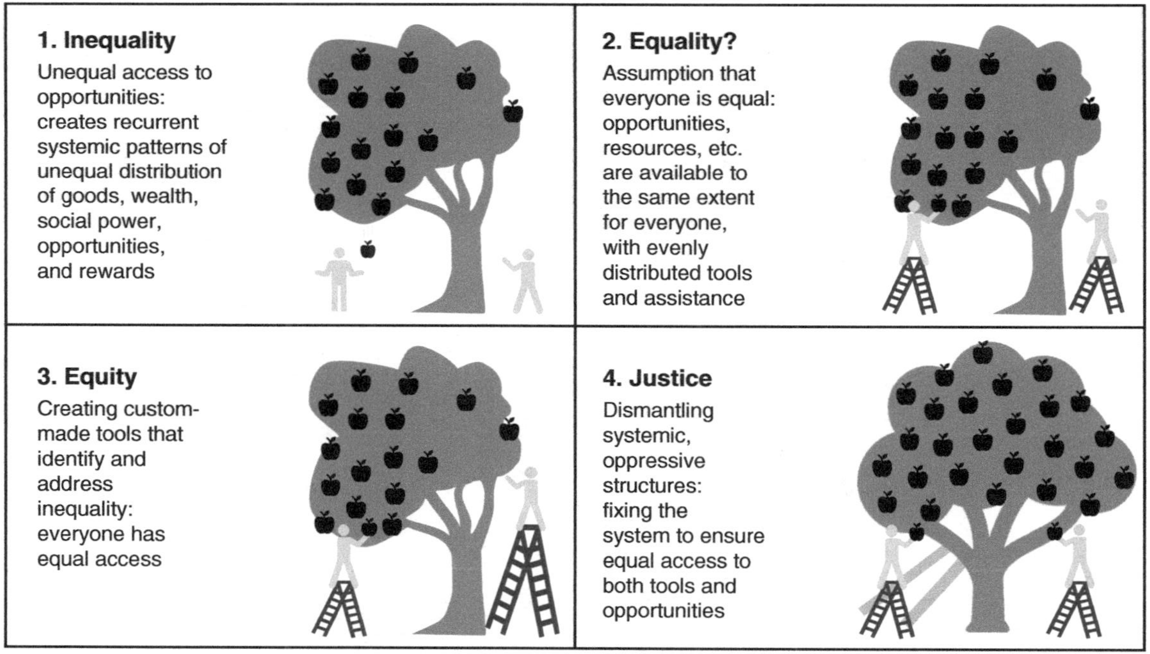

Figure 1.1: Inequality, Equality, Equity, and Justice

Source: Created by author.

Incidence of Asthma: A Root Determinants Example

An important example of root determinants is inequities in the incidence of childhood asthma. In urban areas, ever-increasing rates of childhood asthma are related to damp, mouldy housing, and air pollution (Mukharesh et al., 2023), but what is causing some people to be far more likely to live in these conditions? In the United States, childhood asthma is significantly higher in neighbourhoods with lower socioeconomic status and larger numbers of African-American families (Keet et al., 2015). In Canada, strong evidence supports the key role of structural DoH, such as socioeconomic and political contexts that generate social stratification and inequity in the development and progression of childhood asthma (Trachtenberg et al., 2014). Furthermore, asthma incidence is racialized, as evidenced by "increasing recognition that social DoH, including socioeconomic status, physical environment, and health care, influence racial and ethnic asthma disparities, yet little research has focused on which social DoH and to what degree social DoH are driving these disparities" (Grant et al., 2022, p. 5).

It is important to note that although a significant cause of childhood asthma is related to sub-standard housing conditions and air pollution, these living conditions are also known to be inequitably distributed across social class and **racialization** lines. Racialization is the complex and contradictory process through which some groups come to be categorized as being part of a particular "race" and, on that basis, subjected to differential and/or unequal, often discriminatory, treatment: "racialization [is] the process of manufacturing and utilizing the notion of race in any capacity" (Alberta Civil Liberties Research Centre, n.d.; Dalal, 2002, p. 27). Neighbourhood housing and air pollution rates thus intersect with classism and racism to deepen disparities in asthma incidence. The root causes of inequities in childhood asthma ("causes-of-the-causes") include systemic racism that significantly decreases chances of education and hence employment income, as well as lack of strong public policies to prevent housing insecurity (Gaetz et al., 2016).

Homeless (Unhoused) in Canada: A Root Determinants Example

Homelessness is defined as "the situation of an individual, family or community without stable, safe, permanent, appropriate housing, or the immediate prospect, means and ability of acquiring it" (Canadian

Observatory on Homelessness, n.d.). The term *homeless* is gradually being replaced by *unhoused* for a number of reasons, including the deeply derogatory and discriminatory stereotypes about people with no fixed roof over their heads, as well as the implication that the "homeless" do not have communities or physical spaces they consider to be home (Abrams, 2023). In this discussion, the term *unhoused* is used, unless citing sources that use the word *homeless*.

Rates of the numbers of people in Canada who are unhoused also illustrate the connections between health and well-being and their root causes. A pressing example of how these root determinants operate is the increasing crisis of unhoused people in Canada, where the "crisis" is one of public policy–created poverty and government incapacity to enact an effective national housing strategy. A commonly accepted stereotype about unhoused people and families is that they have caused their own problems—they are lazy and do not have a home because they are irresponsible and do not want to work: "Homeless people are seen as an eyesore, ruining the landscape of the city with their dirty, disheveled appearance" (Cobb, 2020, p. 391). These derogatory stereotypes persist, despite extensive evidence of the root causes of homelessness. According to the authors of the first comprehensive report about homelessness in Canada, the pathways into and out of homelessness are neither linear nor uniform. Individuals and families who become homeless may not share much in common with each other, "aside from the fact that they lack adequate housing, income, and the necessary supports to ensure they stay housed" (Gaetz et al., 2013, p. 4).

The current problem of increasing numbers of unhoused people in Canada is not limited to individual crises. Rather, the crisis was created through neoliberal government decisions to drastically reduce investments in affordable and social housing in the 1990s, decreases in income supports, and the declining spending power of almost half of the Canadian population since that time (Gaetz et al., 2013). In 2013, it was estimated that at least 200,000 Canadians experienced homelessness in any given year; in 2016, the number was estimated to be up to 300,000 (Gaetz et al., 2016). At least 30,000 Canadians were homeless on any given day in 2013 (Gaetz et al., 2013); in 2016, the number increased to 35,000 (Gaetz et al., 2016). As of 2023, these 2016 statistics are the latest estimates of the total, aggregate number of unhoused people in Canada. Currently, many Canadians are at risk of homelessness due to the high cost and unavailability of housing, as well as employment incomes that do not meet the minimal requirements of a living wage (Gaetz et al., 2016).

A **living wage** takes into account country circumstances and is the wage required to afford a decent standard of living for workers and their families (International Trade Union Confederation, 2024). It is not the same as the minimum wage, which is the legislated minimum (set by provincial governments in Canada) that all employers must pay in each province and territory in Canada. "The living wage reflects what people need to earn to cover the actual costs of living in their community, and draws on community-specific data to determine the expenses" (Living Wage Canada, n.d.). Living wage employers voluntarily decide to pay a living wage and maintain their certification as new rates are calculated for their area (Living Wage Canada, n.d.). For example, in Metro Vancouver, as the cost of essentials continues to sharply increase, particularly for housing and food, the living wage climbed to $25.68 per hour in 2023, in stark contrast to the $16.75 per hour legislated minimum wage (Living Wage for Families BC, 2023).

These structural reasons for large numbers of unhoused people may be described as morally indictable in a country that prides itself on having a generosity of spirit and a collective sense of responsibility for each other. In fact, Canada's poverty rates have steadily increased since the 1980s, along with increasing numbers of young people and elderly people facing homelessness due to neoliberal retrenchment in areas such as social housing (Gaetz et al., 2016). In 2016, Organisation for Economic Co-operation and Development (OECD, 2020) data indicated that over 30 percent of people in Canada were estimated to be in danger of falling into poverty. OECD, founded in 1961, is an intergovernmental organization that systematically collates and analyzes globewide data about health and well-being. The OECD goal is to shape policies that foster prosperity, equality, opportunity and well-being for all (OECD, n.d.). In 2018, Canada ranked 24th out of 35 OECD countries in terms of the percent of the population whose income falls below half the country's median income (OECD, 2019). "Social housing policies in Canada have historically faced many political obstacles and the general trend has been free market reliance... Compared to the other advanced capitalist nations, Canada's engagement in social housing began much later and has faced significant neoliberal retrenchments" (Gaetz et al., 2016, p. 92).

Neoliberal policy and governance strategies, described more fully in Chapter 2, have consistently been linked to rising rates of unhoused people in Canada and elsewhere. For example, although the Canadian Government has stated that it is investing $82 billion over 10 years (2017–2027) to expand funding for the homeless (Government of Canada, 2023), Sanger (2019) points out that $200 billion per year in corporate tax evasion could readily fund social support programs, such as free postsecondary tuition and a national pharmacare plan. Over a 10-year period, the time allotted for an $82 billion investment to expand funding for the homeless, and given 2019 taxation statistics, the government could potentially overlook $2 trillion in unlawful corporate tax evasion in Canada—enough for successful elimination of the unhoused crisis in Canada, along with significant other social supports provision. Figure 1.2 illustrates Canadian direct investment abroad, 1987–2023. In 2023, there was over $2.2 trillion in Canadian direct investment abroad. This data represents overall, aggregated investments, and it provides overall contexts for Canadian tax haven use by large multinational corporations.

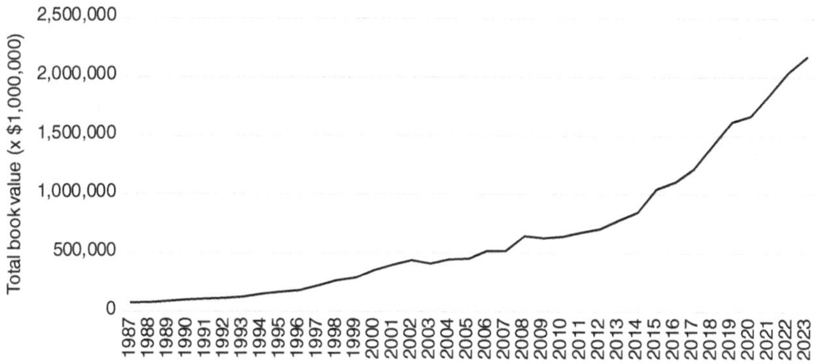

Figure 1.2: Canadian Direct Investment Abroad, 1987–2023

Source: Adapted from Statistics Canada, 2024.

In 2016, the international tax haven leak, known as the Panama Papers (Gibson, 2017), exposed the extent of Canadian firms' corporate tax haven use. At that time, at least 27 percent of Canadian direct investments abroad were found to be diverted to tax havens (The Canadian Press, 2016). In 2018, Canadian corporations held $353 billion in 12 of the world's biggest tax haven destinations (Press Progress, 2019).

Racialization of Heart Disease in Canada: A Root Determinants Example

One of the most common ways to think about health and illness is by linking ill health to its more directly observable causes, such as the relationships among diet, increased body weight, and heart disease. Yes, lack of exercise and diets high in fat and carbohydrates will generally increase weight and tend to cause heart disease, but what are the root-cause factors operating here? For example, in Indigenous (First Nations, Métis, Inuit) Peoples, root determinants of heart disease include intergenerational stress (further detailed in Chapter 3) caused by colonialist, imperialist practices of racism and public-policy decision making that led to land dispossession and destruction of natural habitats that were relied upon for centuries (Battiste & Youngblood Henderson, 2021). It is therefore not a coincidence that Indigenous Peoples and Canadians of African descent have the highest rates of heart disease and diabetes in Canada, when compared to the general population (Schultz et al., 2021). Heart disease rates for Indigenous people are as much as 50 percent higher than in the general Canadian population, and the death rate from stroke is twice as high (Heart and Stroke Foundation of Canada, n.d.). These findings reflect the racialization of disease incidence in Canada, further detailed in Chapter 3.

"Vulnerable and at Risk" or Under Threat?

The above examples about asthma, homelessness, and the racialization of heart disease point to the insidious and often hidden nature of root determinants of health: policy-created poverty in the case of asthma proliferation, policy decisions to avoid addressing root causes of the unhoused crisis in Canada (e.g., lack of sustained attention to affordable housing strategies), and the long-term intergenerational impacts of colonialist policies all operate in a "sly and treacherous manner." Belling the cat, or exposing these root determinants, also involves naming how we use language to hide the everyday realities of increasing disparities across the globe. Many of us, including health practitioners and health, social, and environmental policymakers and researchers, commonly use phrases such as "vulnerable people" or "vulnerable species" in an attempt to identify living things that are particularly "at risk." However, belling the cat involves reframing the concepts of vulnerable and at risk to people and planet under threat:

> The vulnerability discourse implies that individuals, communities, and planet-wide ecosystems are somehow more prone to experiencing ill health, or the damaging impacts of climate crises, in much the same way as one might be more prone to catching a cold. The concept of vulnerability worked well when it first came into common usage to describe human health and illness because it allowed us to name the people who are most oppressed, and thereby attempt to influence public policy in the direction of justice. However, the term is not ultimately effective in ameliorating the physical, spiritual and psychological suffering caused by injustice because it reinforces the idea of a nebulous force that is somehow causing ill health. (McGibbon, 2021a, p. 27)

The vulnerability discourse has become an effective tool to avoid naming how and why inequities in the social DoH are distributed according to the isms. For example, when we refer to groups of people as vulnerable, we support the homogenizing notion that they can be lumped into a vague category, and hence, one that is difficult to measure. Furthermore, experiences of marginalized and racialized peoples are covertly invisibilized through discourses of vulnerability, risk and resilience, individualism, and blame, rather than an acknowledgement that they are instead under threat of systemic oppression (McGibbon et al., 2021). Similarly, the increasingly frequent phrase "equity-seeking groups" is an example of the discursive objectification of injustices and everyday suffering: inequitable health outcomes are reduced to something that happens to "equity-seeking groups," as if they are somehow wandering around looking for equity amidst their experiences of systemic oppression. The more recent characterization of "equity-deserving groups" is similarly problematic because it connotes a hierarchy of worth—who is deserving of health equity and who is not (McGibbon et al., 2021).

SOCIAL, ECOLOGICAL, AND STRUCTURAL DETERMINANTS OF HEALTH

The DoH have gained increasing traction in the midst of the global **polycrisis**, defined as an array of serious, long-term, and interconnected challenges—including (but not limited to) climate change and biodiversity loss, widening economic and social inequalities, and ideological extremism—with its own emergent dynamics (Cascade Institute, n.d.; World Economic Forum, 2023). The following sections describe many of these DoH, focusing on the social DoH, the ecological DoH, the structural DoH, and the overall Root Determinants of Health Framework.

The Root Determinants of Health Framework

Definitions and understandings of the DoH are very difficult to "nail down." When talking about health, there is a strong expectation of singular, "reliable," and relatively static definitions of the social DoH, ecological DoH, and structural DoH. This process is not possible within a politics of health perspective. Mutually exclusive categories do not reflect the contextual realities of the DoH, because the definitions themselves are evolving day-to-day as interest in the politics of health grows amid current global health crises. It is therefore not feasible to create a static list of "what falls into what category" using mutually exclusive groupings. As the evidence in this chapter attests, this definitional strategy would become rapidly outdated. One approach to this conundrum is to consider the social DoH nested within (and interacting with) the ecological DoH. The ecological DoH are then nested within (and interacting with) the structural DoH. For example, people living in circumstances of poverty, a key social DoH, are impacted by climate emergency, a key ecological DoH, in many synergistic and adverse ways when compared to people who do not live in poverty. The ecological DoH are then nested within the structural DoH because evidence now demonstrates that the climate emergency is strongly linked to structural policy and governance approaches, described further in subsequent chapters.

The **Root Determinants of Health Framework** (Figure 1.3) is not meant to be a definitive description. Rather, it is meant as a useful mapping of current critical perspectives on the DoH that can inform action. The diagram has broken, rather than continuous, lines because there is not a rigid separation among the determinants that fall into each of the three categories—their interfaces are porous and synergistic. It is important to note that these synergies are a relatively new area of study,

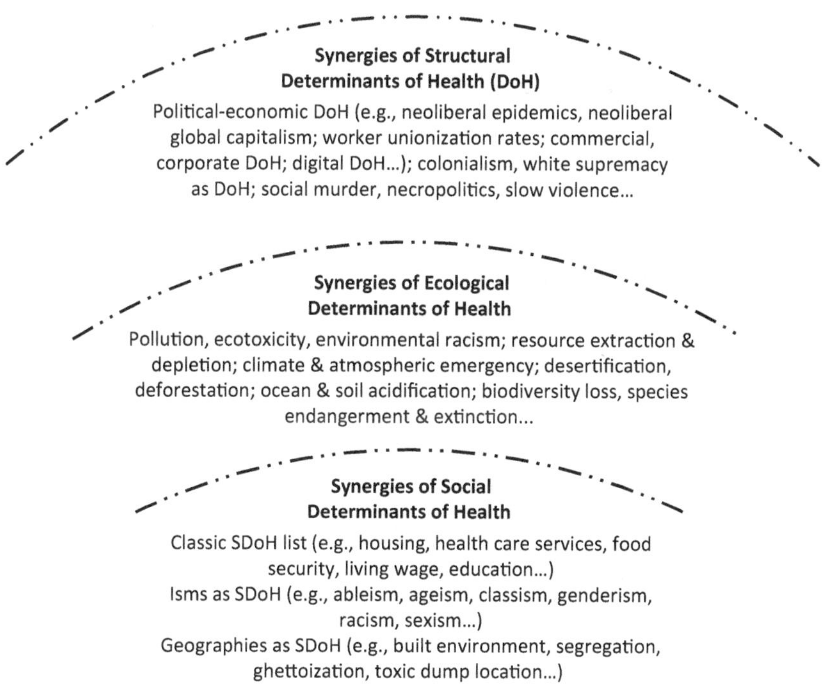

Figure 1.3: Snapshot: Synergies of Social, Ecological, and Structural Determinants of Health

Source: Created by author.

and the categories are in transition. Although it is helpful to make some initial distinctions among the three areas, it is also necessary to integrate synergies: the social DoH are interconnected with the ecological and structural DoH because they are powerfully shaped by these contexts. In much the same way, the ecodeterminants are shaped by the structural determinants because planetary health, and hence the health of all life on Earth, has been shown to be strongly impacted by neoliberal and capitalist imperatives, such as mass-scale natural resource extraction and depletion (Bloomsbury Publishing, 2022). These relationships reflect evolving understandings of the DoH and, most importantly, how the structural DoH cut across all social and ecological DoH areas. The diagram is thus a snapshot of current critical perspectives on the DoH. The following sections introduce a broad overview of the social, ecological, and structural DoH described in the framework. Each of these DoH is more fully described in subsequent chapters.

Social Determinants of Health

The social DoH "are the conditions in which people are born, grow, work, live, and age, and the wider set of forces and systems shaping the conditions of daily life" (WHO, 2008, p. 31). These conditions include economic policies and systems, development agendas, social norms, social policies, and political systems. Unfair, and most importantly, avoidable inequities in the social DoH mean that health and illness follow a social gradient: the lower the socioeconomic position, the worse the health (WHO, n.d.). Although concentration on the social DoH is a relatively recent phenomenon, the notion that social conditions impact health is centuries old. In the 1800s, Rudolf Virchow—a German physician, anthropologist, writer, and politician—wrote, "all diseases have two causes: one pathological and the other political" (Laverack, 2013). At about the same time, Friedrich Engels—a German philosopher, historian, political theorist and revolutionary socialist—linked the everyday living conditions of citizens to the vast impacts of capitalist control of the means of production. He argued that inadequate living conditions, such as lack of safe housing, employment, and access to food, were directly related to decisions made by governments and the ruling elite. The early work of these scholars and activists demonstrates how the modern concept of the social DoH was deeply analyzed over a century ago.

Social DoH were the first globally recognized framework to explicitly name how societal contexts determine health. More recently, characterizations of the social DoH became increasingly known with the World Health Organization's Commission on the Social Determinants of Health (WHO, 2008). In 2002, Raphael, Bryant, and Curry-Stevens created the first pan-Canadian version of the social DoH; the 2002 Toronto Charter designated the social DoH to include early childhood development, education, employment and working conditions, food security, health care services, housing shortages, income and its equitable distribution, social exclusion, sociate safety nets, and unemployment. The Toronto Charter also recognized that Canadian women, Canadians of colour, and new Canadians are disproportionately impacted by inequities in the social DoH, especially income and its distribution, employment and working conditions, housing affordability, and the state of the social safety net (Raphael et al., 2004). These authors explicitly integrated public policy intervention in discussions of the social DoH, calling out the health-damaging impacts of neoliberal retrenchment of social programs as a major factor in the urgency of addressing the social DoH in public policy contexts, analyzed more fully in Chapter 2.

There are numerous iterations of the social DoH, each contributing to a deeper understanding of the complex nature of social, economic, and political contexts of health. For example, Figure 1.4 provides a graphic illustration of key "eco-social" DoH (Canadian Centre for Policy Alternatives [CCPA], n.d.a.). Think Upstream is a national project of the CCPA. It recognizes that social, ecological, and economic conditions shape people's health and the well-being of communities. Upstream's aim is to reframe how governments approach systemic issues, with a focus on whole-of-government policy, upstream solutions to inequities in the social DoH, and community wealth building approaches that produce healthier individuals and healthier communities and nations (CCPA, n.d.b.). Upstream refers to policy and governance solutions that prevent inequities (upstream intervention) rather than attempt to

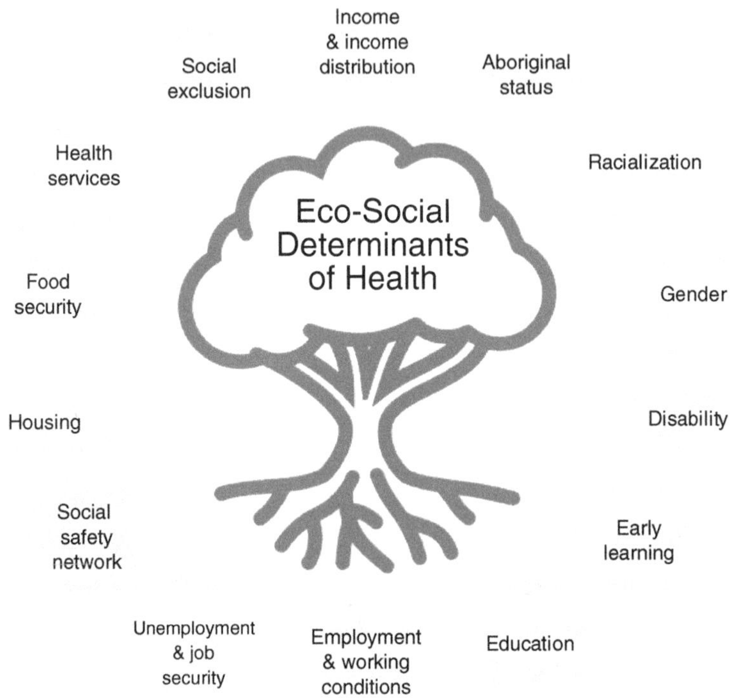

Figure 1.4: Eco-Social Determinants of Health: Canadian Centre for Policy Alternatives

Source: Adapted from Think Upstream, n.d.

mitigate problems after they have already occurred (downstream intervention), the latter being starkly more expensive in terms of financial and human cost (National Collaborating Centre for Determinants of Health, 2014).

Raphael et al. (2020) then integrated systemic political and economic contexts into the original Toronto Charter social DoH: gender, geography, globalization, immigration, Indigenous ancestry, and race. Social DoH contexts create living conditions that deeply influence quality of life. These conditions are determined by government decision making across a broad scope of policy areas. At all levels of government, policies, laws, and directives impact social DoH for Canadians, such as employment income and levels of various social insurance supports, including family benefits, social assistance, and health and social services—all of these supports are also negatively impacted when people lose their jobs due to recurring economic recessions (Raphael et al., 2020).

As demonstrated by Raphael et al.'s (2020) most recent list, the social DoH have historically expanded to include critical social science perspectives that integrate root causes such as globalization. Gender and race were eventually changed to sexism and racism in some social DoH lists (McGibbon & Etowa, 2007). These kinds of changes were pivotal markers in the evolution of new perspectives on the social DoH. For example, it is racism, rather than race, that determines health because race is a social construction—only 0.012 percent of the variation among humans in total genetic material can be attributed to race (Witzig, 1996). An important example of systemic racism as a social DoH is the racialization of COVID-19 pandemic health outcomes (McGibbon, 2021b): 51 percent of people who tested positive for COVID-19 in Manitoba self-identified as BIPOC (Black, Indigenous, People of Colour; Government of Manitoba, 2021). Black people and other people of color made up 83 percent of reported COVID-19 cases in Toronto (Cheung, 2020).

Figure 1.5 deepens existing understandings of the social DoH by applying a First Nations perspective on health and wellness, which is a tool for the First Nations Health Authority (FNHA) and First Nations communities in British Colombia, Canada. The aim is "to create shared understanding of a holistic vision of wellness. This image is just a snapshot of a fluid concept of wellness: it can be adapted and customized freely and is not confined to remain the same" (FNHA, n.d.). The Traditional Wellness Working Group, staff, and advisors from the FNHA first crafted the model as a draft visual concept of wellness. This visual model and description was presented to BC First Nations at *Gathering Wisdom V* for feedback in May, 2012. It was incorporated into the current visual model and description and it is intended to serve as a starting point for discussion by First Nations communities on what they conceptualize as a vision of wellness for themselves and the FNHA (FNHA, n.d.).

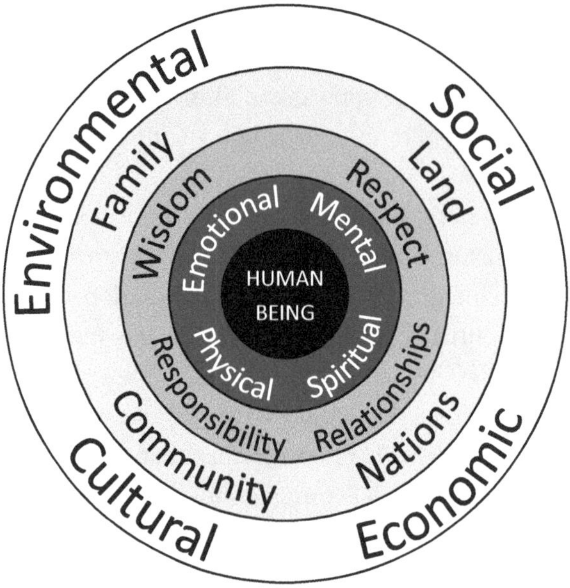

Figure 1.5: First Nations Perspectives on Health and Wellness

Source: Adapted from First Nations Health Authority, n.d.

All of the above examples illustrate how the social DoH developed over time to increasingly integrate the systemic, structural DoH. The evolution of social DoH discussions and debates are described in detail in Chapter 3. Here, it is also necessary to clarify some of the meanings and origins of socioecological models of health, due to their use of the word *ecological*. These models are not necessarily related to considerations of the social, ecological, and structural DoH. The socioecological model was introduced as a conceptual model for understanding human development by Urie Bronfenbrenner in the 1970s. The model states that health is affected by the interactions among the characteristics of the individual, the community, and the environment, which includes physical, social, and political components (Kilanowski, 2017). Socioecological models are sometimes referred to as ecological models, defined as "the interaction between, and interdependence of, factors within and across all levels of a health problem. It highlights people's interactions with their physical and sociocultural environments" (US Department of Health and Human Services, 2005).

Socioecological models do not necessarily imply commonly understood "ecological" considerations, which focus on ecological biosystems, such as human interactions with all life on Earth, including the biosphere, as described in Chapter 4. These discrepancies may be related to the health-field use of the word *environment*, where the word is often used to more generally indicate any contexts that are outside or around the individual, from family and community all the way to political contexts. Socioecological models are also distinct from the concept of social ecology, first introduced by environmental activist Murray Bookchin (1993). He explained the connection between nearly all of our present ecological problems and our deep-seated social problems: "these ecological problems cannot be understood, let alone solved, without a careful understanding of our existing society and the irrationalities that dominate it" (p. 1). Bookchin expanded this thinking, stating that the most serious ecological dislocations we face today are rooted in economic, ethnic, cultural, and gender conflicts, among many others. Bookchin's conceptualization of social ecology is consistent with this book's framing of ecological DoH as directly related to the science of Earth's ecosystems and the structural DoH that impact them.

Ecological Determinants of Health

The social DoH are in turn strongly influenced by their ecological contexts. Where we live, the air we breathe, and our access to safe, ethically produced, and nutritious food, are all examples of ecological DoH. The ecological DoH (ecodeterminants) encompass human health and the health of the whole natural world. "There is a growing recognition that the Earth is itself a living system and that the ultimate determinant of human health, and that of all other species, is the health of the Earth's life-supporting systems" (Hancock et al., 2015, p. 1). Ecodeterminants include pollution and ecotoxicity; resource extraction and depletion; climate and atmospheric emergencies; desertification, deforestation, and acidification; and biodiversity loss, species endangerment, and extinction. Anthropogenic (human) activities contribute vastly to the thinning of the Earth's ozone layer and a higher pollution index across all Earth systems, polluting the global water cycle and hindering the availability of sustainable water supplies (Tijani et al., 2016).

These activities include 300 million metric tons of plastic produced annually, as well as increases in global construction, where more than half of all the concrete ever used was produced in the past 20 years (Waters et al., 2016). Pollution and ecotoxicity are arguably the best-known threats to Earth's life support systems. Ecotoxicology is the science of studying how toxic substances are dispersed and taken up in Earth systems (Fleeger, 2020). For example, endocrine-disrupting chemicals (EDCs), described in more detail in Chapter 4, are one of many prominent examples of ecotoxicity. EDCs in food and consumer products interfere with human and multispecies hormone biosynthesis and metabolism. They are found in pesticides, industrial chemicals, plastics and plasticizers, fuels, and many other chemicals that are in widespread industrial use. The result is a globe-wide deviation from normal control over human reproduction (Diamanti-Kandarakis et al., 2009).

Complex and multiple anthropogenic changes in the Earth's natural systems such as these are captured in the designation of the Anthropocene Epoch, first described by Paul Crutzen (2005) as the current geological age. The term *Anthropocene*, further explored and critiqued in Chapter 4, is characterized by the dominance of humans over the global environment and involves all of the ecological DoH. "Since we depend on [Earth] systems for the most fundamental determinants of our health, these human-induced changes present a profound threat to the health of the world's population in the 21st century" (Hancock et al., 2015, p. 5). As described in Chapter 4, anthropogenic changes have an inequitable and disproportionate impact along social class and racialized lines, and Global North and Global South geographies, to name a few. These impacts in turn powerfully shape inequities in the social DoH because anthropogenic harms are inequitably distributed across systemic injustices such as classism and racism.

Environmental justice studies have long confirmed the relationship between social DoH, such as low-income or racialized status, and the location of environmental health hazards. For example, researchers conducted a large study of health risks from exposure to harmful substances and their toxicological characteristics for populations living near industrial facilities in the City of Toronto (Kershaw et al., 2013). Using the

National Pollution Release Inventory, researchers identified the nature and amount of toxic emissions from specific industrial sites. They then used postal code data to locate racialized and low-income areas near the sites. Results indicated that the proportion of low-income individuals impacted by toxic chemicals was significantly higher when compared to higher income neighbourhoods.

The study also found that the toxin exposure difference was even greater for racialized people, thus proving the double jeopardy of poverty and toxics exposure, and the triple jeopardy of poverty, toxics exposure, and racialization (Kershaw et al., 2013). Municipal, provincial/territorial, and federal governments create policies, laws, and regulations that support environmental harms and produce inequitable distribution of these harms and toxins across the social DoH. At the municipal level, policy decision-making has led to landfills being disproportionately (by far) located near racialized communities in Canada, a preventable situation that is reflected across the globe (Kaufman & Hajat, 2021). **Environmental racism**, further explored in Chapter 4, refers to environmental policies, practices, or directives that disproportionately disadvantage individuals, groups, or communities (intentionally or unintentionally) based on race or colour (Waldron, 2020).

Structural Determinants of Health

Root causes, root determinants, and structural DoH all refer to the politics of health, and they are often used interchangeably. For example, the structural DoH describe the root causes of human and planetary harm. They are called structural because "they are part of the political, economic, and social structure of society and of the culture that informs them" (Navarro, 2007. p. 2). Structural determinants include political DoH, such as neoliberal public policy and governance, colonialism, white privilege and supremacy, capitalism, classism, heterosexism, patriarchy, and racism, to name a few. Politics and power operate in many direct (somewhat measurable) and indirect (hidden) ways to determine health.

For example, if we think of a wharf, the platform or walkway on top of the wharf is mostly what we see (McGibbon et al., 2019; see Figure 1.6). Underneath this surface, multiple large wooden and metal supports provide

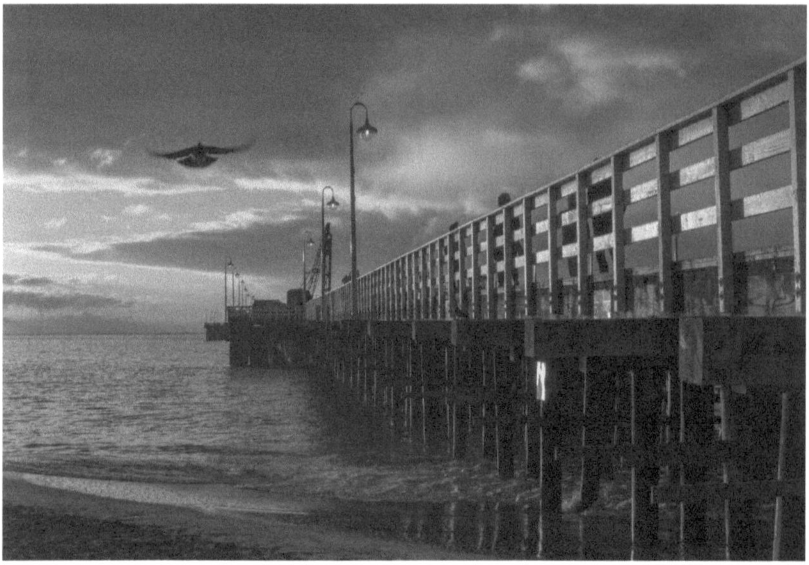

Figure 1.6: Explaining the Structural Determinants of Health: A Seaside Wharf

Source: Photo by Jeff Nissen on Unsplash.

the foundational structures that underpin and support the walking platform of the wharf. In terms of health, on the platform are all the aspects of health that we can "see," such as the statistical incidence of poverty's impacts on the health of families and communities, the physical results of poverty (e.g., childhood malnutrition), and the human and environmental impacts of climate emergency (e.g., desertification, deforestation, species endangerment, and extinction). However, we do not see the root causes because they are hidden below the surface in the systemic structures that support inequitable, unjust health outcomes. The structural determinants include the political DoH, because policy and politics form many of the structures, or root causes, that underpin health outcomes.

Structural Determinants Case Example: Colonialism

Colonialism is a structural or political DoH due to its historical rootedness in Canadian public policy, where federal policies result in ongoing systemic and intergenerational impacts on the health of Indigenous Peoples and peoples of African descent. For example, colonization includes the systematic process of shaping Indigenous subjectivities to reflect and internalize Eurocentric hegemony, creating and reinforcing the **socially constructed** superiority of white Europeans and the inferior, savage, and child- or animal-like nature of Indigenous Peoples (Battiste & Youngblood Henderson, 2021; McGibbon et al., 2013). Socially constructed means that the concept or idea "has been constructed, built, made-up, over time, by society, and by dominant social and cultural systems such as government, education, and health care" (McGibbon & Mbugua, 2018, p. 135). Anne Bishop (2002) described how internalized racism became important in the creation of Indian Residential Schools—a church- and state-sanctioned example of "child abuse being used to force a people to internalize what their conquerors thought to be their rightful place in a racist, sexist, class-stratified society" (p. 72).

SOCIAL, ECOLOGICAL, AND STRUCTURAL DETERMINANTS OF HEALTH: A COMPLEX ADAPTIVE SYSTEM

Previous discussions illustrate that the social, ecological, and structural DoH are interconnected because they synergistically impact each other. They are also emergent, because their focus and content are evolving or emerging as we understand more about how data, Earth, health, and social sciences, and the humanities (to name a few) can together inform public policy change and social change activism. Taken together, the social, ecological, and structural DoH form a complex adaptive system (CAS), a system made up of interrelated components that are constantly changing and unpredictable. Since what is happening in one part of the system impacts other parts of the system, feedback loops are formed. These feedback loops can either enhance solutions to complex problems or increase these problems. The field of CAS evolved within the field of complexity science, where CASs were found to have several main overarching characteristics: 1) they are dynamic, unpredictable, and multidimensional; 2) they have interconnected relationships and parts that are not possible to disentangle; 3) they have positive and negative feedback loops; 4) they self-organize into system-wide coherent patterns; and 5) they demonstrate an overall emergence of control, where processes occurring at the fine scale produce prevailing whole-system patterns over time. In the following chapters, these characteristics and the language of CASs are integrated to more fully explain the politics of the social, ecological, and structural DoH. Chapter 6 is specifically focused on explaining CAS applications in more detail.

CONCLUSION

Politics and power are potent DoH. Despite health promotion concentration on directing Canadians to "improve their lifestyles," the best predictors of health outcomes involve structural power and decision making. In terms of planet health, the best predictors include pollution and ecotoxicity and mass scale resource extraction that is largely related to the dominance of transnational globe-wide corporations. A logical and effective approach for improving health is to name and tackle these policy-created conditions that persistently cause human and planetary health damage and suffering—belling the cat. Yet, despite these already well-documented root causes, public policy progress is slow, and in some cases, actively works against intervening at the structural level. Persistent, and some would say relentless, policy choices to concentrate at the micro, individual level have stymied policy change in the direction of equitable distribution of health outcomes. At the same time, these policy choices serve the hidden and compelling purpose of keeping the public focus away from the structural DoH and the beneficiaries of sustaining health inequities. This chapter and this book provide a roadmap to strengthen our own focus and the focus of public policymakers towards identifying and tackling the systemic, preventable threats to human and planet health.

FURTHER READINGS

Birn, A. (2009). Making it politic(al): Closing the gap in a generation: Health equity through action on the social determinants of health. *Social Medicine*, *4*(3), 166–82.

Canadian Public Health Association. (2015). *Addressing the ecological determinants of health*. https://www.cpha.ca/sites/default/files/assets/policy/edh-discussion_e.pdf
McGibbon, E. (2021). People and planet under threat: The social, ecological and structural determinants of health. In E. McGibbon (Ed.), *Oppression: A social determinant of health* (2nd ed., pp. 25–43). Fernwood Publishing.
Nash, R., Hudson, A., & Luttrell, C. (2006). *Mapping political context: A toolkit for civil society organisations*. Overseas Development Institute.
Raphael, D., Bryant, T., Mikkonen, J., & Raphael, A. (2020). *Social determinants of health: The Canadian facts* (2nd ed.). Ontario Tech University Faculty of Health Sciences and York University School of Health Policy and Management. https://thecanadianfacts.org/

WEBSITES OF INTEREST

Canadian Observatory on Homelessness—https://preventhomelessness.ca/

"The Canadian Observatory on Homelessness (COH) is a non-partisan research and policy partnership between academics, policy and decision makers, service providers and people with lived experience of homelessness. Led by Stephen Gaetz, President & CEO, the COH works in collaboration with partners to conduct and mobilize research designed to have an impact on solutions to homelessness."

Global Inequalities Observatory—https://www.lse.ac.uk/International-Inequalities/Research/Global-Inequalities-Observatory

"The Global Inequalities Observatory seeks to promote rigorous research methods from a wide range of social sciences to foster a greater understanding of the levels, trends, causes, and consequences of economic inequality in multiple countries and regions."

Native Land—https://native-land.ca/

This website offers an interactive map of Indigenous territories and a Territory Acknowledgment Guide, inviting non-Indigenous people to learn more about the lands they inhabit and the history of those lands. Click "Resources" to access the Territory Acknowledgments and search for your region.

Think Upstream—https://www.thinkupstream.ca/

A national project of the Canadian Centre for Policy Alternatives, Think Upstream is "working with a growing network of people who recognize that social, ecological, and economic conditions shape people's health and the wellbeing of our communities... Working at the intersection of the social determinants of health, Think Upstream provides powerful communications tools for policy change, and we want to help you. Through our framing program, we support key change-makers and thought leaders in the social determinants of health universe to help drive compelling narratives that popularize their research findings."

What are Complex Systems?—https://uwaterloo.ca/complexity-innovation/about/what-are-complex-systems

This website is a University of Waterloo primer from the university's Institute for Innovation. It introduces complexity theory, highlighting its strength as an interdisciplinary form of analysis and a tool that can help to understand how complexity science can inform analyzing current complex health and social problems. The website includes nine videos of various specialists answering the question: "What are complex systems?"

GLOSSARY

Complex Adaptive System (CAS): A system made up of interrelated components that are constantly changing, unpredictable, and impossible to disentangle. These systems contain many feedback loops, because what is happening in one part of the system impacts other parts of the system. Feedback loops can either enhance solutions to complex problems or increase these problems.

Ecological Determinants of Health: Encompass human health and the health of the whole natural world. Ecodeterminants include pollution and ecotoxicity; resource extraction and depletion; climate and atmospheric emergencies; desertification, deforestation and acidification; and biodiversity loss, species endangerment, and extinction. Earth systems encompass all ecological systems, such as the atmosphere (the set of layers of gases/air surrounding the planet), the geosphere (solid parts of the Earth, or "the Earth beneath our feet"), the hydrosphere (watersheds, oceans, ice caps), and the biosphere (all global ecosystems of life on Earth; McGibbon, 2021a).

Environmental Racism: Refers to environmental policies, practices, or directives that disproportionately disadvantage individuals, groups, or communities (intentionally or unintentionally) based on race or colour (Waldron, 2020).

Living Wage: Takes into account country circumstances and is the wage required to afford a decent standard of living for workers and their families. A living wage is not the same as the minimum wage, which is the legislated minimum (set by provincial governments in Canada) that all employers must pay in each province and territory in Canada. "The living wage reflects what people need to earn to cover the actual costs of living in their community, and draws on community-specific data to determine the expenses" (Living Wage Canada, n.d.).

Politics of Health: A way to describe factors and influences that determine health, including the political and economic conditions that are powerfully determined by one's social, economic, and political contexts throughout the lifecourse.

Polycrisis: Refers to an array of serious, long-term, and interconnected challenges—including (but not limited to) climate change and biodiversity loss, widening economic and social inequalities, and ideological extremism—with its own emergent dynamics (Cascade Institute, n.d.; World Economic Forum, 2023).

Racialization: The complex and contradictory process through which groups come to be categorized as being part of a particular "race" and, on that basis, subjected to differential and/or unequal, often discriminatory, treatment: "racialization [is] the process of manufacturing and utilizing the notion of race in any capacity" (Alberta Civil Liberties Research Centre, n.d.; Dalal, 2002, p. 27).

Root Causes: Refer to the social, political, economic, and cultural origins of health and social inequities, where health refers to the health-of-all life on Earth, including all aspects of planet Earth itself.

Root Determinants of Health Framework: Depicts the interconnected relationships among social (e.g., housing and food security), ecological (e.g., pollution and ecotoxicity), and structural (e.g., policy and governance systems, colonialism, and the isms) DoH.

Social Determinants of Health (DoH): "The conditions in which people are born, grow, work, live, and age, and the wider set of forces and systems shaping the conditions of daily life" (WHO, 2008, p. 31). These conditions included economic policies and systems, development agendas, social norms, social policies, and political systems. Unfair and, most importantly, avoidable inequities in the social DoH mean that health and illness follow a social gradient: the lower the socioeconomic position, the worse the health (WHO, n.d.).

Socially Constructed: Means that the concept or idea "has been constructed, built, made-up, over time, by society, and by dominant social and cultural systems such as government, education, and health care" (McGibbon & Mbugua, 2018, p. 135).

Structural Determinants of Health (DoH): The root causes, often described as the "cause-of-the-causes," of worsening health outcomes for marginalized and racialized peoples across the globe as well as for planet Earth. Structural determinants are built into/part of societal structures, including policy and governance systems, colonialism, and the isms.

REFERENCES

Abrams, A. (2023, July 20). Is it OK to use the word "homeless"—or should you say "unhoused"? *The Guardian*. https://www.theguardian.com/us-news/2023/jul/20/homeless-unhoused-houseless-term-history

Alberta Civil Liberties Research Centre. (n.d.). *Racialization.* http://www.aclrc.com/racialization

AZQuotes. (n.d.). *Willem de Kooning quotes.* https://www.azquotes.com/author/8208-Willem_de_Kooning

Battiste, M., & Youngblood Henderson, S. (2021). Oppression and the health of Indigenous peoples. In E. McGibbon (Ed.), *Oppression: A social determinant of health* (2nd ed., pp. 85–99). Fernwood Publishing.

Bishop, A. (2002). *Becoming an ally: Breaking the cycle of oppression in people.* Fernwood Publishing.

Blair, E. (2004). *Belling the cat: A retelling of Aesop's fable.* Capstone.

Bloomsbury Publishing. (2022). *Global Health Watch 6: In the shadow of the pandemic.*

Bookchin, M. (1993). What is social ecology? In M. E. Zimmerman (Ed.), *Environmental philosophy: From animal rights to radical ecology.* Prentice Hall.

Canadian Centre for Policy Alternatives (CCPA). (n.d.a). *Social determinants of health.* Think Upstream. https://www.thinkupstream.ca/social-determinants-of-health

Canadian Centre for Policy Alternatives. (n.d.b.). *Services.* Think Upstream. https://www.thinkupstream.ca/services

Canadian Observatory on Homelessness. (n.d.). *Housing first.* https://www.homelesshub.ca/solutions/housing-accommodation-and-supports/housing-first

The Canadian Press. (2016, April 27). *Canadian corporations kept $40 billion more in offshore tax havens last year: Tax group.* https://www.cbc.ca/news/business/canada-corporate-tax-haven-1.3554910

Cascade Institute. (n.d.). *Polycrisis.* https://cascadeinstitute.org/polycrisis/

Cheung, J. (2020, July 30). *Black people and other people of colour make up 83% of reported COVID-19 cases in Toronto.* CBC News. https://www.cbc.ca/news/canada/toronto/toronto-covid-19-data-1.5669091

Cobb, J. (2020). Reflections on working with homeless people. *American Journal of Economics and Sociology, 79*(2), 383–399. https://doi.org/10.1111/ajes.12326

Crutzen, P. J. (2005). Human impact on climate has made this the "Anthropocene age." *New Perspectives Quarterly, 22*(2), 14–16. https://doi.org/10.1111/j.1540-5842.2005.00739.x

Dalal, F. (2002). *Race, colour and the processes of racialization: New perspectives from group analysis, psychoanalysis and sociology.* Routledge.

Diamanti-Kandarakis, E., Bourguignon, J.-P., Giudice, L. C., Hauser, R., Prins, G. S., Soto, A. M., Zoeller, R. T., & Gore, A. C. (2009). Endocrine-disrupting chemicals: An Endocrine Society scientific statement. *Endocrine Reviews, 30*(4), 293–342. https://doi.org/10.1210/er.2009-0002

First Nations Health Authority (FNHA). (n.d.). *First Nations perspective on health and wellness.* https://www.fnha.ca/wellness/wellness-for-first-nations/first-nations-perspective-on-health-and-wellness

Fleeger, J. W. (2020). How do indirect effects of contaminants inform ecotoxicology? A review. *Processes, 8*(12), 1659. https://doi.org/10.3390/pr8121659

Gaetz, S., Dej, E., Richter, T., & Redman, M. (2016). *The state of homelessness in Canada 2016*. Canadian Observatory on Homelessness Press.

Gaetz, S., Donaldson, J., Richter, T., & Gulliver, T. (2013). *The state of homelessness in Canada 2013*. Canadian Homelessness Research Network Press.

Gibson, D. (2017). *Bay Street and tax havens: Curbing corporate Canada's addiction*. Canadians for Tax Fairness. https://www.taxfairness.ca/sites/default/files/2022-07/report-bay-street-and-tax-havens-c4tf.pdf

Gorse, M. (2022). Risk and protective factors to LGBTQ+ youth suicide: A review of the literature. *Child and Adolescent Social Work Journal, 39*(1), 17–28. https://doi.org/10.1007/s10560-020-00710-3

Government of Canada. (2023). *About reaching home: Canada's homelessness strategy*. https://www.infrastructure.gc.ca/homelessness-sans-abri/index-eng.html

Government of Manitoba. (2021). *COVID-19 infections in Manitoba: Race, ethnicity, and Indigeneity: External Report*. https://www.gov.mb.ca/health/publichealth/surveillance/reports.html

Grant, T., Croce, E., & Matsui, E. C. (2022). Asthma and the social determinants of health. *Annals of Allergy, Asthma & Immunology, 128*(1), 5–11. https://doi.org/10.1016/j.anai.2021.10.002

Hancock, T., Spady, D. W., & Soskolne, C. L. (Eds.) (2015). *Global change and public health: Addressing the ecological determinants of health*. Canadian Public Health Association.

Heart and Stroke Foundation of Canada. (n.d.). *Helping to close the gap in Indigenous health*. https://www.heartandstroke.ca/what-we-do/our-impact/helping-to-close-the-gap-in-indigenous-health

International Trade Union Confederation (ITUC). (2024, March 25). *ILO agreement on living wage definition "a leap forward for social justice."* https://www.ituc-csi.org/ILO-agreement-on-living-wage-definition

Kaufman, J. D., & Hajat, A. (2021). Confronting environmental racism. *Environmental Health Perspectives, 129*(5). https://doi.org/10.1289/EHP9511

Keet, C. A., McCormack, M. C., Pollack, C. E., Peng, R. D., McGowan, E, & Matsui, E. C. (2015). Neighborhood poverty, urban residence, race/ethnicity, and asthma: Rethinking the inner-city asthma epidemic. *Journal of Allergy & Clinical Immunology, 135*(3), 655–662. https://doi.org/10.1016/j.jaci.2014.11.022

Kershaw, S., Gower, S., Rinner, C., & Campbell, M. (2013). Identifying inequitable exposure to toxic air pollution in racialized and low-income neighbourhoods to support pollution prevention. *Geospatial Health, 7*(2), 265–278. https://doi.org/10.4081/gh.2013.85

Kickbusch, I. (2015). The political determinants of health—10 years on. *BMJ Clinical Research,* 350, h81. https://doi.org/10.1136/bmj.h81

Kilanowski, J. F. (2017). Breadth of the socio-ecological model. *Journal of Agromedicine, 22*(4), 295–97. https://doi.org/10.1080/1059924X.2017.1358971

Laverack, G. (2013). *Health activism: Foundations and strategies.* SAGE Publications. https://doi.org/10.4135/9781446270004

Living Wage Canada. (n.d.). *What is a living wage?* https://www.livingwage.ca/

Living Wage for Families BC. (2023). *Living Wages in BC and Canada.* Vancity Community Foundation. https://www.livingwageforfamilies.ca/living_wage_rates

Luttrell, C., Bird, K., Byrne, S., Carter, J., & Chakravarti, D. (2007). The power cube explained. *The Poverty-Wellbeing Platform, 3,* 1–5.

Mackenbach, J. P., & McKee, M. (2015). Government, politics and health policy: A quantitative analysis of 30 European countries. *Health Policy, 119*(10), 1298–1308. https://doi.org/10.1016/j.healthpol.2015.08.017

McGibbon, E. (2021a). Embodied oppression: The social, ecological and structural determinants of health. In J. Antony, W. Antony, & L. Samuelson (Eds.), *Power and resistance: Critical thinking about Canadian social issues* (7th ed., pp. 452–492). Fernwood Publishing.

McGibbon, E. (2021b). People and planet under threat: Health impacts of oppression. In E. McGibbon (Ed.), *Oppression: A social determinant of health* (2nd ed., pp. 25–43). Fernwood Publishing.

McGibbon, E., Bailey, A., & Lukeman, S. (2019). Violence and health: A structural perspective. In L. L. Stamler, L. Yiu, A. Dosani, J. Etowa, & C. van Daalen-Smith (Eds.), *Community health nursing: A Canadian perspective* (5th ed., pp. 503–520). Pearson.

McGibbon, E., & Etowa, J. (2007). *Health inequities and the social determinants of health: Spatial contexts of oppression* [Invited keynote presentation], Nova Scotia Health Research Foundation. Health Geomatics Conference, Halifax, NS, Canada.

McGibbon, E., Fierlbeck, K. & Ajadi, T. (2021). Health equity and institutional ethnography: Mapping the problem of policy change. *Witness: The Canadian Journal of Critical Nursing Discourse, 3*(2), 64–80. https://doi.org/10.25071/2291-5796.117

McGibbon, E., Fierlbeck, K., & Ajadi, T. (2022). Institutional ethnography and critical policy analysis: Catalyzing justice in policymaking [Paper accepted for publication]. *Critical Studies: An International and Interdisciplinary Journal.*

McGibbon, E., & Mbugua, J. (2018). Race and racialization in health, health care, and nursing education. In M. McIntyre & C. McDonald (Eds.), *Realities of Canadian nursing* (5th ed.). Wolters Kluwer Health.

McGibbon, E., Mulaudzi, F. M., Didham, P., Barton, S., & Sochan, A. (2013). Toward decolonizing nursing: The colonization of nursing and strategies for increasing the counter-narrative. *Nursing Inquiry, 21*(3), 179–191. https://doi.org/10.1111/nin.12042

Mukharesh, L., Phipatanakul, W., & Gaffin, J. M. (2023). Air pollution and childhood asthma. *Current Opinion in Allergy and Clinical Immunology, 23*(2), 100–110. https://doi.org/10.1097/ACI.0000000000000881

National Collaborating Centre for Determinants of Health. (2014). *Let's talk: Moving upstream.* https://nccdh.ca/resources/entry/lets-talk-moving-upstream

Navarro, V. (2007). Neoliberalism as class ideology; or, the political causes of the growth of inequalities. *International Journal of Social Determinants of Health and Health Services, 37*(1), 47–62. https://doi.org/10.2190/AP65-X154-4513-R520

Organisation for Economic Co-operation and Development (OECD). (n.d.). *Who we are.* https://www.oecd.org/about/

Organisation for Economic Co-operation and Development. (2019). *Society at a glance 2019: OECD social indicators.* OECD iLibrary. https://www.oecd-ilibrary.org/sites/8483c82f-en/index.html?itemId=/content/component/8483c82f-en

Organisation for Economic Co-operation and Development. (2020). *How's life? 2020: Measuring well-being.* OECD iLibrary. https://doi.org/10.1787/9870c393-en

Press Progress. (2019, April 26). *Corporate Canada's pile of cash in offshore tax havens has hit $353 billion for the first time in history.* https://pressprogress.ca/corporate-canadas-pile-of-cash-in-offshore-tax-havens-has-hit-353-billion-for-the-first-time-in-history/

Raphael, D., Bryant, T., & Curry-Stevens, A. (2004). Toronto Charter outlines future health policy directions for Canada and elsewhere. *Health Promotion International, 19*(2), 269–273. https://doi.org/10.1093/heapro/dah214

Raphael, D., Bryant, T., Mikkonen, J., & Raphael, A. (2020). *Social determinants of health: The Canadian facts* (2nd ed.). Ontario Tech University Faculty of Health Sciences and York University School of Health Policy and Management. https://thecanadianfacts.org/

Sanger, T. (2019). *Time to step up for tax justice: Important international reforms to end tax-dodging and tax havens are on the horizon. Why isn't Canada doing more?* Canadian Centre for Policy Alternatives. https://policyalternatives.ca/publications/monitor/time-step-tax-justice

Schultz, A., Nguyen, T., Sinclaire, M., Fransoo, R., & McGibbon, E. (2021). Historical and continued colonial impacts on heart health of Indigenous Peoples in Canada: What's reconciliation got to do with it? *Canadian Journal of Cardiology Open, 3*(12), S149–S164. https://doi.org/10.1016/j.cjco.2021.09.010

Statistics Canada. (2023, April 28). *International investment position, Canadian direct investment abroad and foreign direct investment in Canada, by country, annual (x1,000,000)* [Table 36-10-0008-01]. https://www150.statcan.gc.ca/t1/tbl1/en/tv.action?pid=3610000801

Statistics Canada. (2024, April 29). *International investment position, Canadian direct investment abroad and foreign direct investment in Canada, by country, annual (x 1,000,000).* https://www150.statcan.gc.ca/t1/tbl1/en/tv.action?pid=3610000801

Stevens, P. E., & Hall, J. M. (1992). Applying critical theories to nursing in communities. *Public Health Nursing, 9*(1), 2–9. https://doi.org/10.1111/j.1525-1446.1992.tb00065.x

Think Upstream. (n.d.). *Social determinants of health.* Canadian Centre for Policy Alternatives. https://www.thinkupstream.ca/social-determinants-of-health

Tijani, J. O., Fatoba, O. O., Babajide, O. O., & Petrik, L. F. (2016). Pharmaceuticals, endocrine disruptors, personal care products, nanomaterials and perfluorinated pollutants: A review. *Environmental Chemistry Letters, 14,* 27–49. https://doi.org/10.1007/s10311-015-0537-z

Trachtenberg, A. J., Dik, N., Chateau, D., & Katz, A. (2014). Inequities in ambulatory care and the relationship between socioeconomic status and respiratory hospitalizations: A population-based study of a Canadian city. *Annals of Family Medicine, 12*(5), 402–407. https://doi.org/10.1370/afm.1683

US Department of Health and Human Services. (2005). *Theory at a glance: A guide for health promotion practice.* National Institutes of Health.

Waldron, I. (2020). *Environmental racism in Canada.* Canadian Commission for UNESCO.

Waters, C. N., Zalasiewicz, J., Summerhayes, C., Barnosky, A. D., Poirier, C., Gałuszka, A., Cearreta, A., Edgeworth, M., Ellis, E. C., Ellis, M., Jeandel, C., Leinfelder, R., McNeill, J. R., Richter, D. D., Steffen, W., Syvitski, J., Vidas, D., Wagreich, M., Williams, M., … Wolfe, A. P. (2016). The Anthropocene is functionally and stratigraphically distinct from the Holocene. *Science, 351*(6269). https://doi.org/10.1126/science.aad2622

Witzig, R. (1996). The medicalization of race: Scientific legitimization of a flawed social construct. *Annals of Internal Medicine, 125*(8), 675–679. https://doi.org/10.7326/0003-4819-125-8-199610150-00008

World Economic Forum. (2023). *The global risks report 2023* (18th ed.). https://www3.weforum.org/docs/WEF_Global_Risks_Report_2023.pdf

World Health Organization (WHO). (n.d.). *Social determinants of health.* https://www.who.int/health-topics/social-determinants-of-health

World Health Organization. (2008). *Closing the gap in a generation: Health equity through action on the social determinants of health—Final report of the commission on social determinants of health.* https://www.who.int/publications/i/item/WHO-IER-CSDH-08.1

CHAPTER 2

Critical Policy Analysis Approaches for the Determinants of Health

CHAPTER OBJECTIVES

Using as many examples as possible:

1. Define and describe core concepts about policy.
2. Describe what is meant by the political economy of health, including social democratic political economy and neoliberal political economy.
3. Compare and contrast traditional, social, and materialist epidemiological perspectives on health.
4. Identify and describe key policy analysis approaches and their relationships with addressing inequities in the social DoH.
5. Describe what is meant by a Health in All Policies (HiAP) application for understanding policy.

CRITICAL THINKING QUESTIONS

1. In terms of decreasing health inequities, how might you argue for a social democratic political economy approach? (Include statistics.)
2. How do the various epidemiological approaches to health reflect positivist perspectives and critical perspectives?
3. What are some of the ways that governments can enhance, or stall, climate policy for ecosystem health?

4. What stands out to you in terms of a critical policy analysis approach to understanding policy? How can your understanding contribute to decreasing health inequities?
5. How are the distinct Indigenous-grounded and Afrocentric policy analysis approaches useful in tackling health inequities?

INTRODUCTION

The aim of this chapter is to situate the book's critical policy analysis (CPA) approach within the politics of the social, ecological, and structural determinants of health (DoH). Although health care and health systems politics are relevant in areas such as the population health impacts of health care structures, the inner workings of health care systems are not the focus here. Rather, the focal point is on policy analysis and how CPA, in particular, is a foundation for understanding how health is determined by politics, as described throughout this book. Foregrounding policy and policy analysis supports a deeper understanding of how to navigate the policy change process for redistributive justice in health. Building on the critical perspectives discussion in Chapter 1, this chapter brings social, ecological, and structural DoH into the policy realm because this is a main space where structural change happens, for better or for worse. First, core concepts about policy are described, including public policy, institutional policy, policy analysis, and policy intervention. The foundation is then laid for defining and applying a CPA approach for tackling injustices across the DoH. Although the social DoH are increasingly integrated in language used to describe health in Canada and elsewhere, it is only recently that some sectors of the Canadian public have become aware of the relationships among inequities in the social DoH—such as poverty—or ecological DoH—such as waterway ecotoxicity—and their public policy roots.

Second, the **political economy of health** is explained, since public policies are always influenced by prevailing political and economic authority. Social democratic and neoliberal political economies are compared and contrasted. The human and planet health–damaging impacts that follow neoliberal political economies are illustrated though the case example of austerity measures after the 2008 global financial crisis: neoliberal reforms in New Zealand and Europe. Third, the political economy of health discussions are directly linked to the ideological and practical world of health through explanations and examples from the field of epidemiology. This is a crucial step because any discussion of health is laden with theoretical and political meanings that heavily shape public policy. Extant policy analysis approaches are discussed, including positivist, postmodern, critical feminist and intersectional, post-colonial, Indigenous-grounded, and Afrocentric. The chapter concludes with possibilities of integrating CPA in selected policy for health approaches, with health broadly defined across social, economic, political, and cultural contexts.

CORE CONCEPTS ABOUT POLICY

This section provides a brief overview of important terms in policy studies. Although definitions and descriptions of these terms is necessary for forming a common language to talk about policy, policy analysis, and health, the terms are the subject of much debate across policymakers, researchers, civil society actors, and more. **Policy analysis** refers to the examination and evaluation of available options (existing policies or newly crafted policies) to address various economic, social, or other public issues. The process often includes many areas of data collection, including empirical research and statistical data collection, and the participation of key stakeholders, such as economists, community members, and public officials tasked with enacting policy (Norwich University, n.d.). **Public policy** has many meanings, depending on context and intended use. A public policy is a document drawn up by governmental actors to present their vision of an issue calling for public action and, to some extent, the legal, technical, practical, and operational aspects of this action (Turgeon & Savard, 2012). Public policy may also refer to the processes through which elected representatives decide on a public action designed to deal with an issue, where the issue itself is considered by certain actors, whether governmental or non-governmental, to require some kind of **policy intervention** (Turgeon & Savard, 2012).

Policy intervention refers to the application of a particular policy or series of policies to solve an identified problem or to enhance existing policies to increase their effectiveness.

For example, non-governmental actors in public policy intervention to address violence against women, including femicide, may be local, regional, and international organizations for the advancement of women. These include the Center for Reproductive Rights, a global human rights organization of lawyers and advocates whose work is focused on advocating reproductive rights that are protected by law, and Women for Women International, an international women's rights organization that supports the most marginalized women in countries affected by war and conflict. Other non-governmental actors in policy issues impacting women include directors of non-profit women's centres and shelters, civil society organizations involved in lobbying for women's and gender-centred public policy, and academic partners (e.g., researchers and activists in academic and community settings). Public policy may also refer to public documents approved by publicly elected officials, such as members of parliament (MPs), members of the legislative assemblies in provincial parliaments (MLAs), and members of municipal councils (e.g., mayors, council members). This latter understanding of public policy corresponds with the common meaning held by the general public, the media, and government policymakers. More pragmatically, Thomas Dye (1972) defined public policy as "whatever governments choose to do or not to do."

Institutional policy may be referred to as policy that is developed and implemented within institutional structures, including formally recognized institutions in sectors such as universities and health care, where institutional actors (e.g., boards of directors of universities and hospitals) can be identified. Institutional policy can also refer to systemic or institutionalized structures, where institutional refers to "... a complex of relations forming part of the ruling apparatus, organized around a distinctive function—education, health care, law, and the like" (Smith, 1987, p. 160). Some examples of institutionalized structures are ableism, classism, and genderism. This distinction between different meanings of institutional policy is important. While individual institutions such as universities may fail to create institutional policies to prevent serious problems, such as sexualized violence on university campuses, these processes unfold within institutionalized, systemic structures, such as sexism, misogyny, and patriarchy. All four policy areas described (policy analysis, public policy, policy intervention, and institutional policy) are strongly impacted by the criticality of the various policy analysis approaches described later in this chapter.

Contemporary public policy studies "continue to focus on both the structure of governments and the behaviour of political actors in order to understand and inform what governments actually can and should do, but do so in new ways, having learned and expanded upon the lessons of past work" (Capano & Howlett, 2020, p. 3). Political actors are those affected by, or affecting, a given policymaking issue. Often referred to as players, they can be organizations or individuals (Lah, 2018). For example, common players in health reform politics include

1. Public sector organizations (e.g., government ministries of health and finance, professional regulatory agencies, hospitals, universities)
2. Public sector individuals (e.g., permanent staff who support ministers, provincial and local government leaders)
3. Private sector institutions (e.g., pharmacies, drugs manufacturers)
4. Labour organizations (e.g., medical worker unions, civil service unions, professional associations)
5. Civil society organizations (e.g., nongovernmental foundations, watchdog groups focused on particular health issues)
6. Media organizations (e.g., social media, print and internet news agencies; Lah, 2018).

Knowing who the players are, and where they are situated in the policy issue at hand, is an essential step in promoting or provoking policy change and navigating related power structures. Negotiating pathways to develop relationships with these players is an important process in navigating policy change. In Chapter 6, readers will have the opportunity to apply Gaventa's (2017) power cube to identify key types of power, along with associated players who can influence, support, or obstruct progressive policy change on a given policy problem or issue related to the social, ecological, and structural DoH.

THE POLITICAL ECONOMY OF HEALTH

Building on discussions of critical approaches in Chapter 1, this section describes the political economy of health, a central policy-related perspective for identifying root causes of inequities in health and social outcomes. A political economy perspective analyzes how these inequities are created by public policy and how they can be decreased or eliminated through public policy processes. For example, federal, provincial/territorial, and municipal governments create policies, laws, and regulations that determine how much employment income Canadians receive, the extent of their family benefits and social assistance, the quality and availability of affordable housing, their access to health and social services and recreational opportunities, and what happens when they lose their jobs during economic downturns (Raphael et al., 2020). All of these policies have been shown to strongly determine health (see Ansell et al., 2019; Barnett & Bagshaw, 2020; Navarro, 2007a).

A political economy approach "interrogates economic doctrines to disclose their sociological and political premises... in sum, [it] regards economic ideas and behavior not as frameworks for analysis, but as beliefs and actions that must themselves be explained" (Maier, 1987, p. 3). In other words, political economy perspectives do analyze economic decision-making by governments and other actors; however, the focus is on analyzing sociological and political underpinnings, rather than viewing politics as "neutral." The overall aim is to analyze the role of the economic organization of society in the production and distribution of disease and the burden of illness, and the ways that disease, illness, and wellness are framed (deciding what the problem is perceived to be) and treated (deciding what the policy intervention should be) (Coburn, 2010; McGibbon et al., 2024). Problem framing and deciding on policy interventions vary, sometimes significantly, according to the prevailing political economy of government actors and prevailing political parties. Baer (1982) described the political economy of health as "a critical endeavor that attempts to understand health issues within the context of the class and imperialist relations inherent in capitalist world systems" (p. 1).

Political economy perspectives thus provide a methodological approach for mapping the links among **population health**, politics, economics, and history. Population health refers to health status and health status inequities of the population as a whole, as well as groups within it. These groups may be defined by geography, age, culture, or other defining features. The approach measures health over time, across jurisdictions, and across health and social issues (Public Health Agency of Canada, 2023). The field of economics, in contrast, is largely viewed as consisting of objective and quantifiable sets of measurements and models. Political economy perspectives bring politics and economics together, focusing on how the politics of a nation influences the direction and outcomes of its economic, and hence, any policies that impact health (not only "health" policy) (McGibbon & Hallstrom, 2021).

Materialist political economy approaches are increasingly applied to study health and social injustices. According to Marx (1977), in order to survive and continue existence from generation to generation, it is necessary for human beings to produce and reproduce the material requirements of life. Materialist approaches are based in Marx's assertion that economic factors—the way people produce the necessities of life—determine the kind of politics and ideology a society can have, and also conditions or directs the general processes of social, political, and intellectual life (Marx, 1977). Materialist political economy of health approaches support a systematic understanding of political regimes and related policy interventions, as well as their population health outcomes. The focus is on examination of how the means of production are related to legal, political, religious, and cultural ideologies and institutions (McGibbon & Hallstrom, 2021). The means of production refers to areas such as land, labour, and capital that can be used to produce products (e.g., goods and services). Marx (1977) also emphasized the relationship between social class and access to the means of production, where the ruling classes (e.g., CEOs, corporate shareholders) have control over the means of production. The income inequality model, often referred to as an antecedent of health inequality, acknowledges the relationship between income and health, but it does not connect the poor health of poor people to race and class inequality in capitalist societies (Navarro, 2007b; Raphael, 2021). As Armstrong and Connelly (1989) stated,

> ... class has to be reconceptualized through race and gender within regional, national, and international contexts... Class is dynamic and relational; it is the basis of change. Gender, race/ethnicity, and regionality/nationality interact with class in various ways with one being more salient than another at different points in time. (p. 5)

Political economy of health perspectives are thus an entry point for uncovering sustained, policy-driven inequities in health. More specifically, these perspectives provide a method to connect health and social inequities in people's everyday lives with their political, root causes. The same reasoning applies to the ecological DoH, where environmental damage to the planet can be systematically linked to neoliberal global capitalism, described in Chapter 4.

Political Economy of Social Democratic and Neoliberal Welfare States

The politics of health inequities are most commonly analyzed through a political economy of health lens. Although competence in the area of political economy is generally (and unfortunately) in its nascent state in the health fields, it is often a well-known and recognized area of knowledge across the social and political sciences. With the aim of bridging this gap, the following sections further explain what is meant by a political economy approach and how it is salient in learning about the root causes of health and social inequities. The overall health and social equality of countries is directly associated with its prevailing political economy, both historically and currently (Navarro, 2007a). This discussion focuses on political economies in the **modern welfare state**, which refers to the "extent to which governments or the state use their power to provide citizens with the means to live secure and satisfying lives" (Raphael, 2009, p. 15). The discussion explains two prominent political economies: social democratic political economy and neoliberal political economy, both guided by different sets of structures and interests that shape institutions and policy ideologies (Esping-Andersen, 2015). Differences involve the extent of state intervention required to meet the material and social needs of citizens. Social democratic and neoliberal political economies are not mutually exclusive, and there may be varying combinations of them in any given set of social policies (McGibbon & Hallstrom, 2021).

Social Democratic Welfare States

In **social democratic welfare states**, the ideological inspiration is the reduction of poverty, inequality, and unemployment. Organizing principles are universalism and the socialist ideals of equality, the social rights of all citizens, justice, freedom, and solidarity (Bryant, 2016; Esping-Andersen, 2002; Saint-Arnaud & Bernard, 2003). Social democratic welfare states generally expend more of their national wealth for supports and services, and they are proactive in developing labour, family-friendly, and gender-equity supporting policies (Raphael, 2009). Emphasis is on public policies that increase capacity for collective social, economic, and environmental health and well-being (McGibbon & Hallstrom, 2021). Examples of modern social democratic welfare states are Sweden, Norway, Denmark, and usually Finland (Bambra et al., 2005; Bryant, 2016).

Social support programs provided by the state often include legally guaranteed universal medical and health insurance; unemployment supports, such as retraining and a living wage while looking for work; home care supports; pharmacare; and dental care—in short, a foundation of supports that helps to ensure health and well-being for citizens. The policy case examples in this chapter provide evidence of the immediate population health damage of withdrawing these state-based supports. Social democratic—often referred to as left-leaning—political economies demonstrate consistent policy intervention to ensure universal social supports, including the myriad supports that lift people out of poverty (Bryant, 2016).

Social democratic policies have been shown to have an enduring historical impact on a country's poverty reduction success. Rainwater and Smeeding (2005) analyzed the relationship between left-leaning, or social democratic, cabinet share and people's odds of escaping poverty in 2005. When governments are in power, a set of ministers is appointed by the head of the governing party, such as the prime minister. Ministers have varying portfolios, such as finance; the treasury board; housing, infrastructure, and communities; national defence; science and industry; and Crown-Indigenous relations. This group of ministers is commonly referred to as the cabinet. As such, cabinet ministers have considerable influence on the government's policies and priorities for the country. In 2005, Canada had no cabinet members who represented a left leaning political party and the population had a 7 percent chance of escaping poverty (Rainwater & Smeeding, 2005). In contrast, Sweden had over 30 percent of cabinet members representing a left-leaning political party and the population had corresponding odds of escaping poverty at over 40 percent. Canada does not yet have any cabinet ministers representing a left-leaning political party.

This data, although almost 20 years old, is strongly reflected in current Canadian and global findings regarding population poverty rates. A longitudinal analysis of child poverty in Canada demonstrates that there has been little to no improvement in Canada's OECD (Organisation for Economic Co-operation and Development) rankings as a nation with one of the worst performances in applying social democratic initiatives to decrease child poverty. When compared to more recent figures from the OECD Income Distribution Database for 2015–2016, Canada ranked in the High Range of Child Poverty at 28th out of 43 countries in terms of percentage of children living in poverty, with 17.5 percent of children living in poverty as measured by family income (OECD, n.d.b.). Again, Canada ranked closely with neoliberal governance nations such as the United States. In contrast, Sweden, Norway, Denmark, and Finland ranked in the Low Range of Child Poverty, with less than 10 percent of children living in poverty as measured by family income (OECD, n.d.b.).

Noël (2019) studied minimum income protection in advanced democracies, including Canada, stating that "minimum income protection is the rock-bottom foundation of citizenship rights, and it is a distinctive test of a country's commitment to social justice" (Noël, 2019, p. 243). Findings ranked 18 countries in terms of minimum income. The bottom six countries were the United States (18th), Canada (17th), Spain (16th), France (15th), the United Kingdom (16th), Italy (15th). The top six countries were Finland (6th), Sweden (5th), Ireland (4th), Switzerland (3rd), Netherlands (2nd), Norway (1st). Canada's ranking at second-to-last is an unsettling reminder of the extent of neoliberal governance over time. Noël also concluded that the broader politics of the welfare state are important indicators of minimum income protection, particularly in the politics of their redistribution of wealth—welfare states with a large redistribution budget are more likely to have generous minimum income protection: "as goes the welfare state, so goes minimum income protection" (2019, p. 243). Minimum income protection is strongly associated with social democratic welfare states (Muller & Raphael, 2023). Noël (2019) also found a robust relationship between trade union density and left-cabinet density, noting that the cumulative power of trade unions has a positive influence on minimum incomes.

> Trade unions may think first about their members, but they seem to reinforce what Brady calls 'latent coalitions for egalitarianism'. Trade union density may also be an indirect indicator of the mobilization capacity of collective actors in a given society. It is plausible, for instance, but difficult to demonstrate, that the women's movement or associations defending the rights of the poor are more powerful in countries where the labour movement is stronger. Whatever the case, the poor seem to benefit from the presence of trade unions, even though they are not members. (p. 244)

Neoliberal Welfare States

In contrast, **neoliberal welfare states** are based in the ideology of liberty, with the stated aim of relatively minimal government intervention and a focus on benefits available only through means testing (limiting access through screening), rather than universal availability (McGibbon & Hallstrom, 2021). Social insurance programs are an important example. Social insurance programs are defined differently in various countries. In Canada, social insurance generally refers to a public insurance program (publicly funded) that provides protection against various situations such as loss of income due to unemployment (Employment Insurance benefits), income of seniors (Canada Pension Plan), and health difficulties requiring medically-based intervention (health insurance). Neoliberal welfare strategies underscore the difference between social insurance programs—such as unemployment insurance and state provision of health care services—which are available to all citizens (universally accessible), and social assistance, which is available only to those who are destitute or in danger of becoming destitute (McGibbon & Hallstrom, 2021). "Within [neo]liberal welfare states, liberty, and its close neighbor, self-determination, become available only to a narrow band of the population—those who have sufficient financial resources and cultural capital to define their own living conditions" (Raphael & Curry-Stephens, 2016, p. 366). Neoliberal welfare states ostensibly promote minimal government intervention in the marketplace, a framework that allows for, and often promotes, increasing privatization of services, including education and health care delivery. "Neoliberalism is the belief that that the marketplace should be the arbiter of how economic and other resources are distributed" (Raphael, 2009, p. 32). Modern examples of liberal welfare states are Canada, the United States, the United Kingdom, and Ireland (Bryant, 2016).

There is no universally accepted definition of **neoliberalism**, but one of the fundamental ideas is that the individual is essentially "a piece of capital," to be developed just like any other piece of capital, where commodification and thus profit is the goal. For this purpose, markets are seen to be much better than governments at generating and allocating resources—barriers to the free movement of goods, people, and capital should be as minimal as possible and the entities supplying goods and services should preferably be privately owned (Brown, 2019). Neoliberalism refers to the principles that markets allocate scarce resources, promote efficient growth, and secure individual liberty better than governments. This results in the primacy of economic over social policies (Kickbusch, 2015). Neoliberal mandates include the belief that public welfare systems need to be cut back to eliminate bureaucratic waste, reduce taxation, and allow greater choice through private service provision (Alcock et al, 2022). Neoliberalism generates an inequitable accrual of wealth and opportunity for certain groups. Critics point out that "neoliberalism benefits multinational corporations and the financial sector, as well as particular government agencies and international organizations" (Carlquist & Phelps, 2014, p. 1231).

Schrecker (2016) described three core definitional elements of neoliberalism:

> First, markets are regarded as the normal, natural, and preferable way of organizing most forms of human interaction, not just economic transactions in the conventional sense. Second, the primary function of the state is to ensure the efficient functioning of markets [see roll back and roll out explanation below], although this does not necessarily mean a "rolling back" of state functions. Indeed, the state may need to expand its activities in areas such as policing and interrogation of applicants for state support to which they are legally entitled. Third, those who advocate a variety of redistributive policies must justify their positions against a "base-line" (Sunstein, 1987) outcome that would be generated by a market functioning as markets are supposed to in microeconomics textbooks. (p. 952)

Another hallmark of neoliberalism is its positivist focus on the individual as the unit of analysis and policy intervention, and a concurrent insistence that people are the authors of their own fortune (or misfortune). This stance results in distorted thinking that is not supported by evidence, such as "If I can make the effort to get educated and find a job, then anyone who refuses to do so is lazy and not deserving of state support." Because the market is perceived to be an "impartial and efficient" distributor of resources, wealth and income inequality are considered to be related to moral fortitude (or lack thereof) and the people who accrue more resources deserve their wealth, while the "losers," who have not been able to thrive in a market-driven environment, must simply accept their fate because there is no sustainable alternative to the market-based system (Brunoli, 2017). Due to its global reach, neoliberalism is best understood as a transnational phenomenon rather than as a series of basically unrelated and national developments or unconnected phenomena, seen as "... products of happenstance" rather than as "elements of a complicated but coherent political project" (McGibbon & Hallstrom, 2021; Overbeek & van der Pijl, 1993; Schrecker, 2016). The discourse of neoliberalism is globally dominant, currently and historically. It is therefore normalized and as such, its power operates in a quiet and unseen manner, where it is used to

> ... justify, disguise, or mystify its workings while also preventing objections or challenges to it. In our time, and almost universally, phrases like "the free market," privatization, less (as opposed to more) government, and others like them, which have become the orthodoxy of globalization and counterfeit universals, are the staples of dominant discourse, designed to create consent and tacit approval. (Said, 2001)

The practice of neoliberalism involves two identifiable phases: roll-back and roll-out neoliberalism. These phases have significant implications for public policy to support (or constrain) human and planet health equity.

Roll-Back and Roll-Out Neoliberalism

Neoliberalism in Canada has included at least two phases—roll-back and roll-out neoliberalism (McGibbon & Hallstrom, 2021). This distinction is crucial in understanding how structural DoH create sustained health and social inequities. *Roll-back neoliberalism* involves a withdrawal of the state from providing services and state-based supports, and the deregulation of not only economies but also other sectors, including agriculture, education, and health (Tickell & Peck, 2003). Deregulation refers to reduction of government power, a concrete example being decreases in environmental protection regulations for corporations. It is important to note that this so-called reduction in the government's role in the economy is paradoxically coupled with active public policy intervention to increase government roles in areas such as ensuring corporate tax reduction, privatizing (corporatizing) public assets, and selectively providing massive economic interventions, such as the richest nations' estimated $11.7 trillion in bank bailouts following the financial crisis of 2008 (Labonté & Stuckler, 2016). Corporate and government wealth (profit) accumulation is thus buttressed by austerity measures that are driving the increasing health and social inequalities in neoliberal welfare states and, most importantly from a population health perspective, the selective distribution of those profits: "To be sure, the political project of neoliberalization thrived on the opportunities that arose from economic crisis, but its advance required intellectual leadership and political entrepreneurship, with substantial financial backing" (Schrecker, 2016, p. 3).

In roll-back neoliberalism, the role of the state is reduced in areas of social insurance, and at the same time there is a focus on creating what Heywood (2012) refers to as a "politics of support," with a neoconservative emphasis on "moral conservatism, xenophobia, law-and-order, and the family..." (Ansell, 2019; McGibbon & Hallstrom, 2021; Overbeek & van der Pijl, 1993, p. 15). Throughout this book, evidence is provided about the ways that neoliberal public policy approaches consistently undermine health through policy interventions that damage health, such as hampering worker unionization, which decreases worker rights and hence worker health (Leigh & Chakalov, 2021), and decreasing state-funded social supports related to maternal-child health, thus increasing infant mortality rates (Schrecker, 2016).

The second phase, *roll-out neoliberalism*, is characterized by the consolidation of a state-led project and process; however, rather than focus on national welfare provision (i.e., issues and conditions of equity and equality), it is now focused on international, and in Canada's case, inter-provincial, competitiveness (McGibbon & Hallstrom, 2021; Tickell & Peck, 2003). The stated goal is smaller government, such as reducing industry and corporate regulation, and unconstrained markets. However, roll-out neoliberalism is more about promoting the role of government in any given policy decision making, rather than a focus on the actual size of government role. In other words, large government bureaucracies remain intact, and in some cases expand, despite reduced government roles in provision of state-led programs and services (McGibbon & Hallstrom, 2021), as demonstrated by austerity measures after the 2008 financial crisis.

Policy Case Example: Austerity and the Political Economy of Neoliberal Reforms in New Zealand and Europe

Austerity measures are a pressing example of roll-back neoliberalism as a transnational global project. In terms of political economies, the term *austerity* refers to deficit reduction strategies taken by governments following the financial crisis of 2008. Deficit reduction specifically refers to budget deficit reduction, or reducing the amount of a government's spending so that it matches more closely the government's available monies (e.g., taxes, interest income from governments' business enterprises, and so on). The politics of deficit reduction involves strategic government decisions about just where to cut spending. In 2008, reduction happened primarily though limits to government expenditure, mainly evidenced through reduction in social spending (social supports, social insurance).

These measures were neither homogeneous nor similarly implemented because some public sector programs were protected, while others were targeted for large budget cuts, such as education, health, and other public services (Stuckler et al., 2017). Barnett and Bagshaw (2020) studied the political economy of New Zealand governance for a 10-year period with the aim of determining the impacts of neoliberal austerity-related policy reforms. Results were catastrophic, with over 111,000 jobs lost between 1986 and 1996. Employment loss happened in tandem with welfare benefit reductions, creating severe financial pressures on families with children—child poverty rates rose dramatically after the 1991 budget. Data in 2015 demonstrated that these hardships endured, with 28 percent of children living in poverty, including 20 percent in severe poverty. During this period, New Zealand, previously ranked as a country with low economic inequality, had one of the more significant inequality increases in OECD countries since the 1980s, similar to that of the United States (Barnett & Bagshaw, 2020).

In a systematic review analyzing the impact of austerity measures taken by European governments as a response to the 2008 economic and financial crisis, research focused on the social DoH and child health outcomes (Rajmil et al., 2020). Results of the review demonstrated that

1. High austerity periods, compared to pre-austerity periods, were associated with increased material deprivation, child poverty rates, and low birth weight;
2. Austerity measures had a significant impact on children's health, especially in perinatal indicators and in countries that have significantly reduced their health care budget;
3. The impact of austerity was greater in families with vulnerable children and austerity measures were found to impact deprived groups the most;
4. A significant negative change was detected in the access to, and provision of, services for children with disabilities and in child mental health services; and
5. Austerity consequences included deteriorating social determinants as well as child health outcomes and reduced access to, and quality of, preventive and curative health care services.

Researchers also found an association of government austerity measures with the recent increase in infant mortality caused by rising poverty in the poorest areas of England (Taylor-Robinson et al., 2019). These negative impacts on child health and development have implications for the future adult health of an entire generation (Rajmil et al., 2020). In a 2023 study, researchers studied the height of British children who grew up during the years of austerity and found that the children were falling behind many of their European peers in terms of height (Hill, 2023). In 1985, British girls and boys ranked 69th out of 200 countries for average height at age five. But by 2019, British girls ranked 96th and boys ranked 102nd when compared to other OECD countries. Experts have said that a poor national diet and cuts to the National Health Service

(NHS) are to blame; however, they have also pointed out that height is a strong indicator of general living conditions, including illness and infection, stress, poverty, and sleep quality (Hill, 2023). For example, Tim Cole, an expert in child health, stated that the height of British children growing up in the 2010s during the period of austerity "... tells me that austerity has clobbered the height of children in the United Kingdom (UK)... the last 14 years [since 2008] from age 5 to 19 has been particularly rough for UK children" (Hill, 2023). New Zealand's and Britain's austerity-induced damage to population health outcomes is reflected across the globe in countries such as Canada, where infant mortality rates, an example of social murder further discussed in Chapter 5, continue to be a barometer of neoliberal austerity measures, especially in cuts to social support over time.

CONNECTING POLITICAL ECONOMY OF HEALTH AND EPIDEMIOLOGY

Epidemiology is an important concept within the political economy of health because policymaking across the DoH is guided by deeply entrenched ideologies about the roots of ill health, and hence proposed public policy solutions for achieving health and well-being (McGibbon & Hallstrom, 2021). When governmental, institutional, or other policymakers decide about how to approach health and social issues, they do so within the boundaries of their own differing notions of what constitutes "health" and what constitutes "social." These ideas are, in turn, heavily influenced by larger societal constructs about the nature of health and the nature of its social contexts. Epidemiology is one such construct because it continues to strongly influence health and social policy and it does not necessarily evoke looking for root causes and hence structural policy solutions. Epidemiology may be defined as "the study of the distribution and determinants of health-related states or events (including diseases), and the application of this study to the control of diseases and other health problems" (Canadian Public Health Association, 2017, p. 8). Examining epidemiological perspectives on population health is necessary because decisions about how to "do the looking" are very much determined by whether or not epidemiology and population health are viewed from traditional, social, or materialist perspectives (McGibbon & Hallstrom, 2021).

The field of epidemiology began in 1854 when physician John Snow linked the incidence of cholera in a crowded London district with the location of city wells—the highest incidence of cholera occurred near several contaminated wells. Traditional epidemiology still concerns itself with disease-based public health problems, resulting in significant population health advances in the treatment of communicable diseases across the globe. However, it has been critiqued due to lack of attention to political, economic, and social roots of disease and illness causation (McGibbon & Etowa, 2009). Traditional epidemiology is largely guided by biomedical models of health, with the underpinnings of **positivism**, described later in this chapter, including an identified lack of inclusion of social and political DoH. Traditional epidemiology, focusing on the science of disease causation, is still a crucial aspect of tackling health crises such as the COVID-19 pandemic. Despite these advances, its largely biomedical framing of health provides little capacity for disentangling health crises such as policy-created poverty or the racialization of pandemic illness and death. People living in "ethno-cultural neighborhoods" in British Columbia had an age-adjusted COVID-19 mortality rate 10 times higher than neighborhoods that were less than one per cent visible minority (Carman, 2020).

Social epidemiology, in contrast, focuses on the social production of health and illness, with specific emphasis on health antecedents such as social position, discrimination, racism, power, and privilege (Petteway et al., 2019). Social epidemiology investigates the social, economic, and structural determinants of population health and disease, rather than treating these determinants as simple backgrounds to biomedically-identified conditions (Krieger, 2001). Shaw et al.'s (1999) germinal book, *The Widening Gap: Health Inequalities and Policy in Britain*, related mortality and morbidity statistics to poverty and housing in the United Kingdom. Studying the prevailing political economies of selected jurisdictions across the United Kingdom, the authors found that the social gradient (usually considered an indicator of the various income levels) was the most robust predictor of infant and child mortality and premature adult mortality. "In contemporary Britain, unequal chances of death are interwoven, in social and spatial terms, with unequal chances in life, in terms of education, employment, income, and wealth" (p. 5). Social epidemiologist Nancy Krieger (2003) compared circumstances in 1950, when researchers in the field of social epidemiology first described the relationships among fetal and infant mortality and residential segregation of African Americans to current health injustices:

> Grappling with notions of causation, in turn, raises not only complex philosophical issues but also, in the case of social epidemiology, issues of accountability and agency: simply invoking abstract notions of "society" and disembodied "genes" will not suffice. Instead, the central question becomes: Who and what is responsible for population patterns of disease and well–being, as manifested in present, past and changing social inequalities in health. (p. 677)

Due to its focus on the structural DoH, social epidemiology somewhat overlaps with materialist epidemiology because both approaches target public policy, and thus political analyses to identify and tackle the root causes of social and health inequities.

Materialist epidemiology is based in Marxian analyses that emphasize how the societal hierarchy of class relations "conditions most potently how other variables affect the population's health" (Navarro, 2007a, p. 21). Materialist epidemiological approaches, based in the political economy of health, provide this larger societal context for linking health outcomes across the lifespan with structural, policy-driven ideologies that create and sustain oppression. Navarro et al. (2006) studied how race, gender, and ethnicity impact population health and well-being, analyzing the impacts of these variables as part of a matrix of ruling relations at the core of systems of domination and subordination (McGibbon & Hallstrom, 2021). Not surprisingly, advances in the political economy of health continue to be informed by materialist epidemiology, where there is a resurgence of Marxist models that analyze class division, including the health effects of working-class power

(Muntaner et al., 2011). These models are well-suited for tackling health inequities because they are

> ... particularly broad, sensitive to historical changes, and sociologically relevant through their explicit focus on inequality-generating mechanisms such as social class relations (i.e., relative power between capital and labour), neo-liberal ideology (i.e., private profits vs. public good), and varieties of welfare regimes (i.e., social democratic vs. liberal vs. conservative). (Muntaner et al., 2011, p. 947)

Although materialist epidemiology and social epidemiology have distinct historical and theoretical underpinnings, some of their central ideas are closely similar—both social and materialist epidemiology inform critical perspectives on policy analysis and policy intervention to tackle inequities across the DoH.

POLICY ANALYSIS APPROACHES AND CRITICAL POLICY ANALYSIS

The political economy of health is very much connected to the implementation of policy analysis strategies at any given time. These approaches have many different methods and goals for understanding how policy analysis operates and how to design policy to solve problems, such as the increasing rates of health inequities in Canada and globally. Policy analysis approaches are underpinned by the worldviews or ideological stances of policymakers and all those who inform policy choices, such as policy advisors and policy consultants. Building on the example of unhoused people in Chapter 1, suppose policymakers are asked to develop public policies to address increasing numbers of unhoused people. Since this is a societally and politically contentious social issue, it aptly demonstrates how policy decision making is strongly influenced by the collective worldview of political parties, and hence policymakers, in power (McGibbon et al., 2022).

Depending on the worldview and ideological scaffolding of the prevailing government (and what they claim is the actual "problem"), the resulting policy could include measures such as decreasing or redirecting funding for non-profit community organizations that provide support for homeless people, because the cause of homelessness is framed as lack of motivation and laziness ("the problem") (McGibbon et al., 2022). Importantly, if the problem is perceived to be lack of motivation and the like, then solutions not only fail to address securing safe, dignified housing for unhoused people, they may also result in actually cutting available supports from existing federal and municipal budgets. On the other hand, public policy could include structurally implemented social supports such as basic/guaranteed annual income, based on substantive evidence of the structural causes of homelessness (the "problem") (Gaetz et al., 2016; Peterie et al., 2020). The following sections focus on extant policy analysis approaches: 1) positivist; 2) critical, including postmodern and critical feminist; and 3) postcolonial, Indigenous-grounded, and Afrocentric. It is crucial to note that with the exception of positivist policy analysis, these approaches often have some similar theoretical and practical similarities as well as distinctions regarding their analyses of the centrality of the social relations of power.

Positivist Policy Analysis Approaches

Positivist approaches to policy analysis, based in the tenets of positivism, continue to be the most dominant (see Box 2.1 for more details about positivism). From a positivist policymaker's perspective, the thinking goes something like this: since policy problems must be chosen based on objective, measurable evidence, messy, complex concerns such as classism and racism must be kept outside the policymaking process. To include them would demonstrate subjective bias and therefore would contaminate the value of resulting analyses. Positivist policy analysis approaches are based in reductionism, where the whole can be reduced to the sum of its parts. For example, if policymakers are designing policy to support new immigrants to Canada, they are likely to consider health care needs and housing needs as separate policy challenges that can be addressed separately in the health care sector, and in the housing and immigration sectors. This approach is referred to as "siloing"—separating health, housing, and immigration concerns into three separate government silos. It thus becomes difficult to design and achieve policy interventions because the struggles of people and families are themselves not "separated" or "siloed" in this manner. The same families are then expected to navigate three separate parts of the governance system in their new country.

Objectivity, another cornerstone of positivism, is synergistic with the beliefs of reductionism. Objectivity is related to the belief that policymaking knowledge should be designed solely on measurable, "objective," quantitative data. First-voice, lived experience, and Indigenous (First Nations, Inuit, Métis) and Afrocentric historical knowledges, for example, are at the bottom of the evidence validity scale. Striving for objectivity leads to policy concentration at the micro level because macro political and economic considerations are perceived to eliminate the objectivity so valued in positivist policymaking. For example, say policymakers aim to increase access to healthy food in a particular area. A policy concentration at the micro level might be about the nature and availability of grocery stores and localized transportation. However, these aspects of healthy food access are all inseparably connected to much larger macro societal and political issues, such as culturally relevant food needs and preferences, neighbourhood average income and hence capacity to buy fruits and vegetables, and types and costs of transportation access. Within an objective policy analysis frame, considerations such as lack of culturally appropriate food may ironically be seen to be biased or treating people differently, and hence unequally. So, increasing the number of grocery stores and types of transportation (unless it is cost-free public transportation), without macro considerations, is not likely to solve the problem of access to healthy foods.

Box 2.1: Some of the Main Beliefs Underpinning Positivist Thinking

- **Reductionism:** the belief that the whole can be reduced to the sum of its parts. One of the most prominent examples is the

(continued)

human body, which is separated into many discrete body systems and parts, such as the heart, the brain, the bones, and so on. Teaching in the health fields is still largely organized around these body parts, as are hospitals and most health intervention centres. Policymaking about areas related to health also tends to be based in these assumptions.

- **Objectivity:** the belief that policymaking knowledge should be designed solely on measurable, "objective," quantitative data, rather than "softer," less reliable qualitative data. Under these circumstances, marginalized and racialized voices have little chance of systematically and meaningfully informing public policy.
- **Neutrality:** the belief that a neutral ideological position is not only possible, but desirable. A close cousin to objectivity, neutrality is an ideological position that places one in the "middle" in the face of need. This may include deliberately (or even unintentionally) setting aside the realities of sexism and the historical impacts of patriarchy on the lives of countless people, including women, as well as trans and genderqueer people.
- **Empiricism:** the belief that facts and truths exist and knowledge of these facts or truths may only be developed from that which is directly observable. A prominent example is the dynamic tensions in the field of psychiatry between accepting notions of psychic and intergenerational mental health struggles and yet rejecting these struggles if they cannot be quantified.

Despite claims of objectivity, positivist policymaking oversimplifies complex processes and embeds values into policymaking that are not stated—values are covert and therefore become "givens" rather than being subject to debate (Stanhope & Dunn, 2011). The success of positivist policymaking thus relies on the ability to corral human behavior into manageable measurable constructs (Stanhope & Dunn, 2011). As a result, "social problems are decontextualized and oversimplified in order to generate unambiguous policy solutions. But in a given policy arena, there is rarely one stakeholder or an agreed upon outcome, but instead a myriad of competing demands on policy makers" (p. 277). Positivist policymaking approaches value standardization, objectivity, and simplicity over ambiguity, subjective experience, meaning, and complexity. The dominance of positivist policymaking approaches explain, to a large extent, why it has taken so many decades to introduce the isms into policymaking, a process that is still in its infancy in formal (officially elected) and institutional policy and governance systems.

Critical Policy Analysis Approaches

Postmodern, critical feminist, and critical intersectional policy analysis are critical policy analysis (CPA) approaches that emerged from a critique of the inadequacy of positivist policy analysis in terms of interrogating the social relations of power, and thus designing health equity–centred policy. CPA evolved primarily in the academic field of policy studies and often involves a coalescence of broad-reaching critical scholarship (Fischer et al., 2015), including anthropology, critical health studies, critical policy studies, postcolonial scholarship, and sociology. The lack of methodological sophistication (such as a grounding in positivism) in prevalent policy analysis approaches has also been a catalyst for CPA (Joo & Kwon, 2010). As Marshall (1999) pointed out, the scope for policy research became considerably wider:

> There is room for decades of policy research that asks first, how does this policy or structure exclude certain publics (subordinate nationalities, religions, women, the urban poor, the working class, homosexuals), then asks, what political arrangements support policies and structures that devalue alternative perspectives, that reinforce gender, ethnic/race and class inequities, and asks, who benefits from these arrangements, and finally, what are possible ways to restructure power dynamics and political arrangements to address issues of social justice? (p. 2)

Critical policy studies are also increasingly important as traditional areas of policymaking, such as economic and trade policy, become progressively more complex through "the pressures of globalization and the emergence of new political actors who take advantage of transnational access points and the uncertainty of the locus of power to try to circumvent the state" (Orsini & Smith, 2007, p. 2). CPA draws from the same overarching assumptions as the field of critical policy studies, rejecting the assumption that policy analysis is a neutral, apolitical process. With the exception of positivist policy analysis approaches, the CPA approaches described in this chapter can and do overlap due to their focus on challenging traditional, positivist policy analysis assumptions. Critical analyses of power dynamics and a rejection of the existence of one "objective truth" are core assumptions in each of these CPA approaches. Table 2.1 summarizes central areas of CPA. COVID-19 contexts are applied to more fully describe how these CPA assumptions

Table 2.1: Core Features of Critical Policy Analysis (CPA): COVID-19 Applications

Core Assumptions of CPA Approaches	COVID-19: CPA Applications
1) recognition of hegemonic power structures and the distribution of resources and knowledge (interrogating the roots and development of policy) (Apple, 2019).	Policy to support (or not support) vaccine access during the COVID-19 pandemic demonstrated the already-existing hegemony of multinational pharmaceutical companies in controlling global vaccine access (Chow, n.d.; also see Chapter 6).
2) integration of social stratification and the impact of policy on intersecting relationships of privilege, inequality, differential power and dominance, and subordination (Hankivsky et al., 2014; Shaw, 2004).	Rates of COVID-19 deaths occurred, by far, along social class (classism) and racial (racism) lines (Hankivsky & Kapilashrami, 2020). COVID-19 mortality and morbidity paralleled the devastating impacts of already-existing, public policy–induced social stratification, and still does.
3) the continued hegemony of positivist, rationalist, and individualistic analytic approaches to engaging with policy (Young & Diem, 2017).	Population health approaches to COVID-19 policymaking relied on already existing structures of positivism. The machinery of public health intervention largely rested on traditional epidemiology, which is ill-equipped to translate intergenerational colonial impacts into vaccine access barriers for Indigenous Peoples and Canadians of African descent.

Table 2.1: Core Features of Critical Policy Analysis (CPA): COVID-19 Applications (*Continued*)

Core Assumptions of CPA Approaches	COVID-19: CPA Applications
4) the importance of interdisciplinary, cross-sectoral approaches to methods and theoretical foundations in terms of research and analysis (Young & Diem, 2017).	COVID-19 is a pivotal case study in the importance of collaboration across sectors (health, law, ...) and disciplines (epidemiology, vaccinology, data science, public health, ...) to craft policies for decreasing infection rates as well as mitigating ecosystems implications for zoonoses such as COVID-19 (Centre on Climate Change and Planetary Health, 2020).
5) the role of participatory and emancipatory action and research, with explicit goals of disrupting processes and practices of oppression in local and global spheres (Joo & Kwan, 2010), "seeking to empower participation and enhance democracy" (Fischer et al., 2015, p. 2).	COVID-19 sparked a deepening of public consciousness about the ravages of COVID-19. In order to address infection rates that disproportionately impacted Canadians along classism and racism lines, it became imperative for public and institutional policymakers and researchers to go "out of their way" to listen to marginalized and racialized communities, including their formal leaders and their elders.

Source: Assumptions of CPA adapted from McGibbon et al., 2022.

play out on-the-ground in complex policymaking contexts such as the globe-wide pandemic.

Critical policy analysis derives its theoretical and practical base in perspectives of power and power over and knowledge of the colonial and patriarchal underpinnings of dominant conventional policy analysis. A CPA approach for taking action on the DoH may be guided by theoretical viewpoints from a broad scope of critical perspectives (Diem et al., 2014). McGibbon et al. (2022) summarized some of these perspectives: critical race theory (Atwood & López, 2014; Horsford, 2019), critical quantitative inquiry (Tabron & Ramlackhan, 2019), queer theory (O'Malley & Long, 2017), critical disability studies (Van Aswegen, 2020), cultural political economy (Jessop, 2010), and feminist intersectionality theory (Hankivsky et al., 2014), where feminist theorizing continues to advance the integration of broad acknowledgement of intersecting oppressions across time and across geographies. CPA is accordingly grounded in the belief that it is crucial to understand the complex connections between ruling structures and relations of dominance and subordination in the larger society (Apple, 2019). Exposing embedded power relationships is central to CPA, where policy is always an outcome of historical conditions: "The overall procedure of CPA is assessing the dominant conception of policy and attendant problems that cause and reproduce current structures of policy practice" (Joo & Kwan, 2010, p. 225). Although there are numerous approaches that may fall under the umbrella of CPA, the following section briefly focuses on two important areas: postmodern policy analysis and critical feminist policy analysis.

Postmodern policy analysis is a critical policy approach that supports "a refreshing skepticism toward the full range of things commonly associated with policy: policy itself, the knowledges that support policy and policy proposals, as well as conventional forms of policy analysis" (Bacchi & Goodwin, 2016, p. 3). According to Bacchi and Goodwin, postmodern approaches to policy analysis problematize foundational aspects of policy, including a rejection of the fixed nature of reality and a skepticism about the knowledge bases that support conventional policy formulation and analysis. As aforementioned, the knowledge base supporting policy approaches is limited by where policymakers decide to "do the looking." For example, if mandating institutional policy to accommodate persons with disabilities, resulting policy will be either enhanced or constrained by policymakers' capacity to integrate critical disability perspectives, recognizing that disability is a "social construct, not the inevitable consequence of impairment, and that the social disadvantage experienced by people with disabilities is caused by the physical, institutional and attitudinal (together, the 'social') environment which fails to meet the needs of people who do not match the social expectation of 'normalcy'" (Hosking, 2008, p. 7).

Social relations of power and policymakers' own roles as policy-involved actors are pivotal considerations in postmodern policy analysis, along with how the policy "problem" is represented and what discursive effects are produced by this particular representation (Bacchi & Goodwin, 2016). Although distinct in many of their origins and applications, postmodern policy analysis and critical feminist policy analysis share important methodological and theoretical foundations, including a focus on 1) explaining/exposing structural power relations, 2) analyzing the creation and maintenance of discursive pathways of structural power, and 3) systematic questioning of taken-for-granted historical, political, and cultural notions of "the way things are" and what has come to be known as "truth" (McGibbon et al., 2019).

The main assumptions of CPA are reflected in myriad critical policy approaches, such as *critical feminist policy analysis* (Marshall, 1999; Paterson & Scala, 2020; Shaw, 2004), which integrates theoretical and methodological applications from a broad scope of critical feminist perspectives, such as the CPA examples described previously (e.g., critical race theory, queer theory, critical disability studies, mad studies, and feminist intersectionality theory; McGibbon et al., 2022). At its inception, critical feminist policy analysis integrated critical social theory and feminism to challenge traditional positivist policy analysis that has dominated policy research and design over the last seven decades (Shaw, 2004). Critical feminist intersectional policy analysis focuses on the intersections of isms such as ageism, classism, genderism, heterosexism, racism, and sexism, and the imperative to integrate these identities into policy analysis. Without this explicit integration, policy involves (and hence is targeted towards) only dominant groups. In the case of designing workplace policy for the accommodation of persons with disability, a critical feminist policy analysis approach will deepen the success of the policies because implications for the many forms of access, for example, will be informed by intersections of the isms.

Postcolonial, Indigenous-grounded, and Afrocentric Policy Analysis Approaches

Aspects of CPA approaches are also present within postcolonial, Indigenous, and Afrocentric policy analysis approaches, such as examination of hegemonic power structures. However, these approaches each carry with them distinct theoretical and practical applications that go beyond CPA approaches. Although critiques of historical and ongoing colonial, imperialist systems are embedded in all three of these areas of policy analysis, each area has distinct contributions to the field of policy analysis, including upending settler dominance across macro-level settler policies. Descriptions of the following three approaches to policy analysis are only a brief starting point for readers to get an initial sense of their central importance for innovation in policy analysis approaches that can inform tackling inequities across the DoH.

Postcolonial policy analysis approaches draw from postcolonial theoretical perspectives—including the writings of Leela Gandhi (2019), Bannerji (2004), and Homi Bhabha's (1984) theorizing about the location of culture vis-à-vis colonizers and the colonized—which have all contributed to a robust discourse supporting action to identify, resist and transform the various forms and consequences of colonialism. Grounded in the principles of positivism, it is not possible to use "the settlers' tools," including policymaking tools, to intervene for justice across the policy development, implementation, and evaluation process. Postcolonial policy analysis approaches are as broad-based and varied as the theoretical and practical underpinnings of postcolonial theory itself. For example, Achilleos-Sarll (2018) applied a postcolonial, feminist approach to feminist policy analysis, integrating feminist intersectionality theory (described briefly above). Specifically, this genre of postcolonial policy analysis was used to argue that foreign policy should be re-conceptualized as gendered, sexualized, and racialized. The processes of decolonizing and creating decolonial futures (Grosfoguel, 2007), further described in Chapter 7, are also central considerations in postcolonial perspectives.

Indigenous-grounded policy analysis has its foundations in Indigenous knowledges, more fully described in Chapter 4. It involves analyzing the embeddedness of colonialist policy and its continuing and significant human and planet damage in Canada and globally. As the policy example in Chapter 5 about Indigenous Peoples and the "slow industrial genocide" of the Alberta Tar Sands attests, traditional, settler-driven policymaking does not have the capacity to intervene in Western capitalist systems of human and environmental destruction. Indigenous-grounded policymaking is an important field of knowledge and practice, with significant implications for mainstream policymaking in Canada and elsewhere. This relatively brief introduction provides some of the key ideas as an entry point to further exploration of this pivotal intellectual and practice-based knowledge area for action on the DoH.

In their work on Indigenous-grounded policy analysis, Fleras and Maaka (2010) emphasized that neither policy or policy analysis are neutral or value free. As socially constructed concepts, policy and policymaking are "loaded with dominant values, Eurocentric ideals, and vested interests… A commitment to race neutrality in policymaking serves to bolster White Eurocentricity as the norm, while discrediting Indigenous Peoples' claims to sovereignty status" (Fleras & Maaka, 2009, p. 2). These authors argued that reference to Indigeneity as a policy(making) paradigm is both necessary and overdue. They analyzed and assessed the politics of Māori Indigeneity in Aotearoa New Zealand in constructing an Indigeneity policy agenda model. They further described the development of an Indigenous-grounded analysis (IGA) framework as a policymaking paradigm for Indigenous Peoples of Canada. The IGA framework incorporates five first principles that "inform and legitimize a principled Indigeneity perspective in policy(making)" (p 14): Indigenous difference, Indigenous rights, Indigenous sovereignty; Indigenous belonging, and Indigenous spirituality (including traditional knowledge). The overall goal of the IGA framework is to minimize systemic policy bias while maximizing Indigenous peoples' inputs.

Afrocentric policy analysis approaches reflect the principles and practices of Afrocentricity, a metatheory and a theoretical concept developed and applied by Molefi Kete Asante (1980) who stated that Afrocentricity means "placing African ideals at the center of any analysis that involves African culture and behavior" (p. 2). Afrocentricity involves analyses of the influence of the Eurocentric worldview, which is imbued with a lack of emphasis on values such as spirituality, collectivity, mutual aid, and cooperation (Este & Bernard, 2006; Schiele, 2000), and the sexist and heterosexist assumptions of colonizer countries (Sefa Dei, 1994). Afrocentricity also "embodies a struggle for the total liberation of the African mind from the effects of slavery, colonialism, and neocolonialism" (p. 5).

Afrocentricity is not a unitary theoretical concept and there are multiple voices with many dissenting views and interpretations (Kumah-Abiwu, 2016). Applying Afrocentrism to the policy domain, Kumah-Abiwu argued that "the underlying tenets of the Afrocentric idea have the ability to redefine the widespread negative portrayal of Black identity through concrete policy ideas and initiatives" (p. 167), making the case for an extension of the Afrocentric paradigm to the policy domain. Two main questions guided Kumah-Abiwu's (2016) policy analysis applications of Afrocentricity: how could the core tenets of Afrocentric theoretical perspectives be beneficially applied 1) in shaping policy ideas and solutions to the socioeconomic problems facing communities in the African world? and 2) in teaching and the interpretation of concepts in the general sciences, technology, mathematics, and other fields?

Afrocentric applications for designing, implementing, and analyzing policy have been applied to many and varied policy questions. The following description provides only a few examples. Thompson and Wallner (2011) examined public policy and the establishment of Afrocentric education in Toronto. Although the establishment of Afrocentric schools was recommended in the 1990s by community organizations, a formal working group, and a royal commission, Thompson and Waller analyzed how the tragic death of 15-year-old student Jordan Manners, gunned down in the halls of his school on May 23, 2007, became a focusing event that forced a policy response from the Toronto District School Board. Akua (2017) used an Afrocentric case study policy analysis centred on African-American people, educators, and policymakers in the United States. These participants established that Florida state legislation was needed and necessary for the education of African American students and all students. There are many global examples of Afrocentric policy analysis approaches. An Afrocentric qualitative research methodology was used by Maphaka (2020) to examine shifts in South African foreign policy and, specifically, to determine whether the deepening relations between President Zuma and China led to a shift in South Africa's foreign policy. Each of these authors and researchers applied unique and situation-specific contexts for their Afrocentric policy analysis applications:

> The central argument of Afrocentricity is that an African phenomenon or communities cannot be understood when studied from outside. It requires the researcher to be positioned in African experiences in order to attain valid knowledge about an African phenomenon. (Maphaka, 2020, p. 89)

EXAMPLES OF POLICY ANALYSIS APPLICATIONS

Many broad, overarching policy perspectives and policy analysis applications are used in health, social, economic, and other areas with the goal of addressing inequities and other injustices across the DoH. Three applications are described here: 1) Health in All Policies (HiAP), 2) the National Collaborating Centre for Healthy Public Policy's (NCCHPP) policy analysis model, and 3) the policy briefing process. The aim is to translate some of the main ideas in the chapter into selected aspects of the existing health and policy landscape.

Health in All Policies (HiAP)

The DoH play a major role in the health and well-being of communities and nations. "Many of these factors are beyond the control or influence of the individual or the health sector. These factors form a complex web that is influenced by many sectors, such as local government and transport (Te Whatu Ora, Health New Zealand, n.d.). Health in All Policies (HiAP) is an approach to developing, implementing, and evaluating public policies across sectors and with communities (Te Whatu Ora, Health New Zealand, n.d.). Rather than addressing health exclusively from the health sector, an intersectoral approach means involving relevant policymaking sectors, such as health, labour, community services, education, law, environmental protection, and financial management, to name a few. However, the HiAP approach goes further by acknowledging that health and well-being are impacted by all policies in all governmental sectors, whether or not the policies are formally viewed as having anything to do with health.

The HiAP term was first used in 2006 at the Council of the European Union. The need for cross-sectoral and interdisciplinary action to achieve health-for-all was also emphasized in the WHO's Alma Ata Declaration (WHO, 1978) and the Ottawa Charter (WHO, 1986). HiAP was the theme of WHO's 8th Global Conference on Health Promotion in 2013, where HiAP was defined as an approach to public policies across sectors that systematically takes into account the health and health systems implications of decisions, seeks synergies, and avoids harmful health impacts, in order to improve population health and health equity (WHO, 2013). The HiAP approach is gaining policy-related traction in a broad scope of issues, such as climate crisis (Diallo, 2022), COVID-19 responses (Green et al., 2021), and environmental justice (Bolte et al., 2018). Unfortunately, in most jurisdictions, including Canada, government sectors are still "siloed," each functioning largely with their own separate mandates. This is why a HiAP approach has become prominent when discussing policy related to the DoH. The overall aim is to establish synergistic benefits and to minimize social and health-related harms, taking into account the health implications of all policy decisions (Tonelli et al., 2020). As an intersectoral approach to improving the social DoH and health equity, HiAP and HiAP-inspired approaches have great potential for guiding the post-COVID-19 pandemic recovery efforts at all governance levels in Canada (Poliquin & Carrillo Botero, 2023).

It is also important to note that HiAP approaches also carry with them the application of varied policy analysis and policymaking approaches described earlier. Since positivist policy analysis is still the dominant policymaking approach in most countries, many HiAP applications are also imbued with positivist ideas about how to define "the problem" and hence the choice of policy interventions. So, resulting HiAP policy analyses are not necessarily grounded in critical perspectives, where health and social inequities are understood to be the result of systemic power imbalances, especially those at the structural, policymaking level. Although the idea of HiAP has the potential to be a pivotal paradigm shift in promoting progressive policy reform to tackle health inequities, it can only be as effective as the foundations of its *a priori* theoretical and ideological underpinnings. For example, if the goal is justice in tackling pressing health problems, such as health inequities and environmental destruction, then a HiAP approach will be constricted by the level of criticality in its application. Resulting policymaking will be significantly impacted by whether or not policymakers (and their advisors and the people who produce policy briefs on health and social issues) make the links among climate emergencies and the root causes of damage to Earth's life support systems. As discussed in Chapter 4, decisions to label the problem as "climate change," "climate crisis," or "climate emergency" are also rooted in the level of criticality of HiAP policy applications.

The HiAP approach is evolving to include a broad scope of interpretations of the social DoH, including ecological and structural factors that impact health. For example, HiAP is compatible with the holistic nature of Māori perspectives of health and well-being, recognizing the importance and interconnections among these perspectives (Te Whatu Ora, Health of New Zealand, n.d.). Figure 2.1, adapted from Te Whatu Ora, Health New Zealand (n.d.), illustrates some of the ways that the HiAP concept has evolved. For example, the model demonstrates explicit inclusion and application of political economy influences of health (e.g., markets, wealth creation, macro-economy, politics) and the global ecosystem (e.g., biodiversity and climate change). According to Te Whatu Ora Health (n.d.), HiAP involves work in community and public health areas and aims to reflect the concepts of DoH, equity, and their treaty contexts. Te Whatu Ora Health's work is 1) guided by a social determinants approach that promotes fairness and justice, 2) informed by evidence, and 3) framed by the Treaty of Waitangi. Te Tiriti o Waitangi (known in English as the Treaty of Waitangi) is an agreement made in 1840 between representatives of the British Crown and more than 500 rangatira Māori people. It created the declaration of British sovereignty over New Zealand. The English treaty and the Maori te reo tiriti were interpreted differently—Māori and Pākēha (non-Māori, usually of British ethnic origin or background) therefore had different expectations of the treaty's terms. Ever since, resolution of these differences has presented New Zealand with significant challenges.

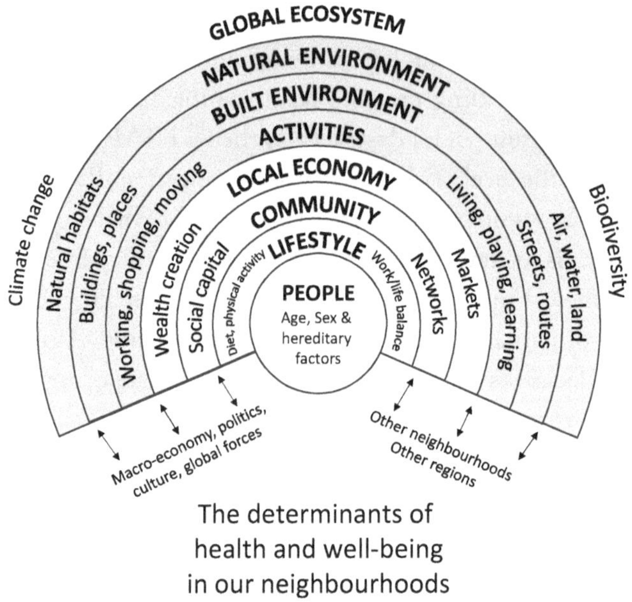

Figure 2.1: Health in All Policies Approach to Community and Public Health

Source: Adapted from Te Whatu Ora, Health New Zealand, n.d.

National Collaborating Centre, Healthy Public Policy: Dimensions of Policy Analysis

The National Collaborating Centre, Healthy Public Policy (NCCHPP) has a mandate to increase the expertise of public health actors across Canada in healthy public policy, which is understood to mean public policy that potentially enhances a populations' health by having a positive impact on the social, economic, and environmental DoH (Poliquin & Carrillo Botero, 2023). The NCCHPP developed an analytical framework for understanding any given public policy under study. The framework is guided by two overall dimensions of analysis: the policy's effects (effectiveness, unintended effects, equity) and its implementation (cost, feasibility, acceptability). The durability of the policy is also considered, capturing assessment of its performance over time. Application of the NCCHPP policy analysis model includes a detailed list of supporting questions for assessing each dimension. This policy analysis application provides a clear roadmap for thinking about complex policy areas. Key aspects of policy analysis have been distilled to provide guided direction for analyzing specific policies. The dimensions could also be strengthened with integration of CPA principles. In addition to the NCCHPP policy-analysis questions, there are crucial questions that can be asked within a CPA lens. Table 2.2 illustrates a few of these kinds of questions, which are added in italics.

For example, equity is a discrete sub-dimension in the framework, rather than an integral aspect throughout all dimensions of any given policy analysis situation. Unless an equity lens is also applied to, say, an analysis of unintended effects, assessment of these effects will be not be systematic across the isms, possibly invisiblizing potential impacts of the policy on already-existing inequities. For example, the COVID-19 pandemic was a natural experiment regarding the crucial need for criticality in policymaking. Largely conventional public health policy was initially implemented regarding vaccine access. High vaccination rates in Canada, the intended outcome of the vaccination policy, were not realized across marginalized and racialized peoples, due, in part, to lack of inclusion of the voices and communities who were already experiencing barriers in access to health and social care (e.g., people living in poverty, Indigenous Peoples, Canadians of African descent, to name a few). Over the first three years of the pandemic, it became clear that a large subgroup of Canadians had relatively little vaccine access, due to many of the health care access barriers that were well in place before the pandemic, including lack of material resources, such as money for transportation to vaccination sites; lack of money for child care; and lack of culturally safe care. Dimensions of policy analysis are thus enhanced or constrained by the overall policy analysis approach that is applied to analyze a particular policy.

The Policy Briefing Process

Policy briefs are an important, practical application of the policy analysis process. They are a key tool to present information from selected sources and to make recommendations to policymakers as well as non-specialized audiences. The result can include analyzing and

Table 2.2: Dimensions for *Critical* Analysis of Public Policies (critical perspective additions in italics)

Effects of Policy	
Effectiveness: What effects does the policy have on the targeted health problem? *Who decided how to frame the problem? Whose voices were included and excluded in the problem framing? What was the worldview/level of criticality of measures/instruments chosen to assess effectiveness? Was effectiveness measured with respect to intersectional policy analysis?*	**Durability of Policy**
Unintended effects: What are the unintended effects of this policy? *Was there a systematic assessment (across the isms) of the distribution of harms and benefits resulting from the new policy? Are these unintended effects ethically acceptable?*	
Equity: What are the effects of this policy on different groups? *Was a recognized equity gauge systematically applied to assess equity effects and impacts of the policy? How does the policy impact Charter rights and treaty rights?*	
Implementation of Policy	
Cost: What is the financial *and human* cost of this policy? *Who decides/designs the dimensions of the cost/benefit analysis? Financial and human cost for whom? Financial and human benefit for whom? Is the projected cost compared to the cost of not implementing the policy? Are costs calculated beyond one election cycle?*	**Durability of Policy**
Feasibility: Is this policy technically feasible? *Does the feasibility team include people with demonstrated content and experiential expertise in the policy area? How are the limits of feasibility decided upon and what is the composition of the team that is chosen to do the deciding (e.g., inclusion across geography, identity, discipline, first-voice, to name a few)?*	
Acceptability: Do the relevant stakeholders view the policy as acceptable? *Who decided which stakeholders are important for this policy issue? What are the tensions and power dynamics among stakeholders (e.g., government, civil society, community) when they disagree about acceptability? How are these tensions processed/resolved?*	

Source: Adapted from *Dimensions of Policy Analysis*, National Collaborating Centre for Healthy Public Policy, 2012.

condensing existing policies as well as making new policy recommendations. Ideally, policy briefs, also known as briefing notes, are a method to provide evidence-based policy advice to help readers make informed policy decisions. "A strong policy brief distills research findings in plain language and draws clear links to policy initiatives. The best policy briefs are clear, concise, stand-alone documents that focus on a single topic" (International Development Research Centre [IDRC], n.d., para. 2). Common sections in a policy brief include 1) a brief overview of the policy problem at hand; 2) an analysis of existing evidence about the problem; 3) a presentation of key policy options for action, including existing policies, if applicable; and 4) conclusions about which option is the best. (See the IDRC website in Website Resources for a more detailed explanation of crafting policy briefs.)

Already, it is apparent that the ideological and theoretical filters used to decide on sources for gathering, assessing, and synthesizing information will determine the criticality of the brief, and hence its usefulness if the goal is equitable policymaking across the various social, ecological, and structural DoH. The criticality of a policy brief may also be assessed with consideration of CPA questions for analyzing public policy in Table 2.2. These questions shape not only the framing of the policy problem but also what kinds of evidence will shape the choice of policy options and ultimately the policy brief recommendations. For example, in Nova Scotia, Canada, after over a half century of first-voice evidence from Indigenous and Black communities, there was still no government action to mitigate environmental racism in the province in areas such as addressing and halting toxic industrial waste in Boat Harbour (further described in Chapter 4). Eventually, due to public pressure from these communities and their allies, as well as international pressure from organizations such as Amnesty International, the provincial government finally held corporate polluters responsible for shutting down industrial pollutant operations and engaging in a clean-up of toxic chemicals in the area. Although the community-based evidence for policy change was systematic and abundant, it was not considered credible or actionable in historical policymaking processes to address environmental racism in Boat Harbour.

CONCLUSION

Policy and politics are foundational ingredients for understanding the hows and whys of injustice across the DoH. Most importantly, without this knowledge it is difficult to make sustainable gains towards equitable redistribution of the social and material supports that we all need to achieve a dignified and health-giving quality of life, one that sustains our happiness and sense of collective well-being. Consequently, strategies are urgently needed to normalize policy and political literacy as interesting and core components across all the disciplines and sectors in formal teaching and learning institutions, such as schools and universities. To isolate these components into "policy" related courses or policy and governance programs is to facilitate a sort of mass unawareness of the tools we need to intervene in the urgent, synergistic humanitarian and climate polycrisis all around us. Compounding lack of public knowledge about the policymaking process is the fact that using existing structures to craft these alternative approaches may slow down progress, possibly to the point of being futile endeavours. Policy and political consciousness must also be somehow reframed within critical policy approaches as well as Indigenous and Afrocentric policy approaches. Community development and civil society groups and organizations have already enacted political literacy for decades and centuries to achieve justice across the globe. There is no need to reinvent the wheel.

FURTHER READINGS

Barnett, P., & Bagshaw, P. (2020). Neoliberalism: What it is, how it affects health and what to do about it. *The New Zealand Medical Journal, 133*(1512), 76–84.

Brunoli, J. (2017, June 24). *This is neoliberalism, part I: The 10 tenets of neoliberalism.* Medium. https://euroyankeeblog.medium.com/10-tenets-of-neoliberalism-ea90f34e51f9

Green, L., Ashton, K., Bellis, M. A., Clemens, T., & Douglas, M. (2021). "Health in All Policies"—A key driver for health and well-being in a post-COVID-19 pandemic world. *International Journal of Environmental Research and Public Health, 18*(18), 9468. https://doi.org/10.3390/ijerph18189468

Krieger, N. (2003). Does racism harm health? Did child abuse exist before 1962? On explicit questions, critical science, and current controversies: An ecosocial perspective. *American Journal of Public Health, 93*(2), 194–199. https://doi.org/10.2105/ajph.93.2.194

Petteway, R. J., Mujahid, M., Allen, A., & Morello-Frosch, R. (2019). Towards a people's social epidemiology: Envisioning a more inclusive and equitable future for social epi research and practice in the 21st century. *International Journal of Environmental Research and Public Health, 16*(20), 3983. https://doi.org/10.3390/ijerph16203983

WEBSITES OF INTEREST

Canadian Centre for Policy Alternatives—https://policyalternatives.ca/

"The Canadian Centre for Policy Alternatives is an independent, non-partisan research institute concerned with issues of social, economic and environmental justice. Founded in 1980, the CCPA is one of Canada's leading progressive voices in public policy debates."

How to Write a Policy Brief (International Development Research Center, IDRC)—https://idrc-crdi.ca/en/funding/resources-idrc-grantees/how-write-policy-brief

This website includes an introduction to writing policy briefs. Drawing on international development projects and policy brief examples, the website walks you through the process of writing an effective policy brief to advocate for your DoH justice issues.

The Human Development Index (HDI)—https://hdr.undp.org/data-center/human-development-index#/indicies/HDI

"The HDI can be used to question national policy choices, asking how two countries with the same level of Gross National Income (GNI) per capita can end up with different human development outcomes."

National Collaborating Centre for Healthy Public Policy—https://ccnpps-ncchpp.ca/

The Centre's mandate is to increase the expertise of public health actors across Canada in healthy public policy through the development, sharing and use of knowledge. The Centre's interest is in healthy public policy, which is understood to mean public policy that potentially enhances populations' health by having a positive impact on the social, economic, and environmental determinants of health.

Te Whatu Ora, Health New Zealand—https://www.tewhatuora.govt.nz/

This website described the details of development and practice applications for Te Whatu Ora's Health in All Policies approach in community and public health, including the principles of community and public health: focusing on the health of communities rather than individuals; influencing health determinants; prioritizing improvements in Māori health; reducing health disparities; basing practice on the best available evidence; building effective partnerships across the health sector and other sectors; and remaining responsive to new and emerging health threats.

GLOSSARY

Institutional Policy: Refers to policy that is developed and implemented within institutional structures, including formally recognized institutions in sectors such as universities and health care, where institutional actors (e.g., boards of directors of universities and hospitals) can be identified. Institutional policy can also refer to systemic or institutionalized structures, where institutional refers to "... a complex of relations forming part of the ruling apparatus, organized around a distinctive function—education, health care, law, and the like" (Smith, 1987, p. 160).

Modern Welfare State: Refers to the "extent to which governments or the state use their power to provide citizens with the means to live secure and satisfying lives" (Raphael, 2009, p. 15).

Neoliberal Welfare State: Refers to countries where the ideological inspiration is liberty, with the stated aim of relatively minimal government intervention and a focus on benefits available only through means testing (limiting access through screening), rather than universal availability (McGibbon & Hallstrom, 2021).

Neoliberalism: Refers to the principle that the marketplace is the best authority regarding how economic and other resources should be distributed (Coburn, 2004). In other words, markets allocate scarce resources, promote efficient growth, and secure individual liberty better than governments. This results in the primacy of economic over social policies (Kickbusch, 2015). Neoliberal mandates include the belief that public welfare systems need to be cut back to eliminate bureaucratic waste, reduce taxation, and allow greater choice through private service provision (Alcock et al, 2022). Critics point out that "neoliberalism benefits multinational corporations and the financial sector, as well as particular government agencies and international organizations" (Carlquist & Phelps, 2014, p. 1231).

Policy Analysis: The examination and evaluation of available options (existing policies or newly crafted policies) to address various economic, social, or other public issues. The process includes many areas of data collection, including empirical research and statistical data collection, and the participation of key stakeholders such as economists, community members, and public officials tasked with enacting policy (Norwich University, n.d.).

Policy Intervention: Refers to the application of a particular policy or series of policies to solve an identified problem or to enhance existing policies to increase their effectiveness.

Political Economy of Health: These perspectives analyze the role of the economic organization of society in the production and distribution of disease and the burden of illness, and the ways that disease, illness, and wellness are framed (deciding what the problem is perceived to be) and treated (deciding what the policy intervention should be; Coburn, 2004; McGibbon et al., 2024).

Population Health: Refers to health status and health status inequities of the population as a whole, as well as groups within it. These groups may be defined by geography, age, culture, or other defining features. The approach measures health over time, across jurisdictions, and across health issues. It captures not only illness and injury, but the positive dimensions of health as well, such as physical fitness levels of the population (Public Health Agency of Canada, 2023).

Positivism: Refers to a way of thinking and analysis that is based in the principles of reductionism, objectivity, neutrality, and empiricism. See Box 2.1 for explanations of these main beliefs underpinning positivist thinking.

Public Policy: A document drawn up by governmental actors to present their vision of an issue calling for public action and, to some extent, the legal, technical, practical and operational aspects of this action (Turgeon & Savard, 2012). Public policy may also refer to the processes through which elected representatives decide on a public action designed to deal with an issue, where the issue itself is considered by certain actors, whether governmental or non-governmental, to require some kind of policy intervention (Turgeon & Savard, 2012).

Social Democratic Welfare State: Refers to countries where the ideological inspiration is the reduction of poverty, inequality, and unemployment. Organizing principles are universalism and the socialist ideals of equality, the social rights of all citizens, justice, freedom, and solidarity (Bryant, 2016; Esping-Andersen, 2002; Saint-Arnaud & Bernard, 2003).

REFERENCES

Achilleos-Sarll, C. (2018). Reconceptualising foreign policy as gendered, sexualised and racialised: Towards a postcolonial feminist foreign policy (analysis). *Journal of International Women's Studies, 19*(1), 34–49.

Akua, C. (2017). *The life of a policy: An Afrocentric case study policy analysis of Florida statute 1003.42(h)* [Doctoral dissertation]. Georgia State University. https://doi.org/10.57709/9465379

Alcock, P., Haux, T., McCall, V., & May, M. (Eds.). (2022). *The student's companion to social policy* (6th ed.). Wiley-Blackwell.

Ansell, A. (Ed.). (2019). *Unraveling the right: The new conservatism in American thought and politics.* Routledge.

Apple, M. W. (2019). On doing critical policy analysis. *Educational Policy, 33*(1), 276–287. https://doi.org/10.1177/0895904818807307

Armstrong, P., & Connelly, M. P. (1989). Feminist political economy: An introduction. *Studies in Political Economy, 30*(1), 5–12.

Asante, M. K. (1980). *Afrocentricity: The theory of social change.* Amulefi Publishing Company.

Atwood, E., & López, G. R. (2014). Let's be critically honest: Towards a messier counterstory in critical race theory. *International Journal of Qualitative Studies in Education, 27*(9), 1134–1154. https://doi.org/10.1080/09518398.2014.916011

Bacchi, C., & Goodwin, S. (2016). *Poststructural policy analysis: A guide to practice.* Springer. https://doi.org/10.1057/978-1-137-52546-8

Baer, H. A. (1982). On the political economy of health. *Medical Anthropology Quarterly, 14*(1), 1–17. https://doi.org/10.1525/maq.1982.14.1.02a00010

Bambra, C., Fox, D., & Scott-Samuel, A. (2005). Towards a politics of health. *Health Promotion International, 20*(2), 187–193. https://doi.org/10.1093/heapro/dah608

Bannerji, H. (2004). Immigrant women: Labour in the North American continent. In M. Bhattacharya (Ed.), *Globalization* (pp. 87–92). Tulika Books.

Barnett, P., & Bagshaw, P. (2020). Neoliberalism: What it is, how it affects health and what to do about it. *The New Zealand Medical Journal, 133*(1512), 76–84.

Bhabha, H. (1984). Of mimicry and man: The ambivalence of colonial discourse. *Discipleship: A Special Issue on Psychoanalysis (Spring), 28*, 125–133. https://doi .org/10.2307/778467

Bolte, G., Bunge, C., Hornberg, C., & Köckler, H. (2018). Environmental justice as an approach to tackle environmental health inequalities. *Bundesgesundheitsblatt-Gesundheitsforschung-Gesundheitsschutz, 61*(6), 674–683. https://doi.org/10.1007/ s00103-018-2739-6

Brown, R. (2019, October 28). *Explaining the neoliberal turn.* TransformingSociety. https://www.transformingsociety.co.uk/2019/10/28/ explaining-the-neoliberal-turn/

Brunoli, J. (2017, June 24). *This is neoliberalism, part I: The 10 tenets of neoliberalism.* Medium. https://euroyankeeblog.medium.com/10-tenets-of-neoliberalism-ea90f34e51f9

Bryant, T. (2016). *Health policy in Canada* (2nd ed.). Canadian Scholars.

Canadian Public Health Association. (2017). *Public health: A conceptual framework.* https://www.cpha.ca/sites/default/files/uploads/policy/ph-framework/phcf_e.pdf

Capano, G., & Howlett, M. (Eds.). (2020). *A modern guide to public policy.* Edward Elgar Publishing.

Carlquist, E., & Phelps, J. (2014). Neoliberalism. In T. Teo, (Ed.), *Encyclopedia of critical psychology* (pp. 1231–1237). Springer.

Carman, T. (2020, November 17). *COVID-19 mortality rate higher in neighbourhoods with more visible minorities: StatsCan.* CBC News. https://www.cbc.ca/news/ canada/british-columbia/covid19-minorities-health-bc-canada-1.5801777

Centre on Climate Change and Planetary Health. (2020). *One health, ecohealth and planetary health: Bridging disciplines for a post-COVID-19 world.* London School of Hygiene and Tropical Medicine. https://www.lshtm.ac.uk/ newsevents/events/one-health-ecohealth-and-planetary-health-bridging -disciplines-post-covid-19

Chow, H. (n.d.). The Moderna vaccine should be a people's vaccine. *Global Justice Now*. https://mailchi.mp/globaljustice/lets-force-big-pharma-to-co-operate-608592?e=18d7ca0c9d

Coburn, D. (2004). Beyond the income inequality hypothesis: Class, neo-liberalism, and health inequalities. *Social Science and Medicine, 58*(1), 41–56. https://doi.org/10.1016/s0277-9536(03)00159-x

Coburn, D. (2010). Health and health care: A political economy perspective. In T. Bryant, D. Raphael, & M. Rioux (Eds.), *Staying alive: Critical perspectives on health, illness, and health care* (2nd ed.). Canadian Scholars.

Diallo, T. (2022). Health in All Policies: For a healthy and equitable post COVID-19 recovery? *Global Health Promotion, 29*(2), 3–4. https://doi.org/10.1177/17579759221092258

Diem, S., Young, M. D., Welton, A. D., Mansfield, K. C., & Lee, P.-L. (2014). The intellectual landscape of critical policy analysis. *International Journal of Qualitative Studies in Education, 27*(9), 106–190. https://doi.org/10.1080/09518398.2014.916007

Dye, T. R. (1972). *Understanding public policy*. Prentice Hall.

Esping-Andersen, G. (2002). *Why we need a new welfare state*. Oxford University Press. https://doi.org/10.1093/0199256438.001.0001

Esping-Andersen, G. (2015). Welfare regimes and social stratification. *Journal of European Social Policy, 25*(1), 124–134. https://doi.org/10.1177/0958928714556976

Este, D., & Bernard, W. T. (2006). Spirituality among African Nova Scotians: A key to survival in Canadian society. *Critical Social Work, 7*(1), 1–22. https://doi.org/10.22329/csw.v7i1.5768

Fischer, F., Torgerson, D., Durnová, A., & Orsini, M. (2015). Introduction to critical policy studies. In F. Fischer, D. Torgerson, A. Durnová, & M. Orsini (Eds.), *Handbook of critical policy studies* (pp. 1–26). Edward Elgar Publishing. https://doi.org/10.4337/9781783472352.00005

Fleras, A., & Maaka, R. (2010). Indigeneity-grounded analysis (IGA) as policy(-making) lens: New Zealand models, Canadian realities. *The International Indigenous Policy Journal, 1*(1), 1–34. https://doi.org/10.18584/iipj.2010.1.1.4

Gaetz, S., Dej, E., Richter, T., & Redman, M. (2016). *The state of homelessness in Canada 2016*. Canadian Observatory on Homelessness Press. https://www.homelesshub.ca/sites/default/files/SOHC16_final_20Oct2016.pdf

Gandhi, L. (2019). *Postcolonial theory: A critical introduction* (2nd ed.). Columbia University Press.

Gaventa, J. (2017, December 18). *What have we learned from the powercube?* Institute of Development Studies. https://www.ids.ac.uk/news/what-have-we-learned-from-the-powercube/

Green, L., Ashton, K., Bellis, M. A., Clemens, T., & Douglas, M. (2021). "Health in All Policies"—A key driver for health and well-being in a post-COVID-19 pandemic world. *International Journal of Environmental Research and Public Health, 18*(18), 9468. https://doi.org/10.3390/ijerph18189468

Grosfoguel, R. (2007). The epistemic decolonial turn: Beyond political-economy paradigms. *Cultural Studies, 21*(2–3), 211–223. https://doi.org/10.1080/09502380601162514

Hankivsky, O., Grace, D., Hunting, G., Giesbrecht, M., Fridkin, A., Rudrum, S., Ferlatte, O., & Clark, N. (2014). An intersectionality-based policy analysis framework: Critical reflections on a methodology for advancing equity. *International Journal for Equity in Health, 13*(1), 119. https://doi.org/10.1186/s12939-014-0119-x

Hankivsky, O., & Kapilashrami, A. (2020). *Beyond sex and gender analysis: An intersectional view of the COVID-19 pandemic outbreak and response.* Global Policy Institute. https://mspgh.unimelb.edu.au/__data/assets/pdf_file/0011/3334889/Policy-brief_v3.pdf

Heywood, A. (2012). *Political ideologies: An introduction* (5th ed.). Macmillan International Higher Education.

Hill, A. (2023, June 21). Children raised under UK austerity shorter than European peers, study finds. *The Guardian.* https://www.theguardian.com/business/2023/jun/21/children-raised-under-uk-austerity-shorter-than-european-peers-study

Horsford, S. D. (2019). School integration in the new Jim Crow: Opportunity or oxymoron? *Educational Policy, 33*(1), 257–275. https://doi.org/10.1177/0895904818810526

Hosking, D. L. (2008, September 2–4). *Critical disability theory* [Presentation]. Disability Studies Conference, Lancaster University, United Kingdom.

International Development Research Centre. (n.d.). *How to write a policy brief.* https://idrc-crdi.ca/en/funding/resources-idrc-grantees/how-write-policy-brief

Jessop, B. (2010). Cultural political economy and critical policy studies. *Critical Policy Studies, 3*(3–4), 336–356. https://doi.org/10.1080/19460171003619741

Joo, K. P., & Kwon, I. T. (2010). *Critical policy analysis: Investigating "missing" values in the lifelong education system of South Korea.* Adult Education Research Conference. https://newprairiepress.org/aerc/2010/papers/37

Kickbusch, I. (2015). The political determinants of health—10 years on. *BMJ Clinical Research, 350.* https://doi.org/10.1136/bmj.h81

Krieger, N. (2001). Theories for social epidemiology in the 21st century: An ecosocial perspective. *International Journal of Epidemiology, 30*(4), 668–677. https://doi.org/10.1093/ije/30.4.668

Krieger, N. (2003). Does racism harm health? Did child abuse exist before 1962? On explicit questions, critical science, and current controversies: An ecosocial perspective. *American Journal of Public Health, 93*(2), 194–199. https://doi.org/10.2105/ajph.93.2.194

Kumah-Abiwu, F. (2016). Beyond intellectual construct to policy ideas: The case of the Afrocentric paradigm. *Africology: The Journal of Pan African Studies, 9*(1), 7–27.

Labonté, R., & Stuckler, D. (2016). The rise of neoliberalism: How bad economics imperils health and what to do about it. *Journal of Epidemiology and Community Health, 70*(3), 312–318. https://www.jstor.org/stable/44017712

Lah, O. (Ed.). (2018). *Sustainable urban mobility pathways: Policies, institutions, and coalitions for low carbon transportation in emerging countries.* Elsevier.

Leigh, J. P., & Chakalov, B. (2021). Labor unions and health: A literature review of pathways and outcomes in the workplace. *Preventive Medicine Reports, 24*, 101502. https://doi.org/10.1016/j.pmedr.2021.101502

Maier, C. S. (1987). *In search of stability: Explorations in historical political economy.* Cambridge University Press.

Maphaka, D. (2020). A shift or priority? An Afrocentric analysis of Zuma's foreign policy towards China. *Strategic Review for Southern Africa, 42(*2), 87–108. https://doi.org/10.35293/srsa.v42i2.75

Marshall, C. (1999). Researching the margins: Feminist critical policy analysis. *Educational Policy, 13*(1), 59–76. https://doi.org/10.1177/0895904899131006

Marx, K. (1977). *A contribution to the critique of political economy.* Progress Publishers. (Original work published 1859)

McGibbon, E. (2016). Oppressions and access to health care: Deepening the conversation. In D. Raphael (Ed.), *The social determinants of health* (3rd ed., pp. 491–520). Canadian Scholars.

McGibbon, E., Bailey, A., & Hendra, S. (2024). Violence and health: Contexts of power and social inequities. In J. Etowa, C. Van Daalen-Smith, & A. Dosani (Eds.), *Community health nursing: A Canadian perspective* (6th ed.). Pearson.

McGibbon, E., & Etowa, J. (2009). *Anti-racist health care practice.* Canadian Scholars.

McGibbon, E., Fierlbeck, K., & Ajadi, T. (2019). *Institutional ethnography as feminist policy analysis: A Canadian case study* [Panel presentation]. International Public Policy Association, 3rd Annual Conference, Montreal, QC, Canada.

McGibbon, E., Fierlbeck, K., & Ajadi, T. (2022). Institutional ethnography and critical policy analysis: Catalyzing justice in policymaking [Paper accepted for publication]. *Critical Studies: An International and Interdisciplinary Journal.*

McGibbon, E., & Hallstrom, L. (2021). Oppression and the political economy of health inequities. In E. McGibbon (Ed.), *Oppression: A social determinant of health* (2nd ed., pp. 85–99). Fernwood Publishing.

Muller, J., & Raphael, D. (2023). Does unionization and working under collective agreements promote health? *Health Promotion International, 38*(4), daab181. https://doi.org/10.1093/heapro/daab181

Muntaner, C., Borrell, C., Ng, E., Chung, H., Espelt, A., Rodriguez-Sanz, M., Benach, J., & O'Campo, P. (2011). Politics, welfare regimes, and population health: Controversies and evidence. *Sociology of Health and Illness, 33*(6), 946–964. https://doi.org/10.1111/j.1467-9566.2011.01339.x

National Collaborating Centre for Healthy Public Policy. (2012). *A framework for analyzing public policies: Practical guide.* http://www.ncchpp.ca/docs/Guide_framework_analyzing_policies_En.pdf

Navarro, V. (2007a). Neoliberalism as class ideology; or, the political causes of the growth of inequalities. *International Journal of Social Determinants of Health and Health Services, 37*(1), 47–62. https://doi.org/10.2190/AP65-X154-4513-R520

Navarro, V. (2007b). What is national health policy? *International Journal of Social Determinants of Health and Health Services, 37*(1), 1–14. https://doi.org/10.2190/H454-7326-6034-1T25

Navarro, V., Muntaner, C., Borrell, C., Benach, J., Quiroga, Á., Rodríguez-Sanz, M., Vergés, N., & Pasarín, M. I. (2006). Politics and health outcomes. *The Lancet, 368*(9540), 1033–1037. https://doi.org/10.1016/s0140-6736(06)69341-0

Noël, A. (2019). The politics of minimum income protection in OECD countries. *Journal of Social Policy, 48*(2), 227–247. https://doi.org/10.1017/S0047279418000351

Norwich University. (n.d.). *What is policy analysis? A critical concept in public administration.* https://online.norwich.edu/what-policy-analysis-critical-concept-public-administration

O'Malley, M. P., & Long, T. A. (2017). Public educational policy as performance: A queer analysis. In M. D. Young & S. Diem (Eds.), *Critical approaches to education policy analysis: Moving beyond tradition* (pp. 63–82). Springer.

Organisation for Economic Co-operation and Development. (n.d.). *Infant mortality rates (indicator).* https://data.oecd.org/healthstat/infant-mortality-rates.htm

Orsini, M., & Smith, M. (Eds.). (2007). *Critical policy studies.* UBC Press.

Overbeek, H., & van der Pijl, K. (1993). Restructuring capital and restructuring hegemony: Neoliberalism and the unmaking of the post-war order. In H. Overbeek (Ed.), *Restructuring hegemony in the global political economy.* Routledge.

Paterson, S., & Scala, F. (2020). Feminist government or government feminism? Exploring feminist policy analysis in the Trudeau era. In A. Dobrowolsky & F. MacDonald (Eds.), *Turbulent times, transformational possibilities? Gender and politics today and tomorrow* (pp. 49–67). University of Toronto Press.

Peterie, M., Bielefeld, S., Marston, G., Mendes, P., & Humpage, L. (2020). Compulsory income management: Combatting or compounding the underlying causes of homelessness? *Australian Journal of Social Issues, 55*(1), 61–72. https://doi.org/10.1002/ajs4.79

Petteway, R. J., Mujahid, M., Allen, A., & Morello-Frosch, R. (2019). Towards a people's social epidemiology: Envisioning a more inclusive and equitable future for social epi research and practice in the 21st century. *International Journal of Environmental Research and Public Health, 16*(20), 3983. https://doi.org/10.3390/ijerph16203983

Poliquin, H., & Carrillo Botero, N. (2023). *Developing a Canadian network for Health in All Policies: Consultations with actors from Canada and abroad.* National Collaborating Centre for Healthy Public Policy. https://ccnpps-ncchpp.ca/docs/2023-Developing-A-Canadian-Network-for-Health-in-All-Policies.pdf

Public Health Agency of Canada. (2023). *Key element 1: Focus on the health of populations.* https://cbpp-pcpe.phac-aspc.gc.ca/population-health-approach-organizing-framework/key-element-1-focus-health-populations/

Rainwater, L., & Smeeding. T. M. (2005). *Poor kids in a rich country: America's children in comparative perspective.* Russell Sage Foundation.

Rajmil, L., Hjern, A., Spencer, N., Taylor-Robinson, D., Gunnlaugsson, G., & Raat, H. (2020). Austerity policy and child health in European countries: A systematic literature review. *BMC Public Health, 20*(1), 564. https://doi.org/10.1186/s12889-020-08732-3

Raphael, D. (2009). Escaping from the phantom zone: Social determinants of health, public health units and public policy in Canada. *Health Promotion International, 24*(2), 193–198. https://doi.org/10.1093/heapro/dap005

Raphael, D. (2021). Raising the volume on the social determinants of health in Canada and elsewhere. In E. McGibbon (Ed.), *Oppression: A social determinant of health* (2nd ed.). Fernwood Publishing.

Raphael, D., Bryant, T., Mikkonen, J., & Raphael, A. (2020). *Social determinants of health: The Canadian facts.* Ontario Tech University Faculty of Health Sciences and York University School of Health Policy and Management. https://thecanadianfacts.org/

Raphael, D., & Curry-Stevens, A. (2016). Surmounting the barriers: Making action on the social determinants of health a public policy priority. In D. Raphael (Ed.), *Social determinants of health: Canadian perspectives* (3rd ed., pp. 361–383). Canadian Scholars.

Said, E. (2001). The public role of writers and intellectuals. In S. Bermann & M. Wood (Eds.), *Nation, language, and the ethics of translation* (Vol. 10, pp. 15–29). Princeton University Press.

Saint-Arnaud, S., & Bernard, P. (2003). Convergence or resilience? A hierarchical cluster analysis of the welfare regimes in advanced countries. *Current Sociology, 51*(5), 499–527. https://doi.org/10.1177/00113921030515004

Schrecker, T. (2016). Neoliberalism and health: The linkages and the dangers. *Sociology Compass, 10*(10), 952–971. https://doi.org/10.1111/soc4.12408

Schiele, J. H. (2000). *Human services and the Afrocentric paradigm.* Haworth Press.

Sefa Dei, G. J. (1994). Afrocentricity: A cornerstone of pedagogy. *Anthropology & Education Quarterly, 25*(1), 3–28. http://www.jstor.org/stable/3195745

Shaw, K. M. (2004). Using feminist critical policy analysis in the realm of higher education: The case of welfare reform as gendered educational policy. *The Journal of Higher Education, 75*(1), 56–79. https://doi.org/10.1353/jhe.2003.0053

Shaw, M., Dorling, D., Gordon, D., & Smith, G. D. (1999). *The widening gap: Health inequalities and policy in Britain*. Policy Press.

Smith, D. (1987). *The everyday world as problematic: A feminist sociology*. Northeastern University Press.

Stanhope, V., & Dunn, K. (2011). The curious case of Housing First: The limits of evidence based policy. *International Journal of Law and Psychiatry, 34*(4), 275–282. https://doi.org/10.1016/j.ijlp.2011.07.006

Stuckler, D., Reeves A., Loopstra, R., Karanikolos, M., & McKee, M. (2017). Austerity and health: The impact in the UK and Europe. *European Journal of Public Health, 27*(Suppl 4), 18–21. https://doi.org/10.1093/eurpub/ckx167

Tabron, L. A., & Ramlackhan, K. (2019). Hypocrisy, state policy, and African American students with disabilities: The guise of access. *Educational Policy, 33*(1), 181–204. https://doi.org/10.1177/0895904818807308

Taylor-Robinson, D., Lai, E. T. C., Wickham, S., Rose, T., Norman, P., Bambra, C., Whitehead, M., & Barr, B. (2019). Assessing the impact of rising child poverty on the unprecedented rise in infant mortality in England, 2000–2017: Time trend analysis. *BMJ Open, 9*(10), e029424. https://doi.org/10.1136/bmjopen-2019-029424

Te Whatu Ora, Health New Zealand. (n.d.). *Health in All Policies approach at community and public health*. https://www.cph.co.nz/your-health/health-in-all-policies/

Thompson, D., & Wallner, J. (2011). A focusing tragedy: Public policy and the establishment of Afrocentric education in Toronto. *Canadian Journal of Political Science/Revue canadienne de science politique, 44*(4), 807–828. https://doi.org/10.1017/S000842391100076X

Tickell, A., & Peck, J. (2003) Making global rules: Globalization or neoliberalization? In J. Peck & H. Yeung (Eds.), *Remaking the global economy: Economic-geographical perspectives* (pp. 163–181). SAGE.

Tonelli, M., Tang, K. C., & Forest, P. G. (2020). Canada needs a "Health in All Policies" action plan now. *CMAJ, 192*(3), E61–E67. https://doi.org/10.1503/cmaj.190517

Turgeon, J., & Savard, J.-F. (2012). Public policy. In L. Côté and J.-F. Savard (Eds.), *Encyclopedic Dictionary of Public Administration* [Online]. https://dictionnaire.enap.ca/Dictionnaire/17/Index_par_mot.enap?by=word&id=14

Van Aswegen, J. (2020). Disabling discourses and charitable model of disability: Labour market activation for people with disabilities, Ireland—A critical policy analysis. *Disability & Society, 35*(3), 435–459. http://dx.doi.org/10.1080/09687599.2019.1634519

World Health Organization (WHO). (1978). *Declaration of Alma-Ata*.

World Health Organization. (1986). *Ottawa Charter for Health Promotion*. The 1st International Conference on Health Promotion, Ottawa, ON, Canada. https://www.who.int/teams/health-promotion/enhanced-wellbeing/first-global-conference

World Health Organization. (2013). *The Helsinki statement on health in all policies*. The 8th Global Conference on Health Promotion, Helsinki, Finland.

Young, M. D., & Diem, S. (2017). Introduction: Critical approaches to education policy analysis. In M. D. Young & S. Diem (Eds.), *Critical approaches to education policy analysis: Moving beyond tradition* (pp. 1–13). Springer.

CHAPTER 3

Critical Perspectives on the Social Determinants of Health

CHAPTER OBJECTIVES

Using as many examples as possible:

1. Describe what is meant by critical perspectives on the social DoH.
2. Identify and explain at least six examples of the relationships among poverty and health.
3. Explain what is meant by intersections of three areas of the social DoH.
4. Describe how oppression "gets under the skin" to deepen disadvantage and create health damage across the lifecourse.
5. Describe the importance of language in the evolution of understandings of the social DoH.

CRITICAL THINKING QUESTIONS

1. What are some of the reasons why people may be resistant to critical perspectives on the social DoH?
2. How is the "lifestyle" perspective on health and wellness perpetuated in our everyday lives?
3. What is the difference between power "to" and power "within"?
4. How is oppression stress related to common, everyday meanings of stress?
5. How would you apply Raphael and Bryant's (2023) eight social DoH discourses to describe the crisis of unhoused people in Canada?

INTRODUCTION

The aim of this chapter is to emphasize the need for criticality in tackling inequities and injustices in the social determinants of health (DoH). Building on Stevens and Hall's (1992) description of the relationships between politics and health in Chapter 1, and critical policy analysis framings in Chapter 2, this chapter begins with a discussion of **critical perspectives** on the social DoH, contrasting them with perspectives that remain focused on the individual and **apolitical** level—the still-dominant perspective. The concept of power is described in more detail regarding the types of power that are important in engaging with critical perspectives: power "over," power "to," power "with," and power "within." An intersectionality lens is then explained, along with how disadvantages and oppression in one area of the DoH are deepened by synergies with other areas (e.g., when ableism, classism, racism, and sexism are experienced at the same time by the same person). Initial understandings of intersections of the isms are then extended to include intersections of the social DoH and intersections of the spatial DoH. The ways that oppression and inequities in the social DoH "get under the skin" are detailed, linking structural, systemic processes with on-the-ground bodily impacts—the embodiment of oppression and the creation and maintenance of oppression stress. The chapter concludes with a discussion of the evolution of the concept of social DoH and the centrality of language in how it is taken up and framed. Some current critiques and debates about the construct of social DoH are explained, emphasizing that definitions and descriptions of the social DoH are contested territory. The chapter concludes with Raphael and Bryant's (2023) eight social DoH discourses, underscoring how choice of language, and hence criticality of social DoH discourses, can identify, or hamper, action points for raising the volume on the social DoH (Raphael, 2021).

CRITICAL PERSPECTIVES ON THE SOCIAL DETERMINANTS OF HEALTH

Although it is generally recognized that health is determined by social factors, there is wide variation on what is meant by "social." On one end of the continuum, social means the micro realm of individual and family influences on health, for example, who you live with, your "lifestyle," and your dietary habits. Since these social factors are generally assumed to be within the control of the individual, the responsibility for maintaining or improving health is also perceived to rest within the individual. In the case of childhood asthma, the dominant view is often that parents have the responsibility to ensure that their children do not live in a damp, and hence moldy, basement apartment. By extension, if they care about their children, they need to take the responsibility to find a higher-paying job, despite facing significant and often insurmountable financial, geographic, and other barriers in the job-access process. Another common example is obesity—people just need to get out more, exercise more, and eat less. Although there is increasing acknowledgement that these micro solutions are simplistic and targeted towards those with the material means to activate these solutions, this thinking still remains dominant. Mental health struggles are often similarly framed in simplistic, micro terms. In this dominant view, people with addictions "just" need to find the willpower to stop (drinking, smoking, vaping, gambling, and so on). If they do not, their addictions are perceived to be a result of their laziness and lack of moral fortitude.

In each of these examples, the social DoH may be likened to a relatively straightforward equation: parents finding a better job = improvement in childhood asthma symptoms and incidence; exercise and healthy eating = decreased obesity; and sufficient willpower = recovery from addiction. These views of the social DoH are stuck in apolitical, acontextual simplicity. Interestingly, "treatment" for each of these health struggles is still also largely stuck within individualized, acontextual simplicity, despite copious long-term evidence to the contrary, such as the crucial role of a livable income (e.g., living wage, guaranteed annual income) for achieving housing and food security (Brown & Tarasuk, 2019). Similarly, Indigenous Peoples' (First Nations, Inuit, Métis) health is heavily determined by the colonialist role of forced separation from traditional lands and foods. These root causes tend to go unacknowledged at the micro level in health and social contexts, as well as in the macro public and institutional policymaking realm.

The facts are clear about the relationships among education, income, poverty, and health (Raghupathi & Raghupathi, 2020), as well as colonialist governance systems (Fleras & Maaka, 2010). For example,

Figure 3.1 depicts the relationship between education level and self-reported health status. In all 33 countries included in the Organisation for Economic Co-operation and Development (OECD, 2019) study, people with a lower level of education considered themselves to be in worse health than those with tertiary education, and there was a 21 percentage points difference between the two groups. Note that Canada

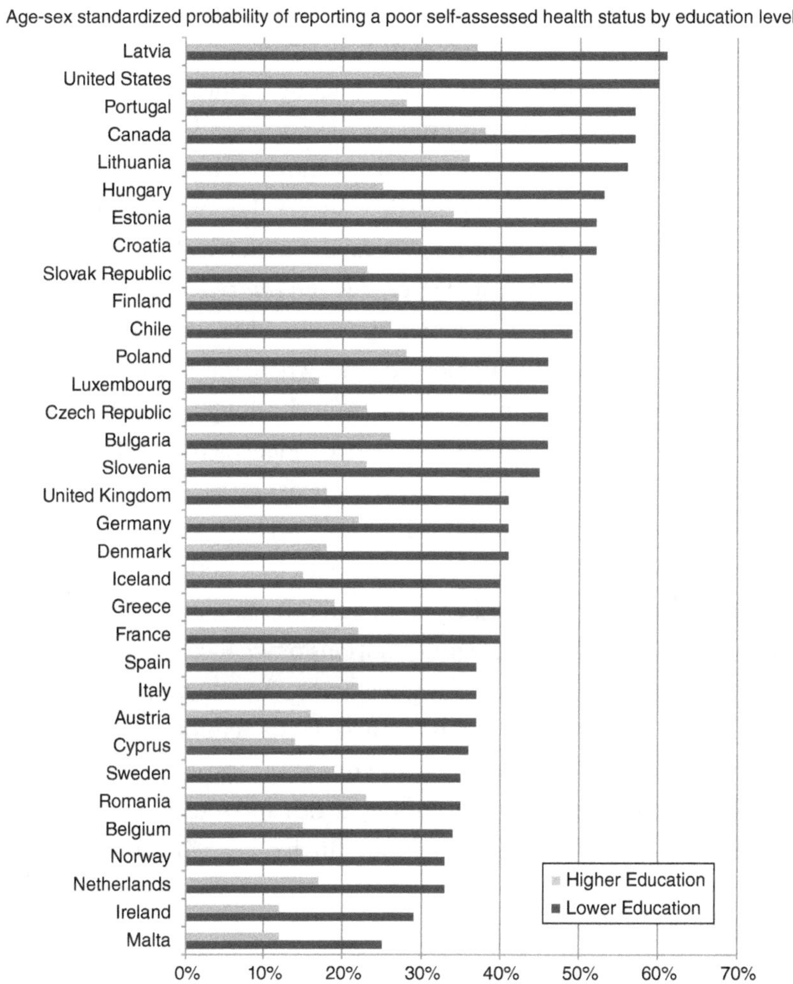

Figure 3.1: OECD Relationship between Education Level and Self-Reported Health Status

Source: Adapted from OECD, 2019.

ranks 30th of the 33 countries included in the study in terms of the highest percentage of people reporting poor health. As analyzed in Chapter 2, these patterns are related to the political economy of health over time, where Canada's increasingly neoliberal political economy is resulting in longitudinal and measurable population health damage. Furthermore, if individuals are blamed for their lack of jobs, education, and the like, then governments ostensibly have little responsibility to legislate social supports (social insurance programs) to lift the population out of poverty.

Individualistic perspectives and associated designations of blame operate in tandem with dominant views about "health" itself. Although the social DoH movement has brought the notion of health into a more complex and nuanced discussion, the word *health* itself still carries significant cultural, political, and moralistic baggage. For example, in a study about the ways that health equity is talked about in Canadian public policy, researchers found that the term *health equity* brought with it the trappings of the word *health*, which draws its ideological and practical applications from the fields of biomedicine, where it is framed within existing philosophical, cultural, and positivist thinking (McGibbon et al., 2022). These meanings of health have been identified as a drawback in descriptions of the social DoH, due to pre-existing health language that is solidly entrenched in biomedical, **Eurocentric**, and colonialist paradigms that are based in positivist and depoliticized notions of individualism and reductionism (described in Chapter 2), "and managerialism, for example the dominance of positivist notions of what counts as efficiency, and standardization of practices across even the most diverse populations" (Sinclaire et al., 2021, p. 60). These views reinforce a sanitization of the brutal realities of people's lives and, at the same time, bypass exposure of the beneficiaries of sustaining health and social inequities (e.g., the ultra-wealthy 1% of the population), further described in Chapter 5.

Pathways for Criticality

In contrast to dominant perspective on the social DoH, critical perspectives lay the foundation for analyzing the "why, how, and who" of worsening health outcomes in Canada and globally. The focus is on naming and analyzing not only inequitable health impacts across the lifecourse but also the beneficiaries of these persistent inequities.

As described in the policy analysis section of Chapter 2, there is not a singular critical perspective, but rather numerous and often synergistic ways to engage in criticality. However, there are foundational ideas that cut across all critical perspectives, such as a direct acknowledgement that power, and its inequitable distribution, are at the root of injustices. Critical perspectives focus on the imperative to systematically critique and expose dominant power structures.

Figure 3.2 describes types of power that are relevant for enacting critical perspectives, particularly in terms of understanding "where power is", how power operates, and how to challenge power. Power, whether it is political, economic, cultural, or social (to name a few), involves power "over," power "to," power "with," and power "within" (Stuart, 2019). *Power "over"* involves the ability of the powerful to impact or constrain the actions and thoughts of the less powerful; *power "to"* involves the material, emotional, and intellectual (for example) capacity to take action and to have agency (for action or intervention); *power "with"* involves the synergy of collective action, social mobilization, and alliance building; and *power "within"* involves a sense of self-dignity and self-awareness that enables agency (e.g., community building and personal/group ownership of political action) (Stuart, 2019).

Core features of a critical perspective, not necessarily in any particular order, involve all of these forms of power: "1) explicit analyses and critique of **hegemonic** power structures and ruling relations (power over)—naming who benefits from injustice; 2) organized public protest and acts of resistance in the face of oppressive, sometimes murderous regimes, and public policies (power to, power with), and the like; and

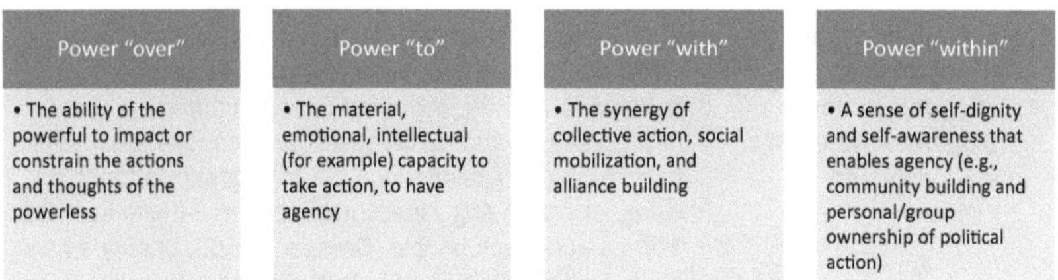

Figure 3.2: Types of Power That Are Central for Enacting Critical Perspectives

Source: Adapted from Stuart, 2019.

3) explicit goals of disrupting, unsettling, and interrupting processes and practices of oppression in local and global spheres, all of which are synergistically connected" (power with, power within) (McGibbon, 2021a, p. 8). As Stevens and Hall (1992) pointed out, understanding the relationship between politics, power, and health involves systematic questioning about "the ways things are." These political contexts refer to political, economic, and policy environments, to name a few, that are relevant to taking action. They include the distribution of power, the range of organizations involved and their interests, and the formal and informal rules that govern interactions among the various players

Table 3.1: Case Applications: Relationships among Politics and Health

Relationships among Politics and Health	**Case Applications**
1. All research, theory, policy, and practice are political because they are intimately affected by the social, economic, and political processes of the society.	"Homosexuality" was considered a psychiatric disease in the American Psychiatric Association's (APA) *Diagnostic and Statistical Manual of Mental Disorders* (DSM) until it was removed in 1973. In the wake of the 1969 Stonewall riots in New York City, gay and lesbian activists, believing psychiatric theories to be a major contributor to anti-homosexual social stigma, disrupted the 1970 and 1971 annual meetings of the APA, a protest action that led to its removal (Drescher, 2015).
2. Oppressive power relations are common in society; usually they operate without much notice and are taken for granted.	Until COVID-19, the general public knew relatively little about the politics of poverty rates in Canada and how they impacted marginalized and racialized peoples in terms of pandemic illness and death rates. Taken-for-granted systemic racism in health systems policies became publicly "unhidden" (through media, etc.) as a direct cause of COVID-19 morbidity and mortality rates.
3. Scientific and practical ways of thinking and getting things done are open to systematic questioning and criticism.	Up until about the early 1960s, much medical research relied on young, white, male participants to develop public and institutional policy interventions for diabetes, heart disease, and numerous other illnesses. Resulting policies, funding allocations, and medical treatment were correspondingly inaccurate for populations such as women and Black people (Dresser, 1992). Changes have been hard-fought by women activists and their allies. For example, the National Institute of Health in the United Kingdom now has a gender and race justice framework for medical research requirements (Baird, 1999).

Table 3.1: Case Applications: Relationships among Politics and Health (*Continued*)

Relationships among Politics and Health	Case Applications
4. Social, economic, and political conditions have a history.	Violence against women, and its health and social impacts, has its roots in historical oppressions, such as public policy decision-making to deny the vote for women. When abundant activism for the enfranchisement of women could no longer be dismissed in Canada, the national right to vote was established for all women, except Indigenous (First Nations, Inuit, Métis) women, who did not receive the right to vote until 1960.
5. One can better understand changing conditions of society's health by studying histories of unsafe physical surroundings, oppressive social arrangements, economic inequities, and political disenfranchisement.	Disproportionately high rates of heart disease in Canadians of African descent can best be understood through the intergenerational and collective impacts of state-based policies of slavery and colonization (rather than "lifestyle deficits")—the stress of racism has been definitively linked to heart disease (Schultz et al., 2021) and even epigenetic make-up (Mulligan, 2021).
6. Liberation from oppressive environmental constraints is an indispensable part of any group's pursuit of well-being and integrity.	A key goal of worker unionization is to eliminate workplace oppression. Workplace unionization rates are positively correlated with better national population health outcomes across the globe: union density and collective agreement coverage reduce the percentage of low-waged workers and the extent of income inequality, as well as decrease low birthweight and infant mortality rates (Muller & Raphael, 2023).

Source: Stevens & Hall, 1992 (first column).

involved (Nash et al., 2006). Naming and understanding political conditions can expose the roots of inequity and injustice. Table 3.1 provides case applications of Stevens and Hall's (1992) analysis of the relationships among politics and health described in Chapter 1.

INTERSECTIONS OF THE SOCIAL DETERMINANTS OF HEALTH

The social DoH were briefly introduced in Chapter 1. This description is deepened with an application of an intersectionality lens, a foundational tool for action on the social DoH. An intersectionality lens supports an understanding of how the social DoH do not happen in isolation. Rather, they combine and overlap to deepen disadvantage. The term ***intersectionality*** was first used by legal scholar Kimberlé Crenshaw (1989) as a result of the antidiscrimination case of *DeGraffenreid v General Motors*. Emma DeGraffenreid was a Black woman who applied for a job at General Motors and was denied employment. She joined four other Black women who were also not hired, and they sued General Motors for discrimination. However, General Motors responded that 1) they hired Black people (Black men worked in industrial and maintenance jobs) and 2) they also hired women (many white women worked as secretaries). Therefore, they were not demonstrating discrimination in employment against Black people or women. Crenshaw argued that in this instance, although discrimination on the basis of race or gender were ruled out *separately*, discrimination on the basis of *race and gender together* had not been taken into consideration (Carbado & Crenshaw, 2019; Palmen, 2021).

An intersectionality lens was taken up by Black feminist scholars such as bell hooks (1990), Patricia Hill Collins (1990, 2003, 2005), and Agnes Calliste and George Sefa Dei (2000). "When feminism is defined in such a way that it calls attention to the diversity of women's social and political reality, it centralizes the experience of all women, especially the women whose social conditions have been least written about, studied, or changed by political movements" (hooks, 1990, p. 52). Collins (1990) described how oppressions in society do not operate independently. Rather, they intersect in complex patterns—models that view each oppression as additive rather than interlocking fail to stress the centrality of power and privilege. Identities, sometimes referred to as identity markers (Hum & Simpson, 2003), intersect to compound oppression. Age, culture, (dis)ability, ethnicity, gender, immigrant status, race, sexual and gender identity, social class, and spirituality all denote social location, a powerful determinant of one's access to the social and material necessities of life. For example, Box 3.1 demonstrates the impacts of intersections of 2SLGBTQIA+ (two-spirited, lesbian, gay, bisexual, trans, queer, intersex, asexual) identity and health care access, an important social DoH.

Box 3.1: Impacts of Intersections of Health Care Access and 2SLGBTQIA+ Identities

- The Wabanaki Two-Spirit Alliance administered an online survey in May 2020 to identify priorities and concerns of Two-Spirit individuals and Indigenous 2SLGBTQQIA+ people in Atlantic Canada during the COVID-19 pandemic. Participants described mental health supports, health supports for Two-Spirit individuals, healing gatherings, and trans-specific supports as effective access interventions for fostering Two-Spirit health (Sylliboy et al., 2022).
- In US health care settings, 33 percent of transgender individuals reported one or more negative experiences related to being transgender such as being refused treatment, being harassed or assaulted, or receiving incompetent care (James et al., 2016).
- In a qualitative study with interviews of 30 women aged 21 to 63 years who defined themselves as lesbian, researchers found that LGBTQ+ people's access to health care treatment and care is characterized by the default assumption that people are heterosexual, cisgender, and not intersex. Avoidance of disclosure was based in fear of reprisal. However, the non-existence of open disapproval towards homosexuality was, for participants, a decisive factor in the creation of a positive relational climate (Marques et al., 2015).
- The historical endurance of discrimination is evident in a 2010 study where LGBTQ participants reported alarming rates of identity-based discrimination in health care settings, with "10% of LGBTQ and 21% of transgender patients experiencing harsh or abusive language (Lambda Legal, 2010) and 8% of LGB patients and 27% of transgender patients having been refused care" (Lambda Legal, 2010, as cited by Rossman et al., 2017).
- American transgender and/or gender diverse individuals reported health care access barriers in terms of probing questions, requests to see genitals, incremental gatekeeping, overt

(continued)

stigmatization, and intentional misgendering, and/or deadnaming while attempting to obtain health care (Meyer et al., 2020).
- In the United States, almost half (48.4%, $n = 108$) of primary care providers had no formal education on transgender and/or gender-diverse health care, yet half (49.7%, $n = 111$) of providers reported previously caring for at least one transgender patient (Stroumsa et al., 2019).

Note: This data uses the 2SLGBTQIA+ terms stated in the various studies.

Application of an intersectional lens to describe the social DoH began over two decades ago, emphasizing "how systems of discrimination such as colonialism and globalization can impact the combination of a person's social or economic status, race, class, gender, and sexuality" (Canadian Research Institute for the Advancement of Women, 2006, p. 7). In 2008, Hankivsky and Christofferson described the relationships between intersectionality and the social DoH, and they argued for an exploration of "the innovative paradigm of intersectionality to better understand and respond to the foundational causes of illness and disease" (p. 7). McGibbon and Etowa (2007) first depicted a model of the social DoH that simultaneously integrated synergies of three areas of social DoH: 1) social DoH as laid out in the Toronto Charter (Raphael et al., 2004) and updated in 2020 (Raphael et al., 2020); 2) the isms as social DoH, based in feminist intersectionality theory about how oppressions such as racism, sexism, and colonialism work together or intersect to deepen disadvantage in social DoH outcomes, and at the same time increase advantage, privilege, wealth, and power for some; and 3) geographies or spatial contexts as social DoH, including segregation, ghettoization, and toxic geographies of disproportionate location of landfills and industrial pollution. Figure 3.3 illustrates how the three areas of social DoH intersect to deepen disadvantage for some and to increase advantage for others. Geographies as DoH are described in more detail in Chapter 4.

The following examples describe some of the ways that Raphael et al.'s (2020) social DoH intersect with each other (e.g., food security,

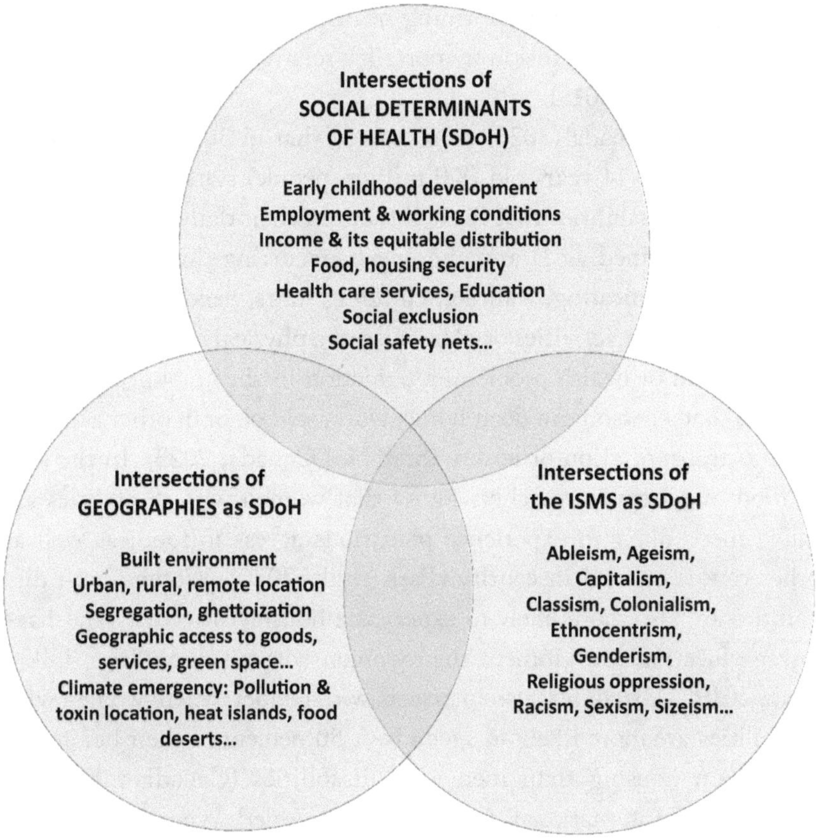

Figure 3.3: Intersections of the Social DoH

Source: Created by author.

education). The examples also describe how these social DoH intersect with the isms as social DoH (e.g., food security, education, disability). For example, social DoH such as education, income, and access to health services are statistically significant predictors of cancer incidence and mortality across various countries in different regions of the world (McDaniel et al., 2019). Researchers also found that education, income, availability of cancer control policies and programs, as well as health system performance in any given country, are accurate predictors of mortality due to lung, breast, cervical, and colorectal cancers. Populations with better education, higher incomes, and lower inequalities, who live in jurisdictions with active cancer control policies and programs and high-performing health systems have better cancer outcomes as reflected in lower mortality relative to other populations (McDaniel et al., 2019).

Statistics Canada (2023) data showed that in 2022, 27 percent of Canadians over 14 years old (8.0 million people) stated that they had one or more disabilities that limited them in their daily activities. Disability was defined as 1) any ongoing or recurring difficulty hearing, seeing, communicating, walking, climbing stairs, bending, learning or doing any similar activities or 2) because of a physical condition or mental condition or health problem, a reduction in the amount or kind of activity that a person can do at home, work, school, or in other activities such as transportation or leisure (Statistics Canada, 2023). In the area of food insecurity, researchers found that women with disabilities are much more likely to experience precarious access to food, as well as other causes of food insecurity (Park et al., 2020). Women with disabilities are also more likely to experience housing insecurity and have lower educational attainment than women without disabilities (Olkin et al., 2019). (Dis)ability also intersects with gender, where women with disabilities are more likely to spend over 50 percent of their before-tax income on housing than men with disabilities (Canadian Feminist Alliance for International Action and DisAbled Women's Network Canada, 2017). In 2022, Canadian employment insecurity intersected with disability status such that persons with a disability were 20 percent less likely to be employed and less than half (42%) of persons with more severe disabilities aged 25 to 64 years were employed (Statistics Canada, 2024). The most common disability type in 2022 was pain-related disability (62%), followed by flexibility (40%), mobility (39%), and mental health-related disabilities (39%) (Statistics Canada, 2024). The prominence of these forms of disabilities indicate a strong likelihood of requiring consistent and complex health care access. However, structural barriers such as lack of disability-specific services in rural areas and, for some, the need for specialized transportation, all intersect with the systemic discrimination of ableism to create significant barriers in access to health care.

Gender intersects with other social locations to impact mental health outcomes as well as access to care. Box 3.2 provides details on how these social DoH intersections play themselves out in people's everyday lives.

Box 3.2: Health Impacts of Intersections of Mental Health, Gender, and Other Identities

- In the United States, women living in poverty, immigrant women, and undocumented women face greater challenges in accessing mental health because of a lack of health insurance, limited transportation, and language barriers (Lauro, 2018).
- A systematic review of longitudinal studies on informal unpaid caregiving and mental health in high income OECD countries, where studies were stratified by gender, found that caregiving had a consistently negative impact on the mental health of women (Ervin et al., 2022).
- In a global narrative review, researchers found that during the COVID-19 pandemic, women who were pregnant, postpartum, miscarrying, or experiencing intimate partner violence were at especially high risk for developing mental health problems (Almeida et al., 2020).
- In Canada, the mental health struggles of Indigenous (First Nations, Inuit, Métis) women involve multiple forms of oppression: complex trauma (Tutty et al., 2020) or intergenerational trauma, associated with serious physical and mental health issues including addictions (Wesley-Esquimaux & Smolewski, 2004).
- In the United States, researchers found that between the ages of 12 and 42, Black women and girls experience more depressive symptoms than white women, and men of any race (Erving et al., 2021).
- In the United States, low-income pregnant women experiencing depressive symptoms encounter significant barriers to receiving mental health care during pregnancy: cost of care, lack of

(*continued*)

insurance, transportation barriers, long waits for treatment, and negative experiences of mental health care in the past discouraged help-seeking during pregnancies (Sacks et al., 2015).

- In a Canadian study, researchers found that young mothers expressed hesitancy in accessing mental health services due to past negative experiences, fears of being judged, being medicated, not being seen as an active partner in care decisions, or experiencing increased child protection involvement (Jack et al., 2022).
- A 2022 global scoping review demonstrated a growing body of research on the impacts of climate change on women's mental health. Women's already-disproportionate caregiving responsibility was identified as being increased during an extreme weather event or climate-related food scarcity. Women's further attachment to land, place, and traditions additionally increases emotional distress when such ties are threatened due to climate change (Stone et al., 2022).

SOCIAL DETERMINANT OF HEALTH INEQUITIES: HOW OPPRESSION "GETS UNDER THE SKIN"

> Oppression is inscribed on the bodies, minds, and spirits of oppressed peoples. These public policy-created injustices generate persistent disparities in physical and mental health and wellbeing. When people experience the mental stress of racism or unjust public and institutional policies that create and sustain poverty, they are impacted persistently over time. (McGibbon, 2021b, p. 134)

The everyday distress of dealing with social DoH adversities, such as poverty and racism, impacts the physiology of the body's stress-handling system, the adrenal system. The following discussion illustrates what is meant by **embodied oppression**. There are complex relationships among the mental and physical stress of intersecting oppressions and their ongoing and measurable bodily impacts. Our bodies are physiologically designed to weather everyday stresses such as traffic jams, missed appointments, and minor health problems, to name a few. Our adrenal system successfully regulates our bodies through these short-term stressful times and helps us maintain overall wellness and physiological balance (homeostasis). The body generally recovers from the ups and downs of these stressors (homeostatic recovery).

The problem arises when individuals and communities experience repeated and sustained exposure to stressors—the body's stress-handling system becomes overburdened and is unable to maintain physiological balance. Chronic, excessive stress then causes cumulative negative impacts on health outcomes through a physiological burden known as **allostatic load**, illustrated in Figure 3.4 (Lee et al., 2015), also known as toxic stress. Toxic stress is the detrimental biological response to living with prolonged and unmediated stress (Shanks & Robinson, 2013). For example, in a systematic review of the association between poverty and biomarkers of toxic stress (Brisson et al., 2020), researchers identified the relationship between poverty, trauma, and toxic stress (Shanks & Robinson, 2013). Carter et al. (2022) studied the biological embedding of racism as a chronic stressor, explaining that when contextual stressors

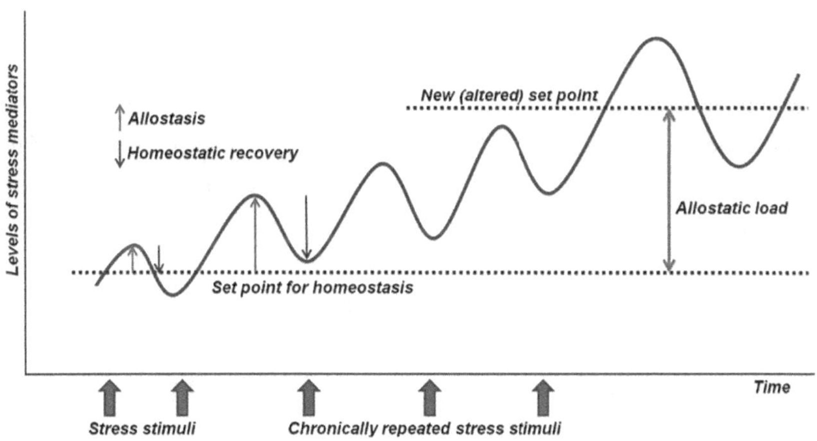

Figure 3.4: Understanding Embodied Oppression Stress: Allostatic Load

Source: Lee et al., 2015.

exceed a person's capacity to cope and maintain homeostasis, there is a resulting harm on a person's body for constantly needing to adapt to unrelenting challenges, such as everyday racism.

The allostatic load concept describes the biological costs of chronic stress, which can lead to many different disease outcomes (Misiak, 2020). Measures of allostatic load demonstrate that exposures to excess stress causes cardiovascular, metabolic, neuroendocrine, and immune system dysregulation, all of which have been found to predict morbidity and mortality (Misiak, 2020). Psychological, spiritual, physical, and physiological health outcomes of adrenal fatigue are thus embodied (McGibbon, in press): increased allostatic load creates changes in the nervous system (e.g., increased blood pressure) and hormonal changes (e.g., increased cortisol, the body's primary stress hormone, and dysregulation of insulin) (Guidi et al., 2020). Results include depression, hypertension, diabetes, cancer, gastric or stomach ulcers and related chronic stomach problems, allergies and eczema, headaches, kidney and liver disease, autoimmune diseases such as arthritis, and overall reduced immunity (Misiak, 2020). As illustrated in Figure 3.4, allostatic load then increases over time, creating new (altered) and higher set points for physiological balance or homeostasis (McGibbon, in press).

Impacts of chronic stresses—such as experiencing everyday racism, sexism, and/or homophobic hatred, or worrying about food and shelter—explain the significantly disproportionate rates of heart disease and diabetes in Indigenous Peoples and Canadians of African descent, as detailed in Box 3.3. Chronic income insecurity and the intergenerational perniciousness of poverty have also been found to overtax the adrenal system and result in heart failure (Ahmad et al., 2019) and depression (Ridley et al., 2020). When poverty intersects with racism and already-existing illnesses, the adrenal impact is compounded. For example, there is increasing evidence that COVID-19 disproportionately impacted racialized people and people with low socioeconomic status—these impacts are even greater for people experiencing rheumatic (autoimmune) diseases such as arthritis (Mehta et al., 2020).

The **cycle of oppression**, illustrated in Figure 3.5, supports an understanding of how oppression stress "gets under the skin" through

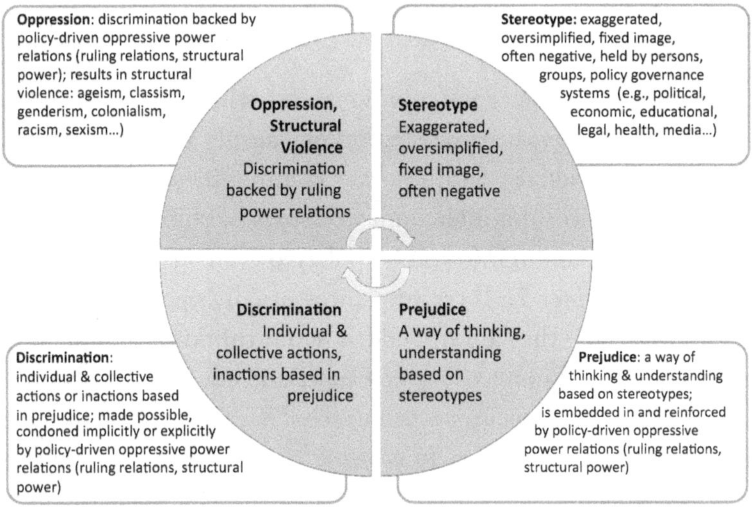

Figure 3.5: The Cycle of Oppression: Stereotyping, Prejudice, Discrimination, Oppression

Source: Adapted from McGibbon, 2021a.

the process of experiencing everyday stereotyping and prejudice, which are rooted in systemic oppressions, including ableism, ageism, classism, genderism, heterosexism, racism, and sexism. A stereotype is an exaggerated, oversimplified, often negative, fixed image held by persons, groups, and systems (e.g. actors in political, economic, health, education, and legal governing systems; the media). We have all grown up exposed to countless embedded stereotypes through processes such as our upbringing and our formal education experiences, as well as through news, social, and entertainment media. We absorb these stereotypes whether we want to or not. For example, since we have all grown up in a sexist and racist society, we have all absorbed some of these stereotypes, such as girls are not good at math (McGuire et al., 2021) and Indigenous women (Turpel-Lafond & Johnson, 2021) and women of African descent (Boyd, 2019) have a higher pain tolerance than white Euro-Canadian women. The latter findings mean that Indigenous women and women of African descent have been found to be less likely to receive adequate pain medication in clinical settings. We are largely unaware of the everyday ways that our thinking is distorted by this basket of stereotypes.

Prejudice is preconceived opinions and whole ways of thinking based on stereotypes, because stereotypes deeply impact the way we think about individuals, families, and communities, and even whole countries. Prejudices are interconnected ways of thinking and understanding, created and reinforced by policy-driven structural power, as described in Chapter 2. These prejudices usually operate without our direct knowledge—they are embedded in our thinking, and in order to "see" them, we need to make a specific effort to educate ourselves about the isms and related unearned privileges. Discrimination is action or inaction based on prejudice. It is made possible and condoned, implicitly or explicitly by policy-driven, structural power (McGibbon, 2021a). It is crucial to note that when we engage in discriminatory practices, we are usually not aware of our discrimination. Oppression is discrimination backed up by systemic, structural power relations (e.g., public and institutional policies; the media; political, economic, health, education, and legal governing systems). Prominent examples of systemic oppression are ageism, classism, racism, sexism, and colonialism. Oppression is the area of the cycle that is most often difficult to understand because it involves thinking about the very underpinnings of society and how they influence our own actions/inactions and the actions/inactions of those with systemic power, such as public and institutional policymakers.

A pressing example of the cycle of oppression is the tragic death of Joyce Echaquan, a 37-year-old Atikamekw woman and mother of seven. Ms. Echaquan's story is one of abuse, trauma, and ultimately death at the hands of staff in the health care system. Although the telling of her experience involves repugnant actions and inactions, it is important to name and publicly honour Ms. Echaquan's story. She went to the Joliette Hospital in Montreal, Quebec, with complaints of stomach pains and a history of heart problems. She died on September 28, 2020 (Banerjee, 2021). Before her death, Ms. Echaquan recorded a Facebook Live video where two staff members were in her room and can be heard saying to her, in French: "You're stupid as hell." Another staff member told her that she made bad choices in life and asked what her children would think of her behaviour (Banerjee, 2021).

These *stereotypes* about Indigenous women led to *prejudice* when health care staff incorrectly assumed that Ms. Echaquan was suffering from narcotics withdrawal. *Discrimination* (action) occurred when they labelled her as a drug abuser despite there being no evidence to support this claim (Banerjee, 2021). Discrimination (inaction) occurred when care staff failed to assess and intervene according to Ms. Echaquan's clinical symptoms. In her report, coroner Géhane Kamel found that Ms. Echaquan had died of excess fluid in her lungs and that her death was preventable and an "undeniable" case of racism (Banerjee, 2021). Ms. Echaquan's death resulted in nation-wide calls for political leaders in Quebec to acknowledge the presence of systemic racism in the province. Systemic *oppression* was demonstrated by Quebec Premier François Legault, who acknowledged that the incident was "totally unacceptable" but denied that racism existed in the province and hence took no action to address racism and discrimination that resulted in Ms. Echaquan's death (Banerjee, 2021). Box 3.3 further details how oppressions such as racism become embodied and eventually result in health damage.

Box 3.3: Embodied Racism: Some Facts about How Racism "Gets under the Skin"

Cardiovascular Disease

- For racialized women, barriers to optimal cardiovascular health begin early in life—with inadequate access to effective contraception, postpartum follow-up, and maternity leave—and result in excess rates of myocardial infarction, stroke, and cardiovascular death (Lindley et al., 2021).
- When researchers studied prevalence of diabetes and heart disease in the province of Ontario, Canada from 2001 to 2012, they found that rates of diabetes had almost doubled among Black women. Prevalence of hypertension increased by 30 percent from

(continued)

2009 to 2012 among Black women—the highest increase, by far, of any of the groups studied (Chinese, white, South Asian, Black; Chiu et al., 2015).

- In a 2016–2019 study of health outcomes and follow-up care differences between First Nations (FN) and non-FN coronary angiogram (heart disease diagnostic test) patients, researchers found that FN people had significantly worse overall health and significantly less follow-up care than non-FN patients (Schultz et al., 2018).
- Heart disease is the leading cause of death for people of most racial and ethnic groups in the United States (National Center for Health Statistics, 2020).

Diabetes

- A US study found that non-Hispanic Black children have higher rates of ketoacidosis when diagnosed with diabetes, higher rates of subsequent hospital admissions, and lower rates of technology use in managing their disease (Lipman et al., 2020). As technology has evolved to play a more central role in the management of this disease, these devices have not been distributed or used equitably across populations at risk for childhood onset diabetes (Lipman et al., 2020).
- A Canadian study found that the lifetime risk of Type 2 diabetes at 20 years of age was 75.6% among men and 87.3% among women in the First Nations group, compared with 55.6% among men and 46.5% among women in the non–First Nations group. The risk was higher among First Nations people than among non–First Nations people for all index ages and for both sexes (Turin et al, 2016).
- In Canada, diabetes rates are increasing more rapidly among First Nations (FN) when compared to the general population and FN are more likely to develop complications: women are at higher risk of cardiovascular disease complications and men are at higher risk of kidney problems, hypertension, limb complications, and retinopathy (Cheran et al., 2023).
- A US study found that diabetes prevalence was almost twice as prevalent for Black Americans overall (20.4%) when compared to white Americans (12.1%; Cheng et al., 2019).

- A Canadian study found that individuals from South Asian communities are known to have a higher likelihood of developing Type 2 diabetes than people of Western European and North American descent, a finding that is often attributed to individual lifestyle and behavioural factors. This focus on individual responsibility can position communities as complicit in their illness, compounding stigmatization, systemic discrimination, and racism (D'Silva et al., 2022).

Note: This table cites authors' terms in the studies (i.e., Chinese, Black Americans, white Americans, First Nations, Hispanic, Indigenous, etc.).

EVOLUTION OF THE SOCIAL DETERMINANTS OF HEALTH: THE IMPORTANCE OF LANGUAGE

In the evolution of the term *social DoH*, choices to include or omit certain words, and the framings of the words, are themselves determinants of health. For decades, social scientists and others explicitly used language that pointed to evidence linking politics and health (see Dahlgren & Whitehead, 1991). However, it was not until the WHO report of the Commission on the Social Determinants of Health (2008) that these decades-old arguments began to more fully enter mainstream consciousness and hence become more broadly acceptable. In this section, the importance of language, and the particular words we choose, is emphasized with an explanation of some of the current critiques and debates about language and the social DoH. Raphael and Bryant's (2023) eight discourses are then discussed, underscoring the centrality of language, not only in how the social DoH are described but also in terms of how the various discourses directly impact political, public policy action (or inaction) for tackling inequities in the social DoH.

Language and the Social Determinants of Health: Some Current Critiques and Debates

Historically important social DoH models and frameworks demonstrate that these models continue to evolve over time and therefore have no static definition. As detailed below, each of these models has ultimately informed the various social DoH models, such as the one used for this book (see Figure 3.3). Meanings and understandings of the social DoH are increasingly contested, leading to rich debates about their very utility as an analytic lens to guide knowledge and policy change for justice in human and planet health. For example, the use of lists to describe the social DoH has been critiqued as overly linear, deterministic, and apolitical (Mishori, 2019).

Some argue that lists of social DoH have become so long as to be not useful (Islam, 2019). Furthermore, critiques of the list approach have also led to conclusions that the list approach is what is causing lack of public policy uptake of the social DoH because the lists are too dissimilar (Islam, 2019). This claim is also contested, and authors applying critical perspectives point to the dominance of policymaking grounded in neoliberal political economies of health (described in more detail in Chapter 2) as the most prominent barrier to social DoH uptake in public policy and governance. Critiques of the list approach tend to assume an *a priori* lack of criticality and root-cause analyses in conceptualizing the social DoH. Nonetheless, creating a list is a practical strategy to include various complex social DoH, such as food insecurity. However, in the absence of narrative explanations of policy-created poverty, "listing" food insecurity as a social DoH is of limited utility. Listing and concurrently naming root causes of food insecurity (e.g., lack of a federal living wage policy) introduces a centrally important criticality to the "list."

In the area of health equity and the social DoH, the list approach has also been described as an outcome of persistent biomedical, reductionist framings of health (McGibbon et al., 2019). Problematizing the word *health* in social DoH explains, in part, why explicitly political meanings of the social DoH became depoliticized in some contexts, especially in the area of health and health care, where they were, and often still are, reduced to a list reflecting the ideological power of individualism, reductionism, and positivism that still dominate the health fields. In discussions of the Ottawa Charter, Ratima et al. (2019) explain how the discipline of health promotion has not made the shift from reductionist Western worldviews towards "(w)hol(e)istic and relational ways of many Indigenous paradigms" (p. 35) and worldviews that have developed over millennia of human experience. Since the word *health* is included in the social DoH phrase, framings have the strong potential to be automatically rooted in the historical scaffoldings of biomedical positivism.

McGibbon et al.'s (2021) empirical analysis of the discursive organization of the word *health* found that the word itself serves to ideologically and culturally confine discourses within biomedical and imperialist dominance. "Once the concept of health enters into texts and talk, the ideological framing of the issue at hand becomes encrusted within a narrow orbit of analysis, relying overwhelmingly on Eurocentric and biomedical paradigms" (McGibbon et al., 2021, p. 69). Critical discourse analysts have consistently emphasized "the way social power abuse, dominance and inequality are enacted, reproduced and resisted by text and talk in the social and political context" (Van Dijk, 2015, p. 352). Smith (1990) refers to these processes as the textual organization of power, where texts themselves are central instruments for maintaining authority and supremacy. More specifically, health talk is situated within the dominance of biomedical imperialism and the historical violences of colonialism (McGibbon et al., 2021). Biomedical imperialism involves attention to both biological and genealogical respectability, with racial and national hierarchy as an organizing and ranking mechanism. This includes the dynamic tension "between the sociologies of race, ethnicity and post-colonialism, on the one hand, and the sociologies of science, biomedicine, and genetics, on the other" (Fitzgerald et al., 2020, p. 1171).

Studies have shown that documentation within public health practice indicates that there may be a lack of clear understanding of social DoH on the front lines of public health intervention (Morrison et al., 2014). In consideration of initiatives to address health equity, administrative and managerial tensions have also been found with the ideological and paradigmatic shift from biomedical approaches to a justice-based focus for the social DoH (McPherson et al., 2016). As can be expected, descriptions of social DoH frameworks in terms of actionable concepts rests, in part, on the level of criticality of the framework under consideration—in other words, whether the knowledge base informing the framework is mechanistic, with biomedical, reductionist theoretical lenses, or whether it is interpretive and critical. The former approach results in list-like depictions of the social DoH in the absence of accompanying explanations of their political and social contexts.

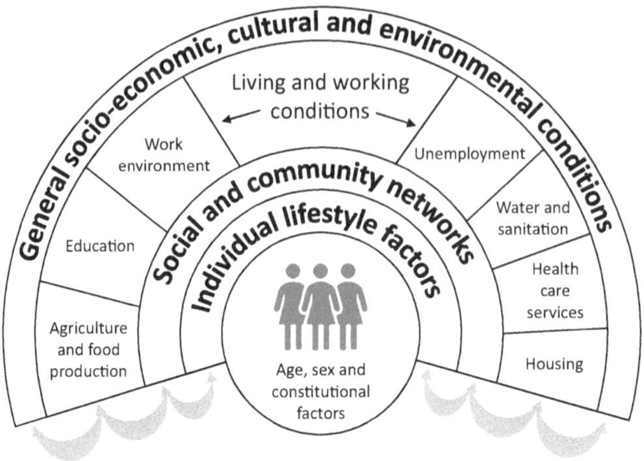

Figure 3.6: The Dahlgren-Whitehead Model Rainbow Model of the Determinants of Health

Source: Adapted from Dahlgren & Whitehead, 2021.

The latter results in critical social science and health sciences perspectives that name and tackle the root causes of health inequity. Some authors have provided methodological and theoretical clarity by linking social DoH descriptions to ruling relations about those who create and benefit from social and health inequalities (McGibbon, in press; Raphael, 2021). The *Dahlgren-Whitehead Rainbow Model* (Figure 3.6), originally published in 1991, demonstrates how the social, ecological, and structural DoH have historically been synthesized to cut across social, economic, cultural, and environmental conditions.

Politics and Health: How Language Can Identify Action Points

Chapter 1 described how the language that we use, including the language used by policymakers, can constrain action (individualistic, micro language results in scant or absent evidence of tackling of root causes) or promote action (critical perspectives take aim at the public policy causes, and hence promote structural solutions). Raphael (2021) and Raphael and Bryant (2023) described degrees of criticality of social DoH perspectives within eight social DoH discourses (see Figure 3.7). In the micro, individualistic area of the discourse spectrum, social DoH are viewed as identifiers of people requiring specific health and social services or people with modifiable medical and behavioural risk factors. As the criticality of discourses increases, social DoH are seen as indicators of material living conditions that shape health, and then as living conditions that have been found to differ as a function of belonging to a particular group

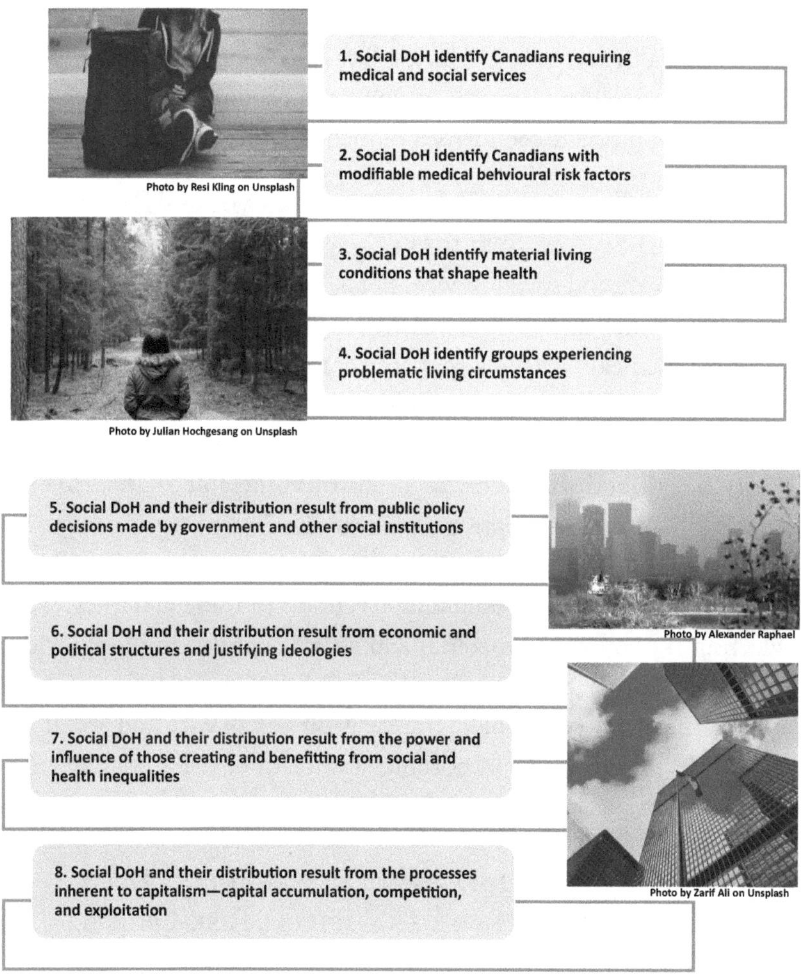

Figure 3.7: Raphael and Bryant's Eight Social DoH Discourses

Source: Adapted from Raphael & Bryant, 2023.

(e.g., Indigenous Peoples, Canadians of African descent, 2SLGBTQIA+ people, im/migrant communities). Here, criticality deepens to name inequitable social DoH outcomes across the isms. The last four discourses situate the social DoH in public policy decision making by governments and other social institutions. They are the results of structural, economic decision making and underlying justifying ideologies such as neoliberalism. In the seventh discourse along the social DoH continuum, Raphael and Bryant (2023) name the unequal distribution of the social DoH as the result of the power and influence of those who create and benefit from social and health inequalities. In the last discourse, overarching global structures of capitalism—capital accumulation, competition, and exploitation—are the ultimate root drivers of inequities across the social DoH.

Discourse 1: Social DoH Identify Canadians Requiring Health and Social Services

In the health care and social services fields, authorities recognize that individuals, families, and communities who experience unfavorable social DoH have medical problems that are more severe and varied in scope (Raphael, 2021). In this first discourse, the social DoH represent a set of living conditions that can help to aim the targeting of services and identify health and social service needs of vulnerable individuals and groups (e.g., unhoused people, people who live in poverty, im/migrants) (Raphael, 2021). Although the provision of health and social services is important, limiting analyses and intervention to these activities, while neglecting the sources of material and social deprivation, does little to reduce the need for these services (Raphael, 2021). This discourse can reinforce the already dominant emphasis on health care and social services, while obscuring the importance to health of the inequitable distribution of social DoH (Raphael, 2021).

Discourse 2: Social DoH Identify Canadians with Modifiable Medical and Behavioural Risk Profiles

Similarly, "healthy lifestyles" interventions recognize that individuals and communities who experience adverse social DoH are more likely to exhibit a range of medical (e.g., high blood sugar and "bad" cholesterol levels) and behavioural (e.g., poor diet, lack of physical activity, tobacco, and excessive alcohol use) risk factors (Raphael, 2021). Interventions are thus directed at improving lifestyle choices, which have been shown to have little impact on improving the health outcomes of marginalized and racialized peoples (McGibbon et al., 2024).

Discourse 3: Social DoH Identify Material Living Conditions That Shape Health

In this discourse, there is clear recognition that adverse social DoH themselves are important influences upon health and they impact health through various pathways (Raphael, 2021). Here, there is an acknowledgement that health is shaped by the conditions in which people are born, grow, work, live, and age, as well as the conditions shaping everyday life: economic policies and systems, development agendas, social norms, and social policies and political systems (WHO, n.d.). It is these conditions that cause inequities in health and well-being, not "poor lifestyle" (Raphael, 2021). "The plethora of feeding programs, clothing and food drives, and coping or anger-management classes are other examples of the distortion of this discourse" (Raphael, 2021, p. 52).

Discourse 4: Social DoH Identify Those Groups Experiencing Problematic Material Living Circumstances

As explained earlier in this chapter, social DoH intersect across the isms to deepen inequities in health and social outcomes. "Identifying groups experiencing health-threatening living conditions can mobilize Canadians to address issues of discrimination and marginalization. But if the public-policy antecedents of the inequitable distribution of social DoH are deemphasized, action may be limited to literacy and counselling programs, and anti-discrimination training, rather than altering the societal structures and processes creating these inequities" (Raphael, 2021, p. 53).

Discourse 5: Social DoH and Their Distribution Result from Public Policy Decisions Made by Governments and Other Societal Institutions

As discussed in Chapter 2, inequities and injustices in the social and ecological DoH are traceable to public policy decisions over time. For example, austerity measures after the 2008 global financial crises resulted in severe cuts to social insurance programs in New Zealand, resulting in measurable and significant increases of children living in poverty (28%), including in severe poverty (20%) (Barnett & Bagshaw, 2020). Achieving and sustaining equitable distribution of social DoH over time thus requires identifying health damaging public policies, such as these austerity measures.

Discourse 6: Social DoH and Their Distribution Result from Economic and Political Structures and Justifying Ideologies

This discourse involves openly acknowledging the links among economic and political structures, and the ideologies that justify them. As discussed in Chapter 2, neoliberal political economies cause health-damaging impacts that are driven by justifying ideologies, such as the market as an "impartial and efficient" distributor of resources. This thinking is based in the ideology of **meritocracy**—wealth and income inequality are related to moral fortitude (or lack thereof) and the people who accrue more resources deserve their wealth, while the "losers," who have not been able to thrive in a market-driven environment, must simply accept their fate because there is no sustainable alternative to the market-based system (Brunoli, 2017).

Discourse 7: Social DoH and Their Distribution Result from the Power and Influence of Those Creating and Benefiting from Social and Health Inequalities

"This discourse identifies the individuals and groups in Canada who, through their undue power and influence upon governments, create and benefit from social and health inequalities, and in the process skew the distribution of [social DoH]" (Raphael, 2021, p. 56). The corporate and business sector exert massive influence on governments by actions or inactions, such as 1) successfully lobbying for tax structures that favour the corporate sector and the wealthy, thereby reducing public expenditures (Raphael, 2021) in areas such as affordable housing, and the promise of universal dental care and pharmacare in Canada; and 2) advocating for controlling wages and employment benefits, and relaxing labour standards and protections (Carroll & Sapinski, 2018; Langille, 2016, as cited in Raphael, 2021). As detailed in Chapter 1, it is estimated that over a 10-year period, the Canadian government allowed (lack of action) $2 trillion in corporate tax evasion, while offering $82 million over a 10-year period to address homelessness (Sanger, 2019)—a very small fraction of the cash diverted from lawful taxation rules to benefit mega-corporations.

Discourse 8: Social DoH and Their Distribution Result from the Processes Inherent to Capitalism—Capital Accumulation, Competition, and Exploitation

This discourse identifies the problems caused by capitalism, especially inequality, exploitation, and alienation (Raphael & Bryant, 2023), where alienation refers to the estrangement of people from aspects of their human nature as a consequence of the division of labour and living in a society of stratified social classes (Marx, 2016). The practical implications of this discourse is the identification of problems "caused by capitalism of inequality, alienation, and exploitation and [development of] visions of a post-capitalist socialist society, building on social and political movements that can erode capitalist structures and strengthen alternative citizen-controlled institutions" (Raphael & Bryant, 2023, p. 3). (Also see Chapter 7, alternative political economies.)

Mapping these discourses is an example of belling the cat—exposing how language and discourse can be used to prevent action on the social DoH (keeping the focus on individual needs and shortcomings) or to provoke action (keeping the focus on beneficiaries of sustaining public policy that promotes child poverty, infant mortality, and other preventable inequities across the social DoH). The tracing of social DoH discourses demonstrates the powerful impact of how policy and governance structures and processes use language that frames these determinants as largely individual problems. This focus not only obfuscates any real solutions over time, it also hides the perpetrators and beneficiaries of keeping people poor and hungry. Table 3.2 applies the eight discourses to the problem of food insecurity. Food insecurity is an apt example because this pivotal social DoH does require urgent intervention in the short term—people need to eat and to feed their families. The problem is that interventions get stuck there (e.g., proliferation of food banks) in the absence of focusing on the root problems causing food insecurity.

Table 3.2: Raphael and Bryant's Eight Discourses: Applying Public Policy Framings of Food Insecurity

Social DoH Discourse	Policy Framing of the Problem of Food Insecurity
Discourse 1: Social DoH Identify Canadians Requiring Health and Social Services	Food insecurity causes sustained hunger, as well as lack of financial capacity to buy healthy foods. Service providers can assist with locating a food bank.
Discourse 2: Social DoH Identify Canadians with Modifiable Medical and Behavioural Risk Profiles	People living with food insecurity often have high fat (cheaper food) diets lacking in fruits and vegetables. These diets cause health damage over time. Therefore, healthy eating and healthy lifestyle coaching can offer a solution.
Discourse 3: Social DoH Identify Material Living Conditions That Shape Health	Food insecurity is caused by the conditions in which people are born, live, and so on. These conditions are what cause health inequities related to food security.
Discourse 4: Social DoH Identify Those Groups Experiencing Problematic Material Living Circumstances	Food insecurity differs among Canadians occupying different social locations. Identifying how these social locations may intersect (e.g., gender identity, disability, age) can improve barriers in access to healthy food. However, if interventions are limited to counselling programs (for those experiencing discrimination in food access) and anti-discrimination training (for service providers), then addressing structural barriers will be limited or absent.
Discourse 5: Social DoH and Their Distribution Result from Public Policy Decisions Made by Governments and Other Societal Institutions	Food insecurity in OECD countries is created by policymaking decisions that can be directly linked to governments' budget austerity measures causing increasing and severe family poverty (e.g., see Barnett & Bagshaw, 2020).
Discourse 6: Social DoH and Their Distribution Result from Economic and Political Structures and Justifying Ideologies	Food insecurity is rooted in the economic and political structures of neoliberal capitalism and ideologies such as belief in meritocracy, where wealth is related to the merits of moral fortitude (rather than cultural and class privilege)—people who accrue more resources are deserving of their wealth (Brunoli, 2017).

Table 3.2: Raphael and Bryant's Eight Discourses: Applying Public Policy Framings of Food Insecurity (*Continued*)

Social DoH Discourse	Policy Framing of the Problem of Food Insecurity
Discourse 7: Social DoH and Their Distribution Result from the Power and Influence of Those Creating and Benefiting from Social and Health Inequalities	Food insecurity is significantly deepened by Big Food (a globe-wide industrial consortium of mega-corporations) that heavily controls agricultural food production, industrial processing, and distribution of food to ensure multi-billion-dollar yearly profits.
Discourse 8: Social DoH and Their Distribution Result from the Processes Inherent to Capitalism—Capital Accumulation, Competition, and Exploitation	Food insecurity is rooted in capitalism's mandate to exploit planetary food availability through processes such as monoculturing Earth's food supply by Monsanto Agricultural Co. and Amazon Rainforest deforestation by JBS meatpacking megacorporation with net sales of 209 billion (USD) from 2021–2023 (Maisonnave, 2024).

Source: Adapted from Raphael & Bryant, 2023.

CONCLUSION

The construct of the social DoH has served us well in terms of enlightening the complex pathways of injustice in social and health inequity. Framings of the social DoH are more and more likely to integrate the root causes of the polycrisis, such as the synergies among neoliberalism, globalization, and capitalism. Beyond definitional debates about the social DoH lie the more foundational and elusive problem: inequities are skyrocketing because the social DoH as a construct have yet to even be integrated in public policy in any systematic or measurable manner. If inequities are to be successfully tackled, attention needs to shift to these hidden processes—the public policy drivers of human and planet health damage. Debating definitions of the social DoH amid the current polycrisis is perhaps akin to "scrambling for deck chairs on the Titanic." Instead, refocusing on core impacts of oppression, and its structural precursors, is a necessary solution-based strategy to address and tackle the inequitable politics of the DoH.

FURTHER READINGS

Almeida, M., Stresha, A. D., Stojanac, D., & Miller, L. J. (2020). The impact of COVID-19 pandemic on women's mental health. *Archives of Women's Mental Health, 23*(6), 741–748. https://doi.org/10.1007/s00737-020-01092-2

Barnett, P., & Bagshaw, P. (2020). Neoliberalism: What it is, how it affects health and what to do about it. *The New Zealand Medical Journal, 133*(1512), 76–84.

Drescher, J. (2015). Out of DSM: Depathologizing homosexuality. *Behavioral Sciences, 5*(4), 565–575. https://doi.org/10.3390%2Fbs5040565

Hankivsky, O., & Christoffersen, A. (2008). Intersectionality and the determinants of health: A Canadian perspective. *Critical Public Health, 18*(3), 271–283. https://doi.org/10.1080/09581590802294296

Marques, A. M., Nogueira, C., & de Oliveira, J. M. (2015). Lesbians on medical encounters: Tales of heteronormativity, deception, and expectations. *Health Care for Women International, 36*(9), 988–1006. https://doi.org/10.1080/07399332.2014.888066

WEBSITES OF INTEREST

Campaign 2000: End Child and Family Poverty—https://campaign2000.ca/

"Campaign 2000 is a cross-Canada public education movement to build Canadian awareness and support for the 1989 all-party House of Commons resolution to end child poverty in Canada by the year 2000. Campaign 2000 began in 1991 out of concern about the lack of government progress in addressing child poverty. Campaign 2000 is non-partisan in urging all Canadian elected officials to keep their promise to Canada's children."

Feminist Frequency—https://feministfrequency.com

This Peabody award-winning website offers access to Anita Sarkeesian's mini-documentaries about the representation of women in the digital world. Feminist Frequency originated as a non-profit dedicated to ending toxicity and abuse in the games industry and gaming spaces at large. Click "Videos" or "Resources" to explore.

National Collaborating Centre for the Determinants of Health (NCCDH)—https://nccdh.ca/

The NCCDH supports the Canadian public health community with knowledge and resources to act on the structural and social determinants of health to achieve health equity. The centre achieves this by translating emerging research and evidence, defining concepts, exchanging promising practices, and bringing people together.

National Collaborating Centre for Indigenous Health (NCCIH)—https://www.nccih.ca/en/

"The NCCIH is a national Indigenous organization established in 2005 by the Government of Canada and funded through the Public Health Agency of Canada to support First Nations, Inuit, and Métis public health renewal and health equity through knowledge translation and exchange. The NCCIH is hosted by the University of Northern BC in Prince George, BC."

GLOSSARY

Allostatic Load: Refers to the biological costs of chronic stress, which can lead to many different disease outcomes (Misiak, 2020). Measures of allostatic load demonstrate that exposures to excess stress causes cardiovascular, metabolic, neuroendocrine, and immune system dysregulation, all of which have been found to predict morbidity and mortality (Misiak, 2020).

Apolitical: Refers to a way of thinking that does not consider the politics of why things "are the way they are." This approach can be unintentional, such as when people are not, for a number of reasons, aware of broader historical, social, political, and economic contexts, and hence lack the capacity to analyze the politics of areas such as the social DoH. It can also be intentional, such as when policymakers are aware of some of the structural causes of poverty, yet fail to integrate these causes into their policy interventions to address poverty.

Critical Perspectives: Refer to acknowledgement and analysis of forms of power and involves "1) critiques of hegemonic power structures and ruling relations (power over)—naming who benefits from injustice; 2) organized public protest and acts of resistance in the face of oppressive, sometimes murderous regimes, public policies (power to, power with), and the like; and 3) explicit goals of disrupting, unsettling, and interrupting, processes and practices of oppression in local and global spheres, all of which are synergistically connected" (power with, power within; McGibbon, 2021a, p. 8).

Cycle of Oppression: Refers to the cyclic process of how stereotyping (oversimplified, fixed images, often negative) leads to prejudice (ways of thinking based on stereotypes). Prejudice then causes discrimination (action or inaction based in prejudicial thinking). Finally, oppression is when discrimination is backed up by systemic power, such as the power of educational institutions to often "look the other way" in the face of sexualized violence on campus.

Embodied Oppression: Refers to the process whereby oppressive social and living circumstances eventually cause changes in the body's stress handling systems. These changes have been shown to result in serious bodily impacts over time, such as heart disease, diabetes, and compromised immune system capacity. Oppressive psychological and spiritual circumstance happen in tandem with physical stresses (e.g., food insecurity) and also become embodied through the physiological impacts of depression and trauma.

Eurocentric: Refers to an attitude or set of empirical beliefs that frame Europe as "the primary engine and architect of world history, the bearer of universal values and reason, and the pinnacle and therefore model of progress and development" (Sundberg, 2009). It involves belief in the superiority of Eurocentric thinking and ways of approaching many areas, such as countries' governance systems, approaches to health and well-being, and education, and so on. Eurocentrism resulted in the advance and justification of colonialism across the globe.

Hegemonic: Refers to the process by which the dominant culture maintains its overarching authority and dominance. Examples include Eurocentric culture and biomedical dominance. Hegemonic ideas and processes are reinforced by the dominant group through education, advertising, publication, and the mobilization of a police force as well as military personnel to subdue opposition (Felluga, 2015).

Intersectionality: Refers to the ways in which systems of inequality based on gender, race, ethnicity, sexual orientation, gender identity, disability, class, and other forms of discrimination "intersect" to deepen disadvantage. Oppressions in society do not operate independently. Rather, they intersect in complex patterns—models that view each oppression as additive rather than interlocking fail to stress the centrality of power and privilege. Identities, sometimes referred to as identity markers (Hum & Simpson, 2003), intersect to compound oppression.

Meritocracy: Refers to the belief that wealth and income inequality are related to moral fortitude (or lack thereof) and the people who accrue more resources deserve their wealth, while the "losers," who have not been able to thrive in a market-driven environment, must simply accept their fate (Brunoli, 2017). "Merit" has been analyzed as a popular myth that legitimizes social order (Hearn, 2021), such as social stratification.

REFERENCES

Ahmad, K., Chen, E. W., Nazir, U., Cotts, W., Andrade, A., Trivedi, A. N., Erqou, S., & Wu, W.-C. (2019). Regional variation in the association of poverty and heart failure mortality in the 3135 counties of the United States. *Journal of the American Heart Association, 8*(18), e012422. https://doi.org/10.1161/jaha.119.012422

Almeida, M., Shrestha, A. D., Stojanac, D., & Miller, L. J. (2020). The impact of the COVID-19 pandemic on women's mental health. *Archives of Women's Mental Health, 23*(6), 741–748. https://doi.org/10.1007/s00737-020-01092-2

Baird, K. L. (1999). The new NIH and FDA medical research policies: Targeting gender, promoting justice. *Journal of Health, Politics, Policy and Law, 24*(3), 531–565. https://doi.org/10.1215/03616878-24-3-531

Banerjee, S. (2021, October 1). Coroner's report into Joyce Echaquan death urges Quebec to recognize systemic racism. *The Canadian Press.* https://globalnews.ca/news/8235822/quebec-coroner-report-joyce-echaquan-systemic-racism/

Barnett, P., & Bagshaw, P. (2020). Neoliberalism: What it is, how it affects health and what to do about it. *The New Zealand Medical Journal, 133*(1512), 76–84.

Boyd, E. L. (2019). *Gendered racism and pain: The intersection of racism and sexism on pain outcomes* [Doctoral dissertation]. University of Maryland.

Brisson, D., McCune, S., Wilson, J. H., Speer, S. R., McCrae, J. S., & Hoops Calhoun, K. (2020). A systematic review of the association between poverty and biomarkers of toxic stress. *Journal of Evidence-Based Social Work, 17*(6), 696–713. https://doi.org/10.1080/26408066.2020.1769786

Brown, E. M., & Tarasuk, V. (2019). Money speaks: Reductions in severe food insecurity follow the Canada Child Benefit. *Preventive Medicine, 129*, 105876. https://doi.org/10.1016/j.ypmed.2019.105876

Brunoli, J. (2017, June 24). *This is neoliberalism, part I: The 10 tenets of neoliberalism.* Medium. https://euroyankeeblog.medium.com/10-tenets-of-neoliberalism-ea90f34e51f9

Calliste, A., & Sefa Dei., G. (Eds.). (2000). *Anti-racist feminism: Critical race and gender studies.* Fernwood Publishing

Canadian Feminist Alliance for International Action and DisAbled Women's Network Canada—Réseau D'Action des Femmes Handicapées du Canada (FAFIA). (2017). *Women with disabilities in Canada: Report to the Committee on the Rights of Persons with Disabilities on the occasion of the committee's initial review of Canada.* https://fafia-afai.org/wp content/uploads/2017/02/FAFIA_DAWN_CRPD2017.pdf

Canadian Research Institute for the Advancement of Women. (2006). *Intersectional feminist frameworks: A primer.* https://www.criaw-icref.ca/publications/intersectional-feminist-frameworks-a-primer/

Carbado, D. W., & Crenshaw, K. W. (2019). An intersectional critique of tiers of scrutiny: beyond "either/or" approaches to equal protection. *Yale Law Journal Forum, 129*, 108–129. https://www.yalelawjournal.org/pdf/CarbadoCrenshaw_AnIntersectionalCritiqueofTiersofScrutiny_t1657eh9.pdf

Carroll, W., & Sapinski, J. P. (2018). *Organizing the 1%: How corporate power works.* Fernwood Publishing.

Carter, S., Mekawi, Y., Sheikh, I., Sanders, A. S., Packard, G., Harnett, N. G., & Metzger, I. W. (2022). Approaching mental health equity in neuroscience for Black women across the lifespan: Biological embedding of racism from Black feminist conceptual frameworks. *Biological Psychiatry: Cognitive Neuroscience and Neuroimaging, 7*(12), 1235–1241. https://doi.org/10.1016/j.bpsc.2022.08.007

Cheng, Y. J., Kanaya, A. M., Araneta, M. R. G., Saydah, S. H., Kahn, H. S., Gregg, E. W., Fujimoto, W. Y., & Imperatore, G. (2019). Prevalence of diabetes by race and ethnicity in the United States, 2011–2016. *JAMA, 322*(24), 2389–2398. https://doi.org/10.1001/jama.2019.19365

Cheran, K., Murthy, C., Bornemann, E. A., Kamma, H. K., Alabbas, M., Elashahab, M., Abid, N., Manaye, S., & Venugopal, S. (2023). The growing epidemic of diabetes among the Indigenous population of Canada: A systematic review. *Cureus, 15*(3), e36173. https://doi.org/10.7759%2Fcureus.36173

Chiu, M., Maclagan, L. C., Tu, J. V., & Shah, B. R. (2015). Temporal trends in cardiovascular disease risk factors among white, South Asian, Chinese and Black groups in Ontario, Canada, 2001 to 2012: A population-based study. *British Medical Journal Open, 5*(8), e007232. https://doi.org/10.1136/bmjopen-2014-007232

Collins, P. H. (1990). *Black feminist thought: Knowledge, consciousness, and the politics of empowerment.* Unwin Hyman.

Collins, P. H. (2003). The politics of Black feminist thought. In C. R. McCann, S.-K. Kim, & E. Ergun (Eds.), *Feminist theory reader: Local and global perspectives* (pp. 318–333). Routledge.

Collins, P. H. (2005). *Black sexual politics: African Americans, gender, and the new racism.* Routledge.

Crenshaw, K. (1989). Demarginalizing the intersection of race and sex: A Black feminist critique of antidiscrimination doctrine, feminist theory and antiracist politics. *University of Chicago Legal Forum, 1989*(1), 139–166.

Dahlgren, G., & Whitehead, M. (1991). *Policies and strategies to promote social equity in health.* Institute for Futures Studies.

Dahlgren, G., & Whitehead, M. (2021). The Dahlgren-Whitehead model of health determinants: 30 years on and still chasing rainbows. *Public Health, 199*, 20–24. https://doi.org/10.1016/j.puhe.2021.08.009

D'Silva, C., Hafleen, N., Mansfield, E., Martel, S., Fierheller, D., Banerjee, A., Malhotra, G., Mutta, B., Dhillon, P., Hasan, Z., Parikh, A., Nooraie, R. Y., Chaze, F., & Zenlea, I. (2022). Service provider perspectives on exploring social determinants of health impacting Type 2 diabetes management for South Asian adults in Peel Region, Canada. *Canadian Journal of Diabetes, 46*(6), 611–619. https://doi.org/10.1016/j.jcjd.2022.05.011

Drescher, J. (2015). Out of DSM: Depathologizing homosexuality. *Behavioral Sciences, 5*(4), 565–575. https://doi.org/10.3390%2Fbs5040565

Dresser, R. (1992). Wanted single, white male for medical research. *The Hastings Center Report, 22*(1), 24–29. https://doi.org/10.2307/3562720

Ervin, J., Taouk, Y., Alfonzo, L. F., Peasgood, T., & King, T. (2022). Longitudinal association between informal unpaid caregiving and mental health amongst working age adults in high-income OECD countries: A systematic review. *eClinicalMedicine, 53*, 101711. https://doi.org/10.1016/j.eclinm.2022.101711

Erving, C. L., Patterson, E. J., & Boone, J. (2021). Black women's mental health matters: Theoretical perspectives and future directions. *Sociology Compass, 15*(9), e12919. https://doi.org/10.1111/soc4.12919

Felluga, D. (2015). *Critical theory: The key concepts*. Routledge.

Fitzgerald, D., Hinterberger, A., Narayan, J., & Williams, R. (2020). Brexit as hereditary redux: Imperialism, biomedicine and the NHS in Britain. *The Sociological Review, 68*(6), 1161–1178. https://doi.org/10.1177/0038026120914177

Fleras, A., & Maaka, R. (2010). Indigeneity-grounded analysis (IGA) as policy(-making) lens: New Zealand models, Canadian realities. *The International Indigenous Policy Journal, 1*(1). https://doi.org/10.18584/iipj.2010.1.1.4

Guidi, J., Lucente, M., Sonino, N., & Fava, G. A. (2020). Allostatic load and its impact on health: A systematic review. *Psychotherapy and Psychosomatics, 90*(1), 11–27. https://doi.org/10.1159/000510696

Hankivsky, O., & Christoffersen, A. (2008). Intersectionality and the determinants of health: A Canadian perspective. *Critical Public Health, 18*(3), 271–283. https://doi.org/10.1080/09581590802294296

Hearn, J. (2021). Reframing the history of the competition concept: Neoliberalism, meritocracy, modernity. *Journal of Historical Sociology, 34*(2), 375–392. https://doi.org/10.1111/johs.12324

hooks, b. (1990). *Yearning: Race, gender and cultural politics*. Between the Lines.

Hum, D., & Simpson, W. (2003). Labour market training of new Canadians and limitations to the intersectionality framework. *Canadian Ethnic Studies, 35*(3), 56–69.

Islam, M. M. (2019). Social determinants of health and related inequalities: Confusion and implications. *Frontiers in Public Health, 7*, 11. https://doi.org/10.3389%2Ffpubh.2019.00011

Jack, S. M., Duku, E., Whitty, H., Van Lieshout, R. J., Niccols, A., Georgiades, K., & Lipman, E. L. (2022). Young mothers' use of and experiences with mental health care services in Ontario, Canada: A qualitative descriptive study. *BMC Women's Health, 22*(1), 214. https://doi.org/10.1186/s12905-022-01804-z

James, S. E., Herman, J. L., Rankin, S., Keisling, M., Mottet, L., & Anafi, M. (2016). *The report of the 2015 U.S. Transgender Survey: Executive summary*. National Center for Transgender Equality. https://transequality.org/sites/default/files/docs/usts/USTS-Full-Report-Dec17.pdf

Lauro, A. P. (2018). *Access to mental health care for depression among Latina women in Adams County* [Student publication]. The Cupola, Gettysburg College.

Lee, D. Y., Kim, E., & Choi, M. H. (2015). Technical and clinical aspects of cortisol as a biochemical marker of chronic stress. *BMB Reports, 48*(4), 209–216. https://doi.org/10.5483/bmbrep.2015.48.4.275

Lindley, K. J., Aggarwal, N. R., Briller, J. E., Davis, M. B., Douglass, P., Epps, K. C., Fleg, J. L., Hayes, S., Itchhaporia, D., Mahmoud, Z., De Oliveira, G. M. M., Ogunniyi, M. O., Quesada, O., Russo, A. M., Sharma, J., Wood, M. J., & American College of Cardiology Cardiovascular Disease in Women Committee and the American College of Cardiology Health Equity Taskforce. (2021). Socioeconomic determinants of health and cardiovascular outcomes in women: JACC review topic of the week. *Journal of the American College of Cardiology, 78*(19), 1919–1929. https://doi.org/10.1016/j.jacc.2021.09.011

Lipman, T. H., Willi, S. M., Lai, C. W., Smith, J. A., Patil, O., & Hawkes, C. P. (2020). Insulin pump use in children with Type 1 diabetes: Over a decade of disparities. *Journal of Pediatric Nursing, 55*, 110–115. https://doi.org/10.1016/j.pedn.2020.08.007

Maisonnave, F. (2024, January 18). *Bid by meatpacker JBS to join New York Stock Exchange faces opposition over Amazon deforestation*. Toronto City News. https://toronto.citynews.ca/2024/01/18/bid-by-meatpacker-jbs-to-join-new-york-stock-exchange-faces-opposition-over-amazon-deforestation/

Marques, A. M., Nogueira, C., & de Oliveira, J. (2015). Lesbians on medical encounters: Tales of heteronormativity, deception, and expectations. *Health Care for Women International, 36*(9), 988–1006. https://doi.org/10.1080/07399332.2014.888066

Marx, K. (2016). Economic and philosophic manuscripts of 1844. In W. Longhofer & D. Winchester (Eds.), *Social theory re-wired: New connections to classical and contemporary perspectives* (2nd ed.). Routledge.

McDaniel, J. T., Nuhu, K., Ruiz, J., & Alorbi, G. (2019). Social determinants of cancer incidence and mortality around the world: An ecological study. *Global Health Promotion, 26*(1), 41–49. https://doi.org/10.1177/1757975916686913

McGibbon, E. (2021a). People and planet under threat: The social, ecological, and structural determinants of health. In E. McGibbon (Ed.), *Oppression: A social determinant of health* (2nd ed). Fernwood Publishing.

McGibbon, E. (2021b). The politics of mental health: Pathologizing the impacts of injustice. In E. McGibbon (Ed.), *Oppression: A social determinant of health* (2nd ed.). Fernwood Publishing.

McGibbon, E. (In press). Classism and health: What the body remembers. In T. Bryant (Ed.), *Handbook of the social determinants of health*. Edward Elgar Publishing.

McGibbon, E., & Etowa, J. (2007). *Health inequities and the social determinants of health: Spatial contexts of oppression* [Invited keynote presentation]. Nova Scotia Health Research Foundation Health Geomatics Conference, Halifax, NS, Canada.

McGibbon, E., Fierlbeck, K., & Ajadi, T. (2019). *Mapping health equity in Canadian public policy: Ruling relations and the dynamics of oppression* [Panel presentation]. International Public Policy Association, 3rd Annual Conference, Montreal, QC, Canada.

McGibbon, E., Fierlbeck, K., & Ajadi, T. (2021). Health equity and institutional ethnography: Mapping the problem of policy change. *Witness: The Canadian Journal of Critical Nursing Discourse, 3*(2), 64–80. https://doi.org/10.25071/2291-5796.117

McGibbon, E., Fierlbeck, K., & Ajadi, T. (2022). Institutional ethnography and critical policy analysis: Catalyzing justice in policymaking [Paper accepted for publication]. *Critical Studies: An International and Interdisciplinary Journal.*

McGibbon, E., Sheppard, D., & Jubin, M. (2024). Community mental health practice. In. A. Dosani, J. Etowa, & C. van Daalen-Smith (Eds.), *Community health nursing: A Canadian perspective* (6th ed.). Pearson.

McGuire, L., Monzavi, T., Hoffman, A. J., Law, F., Irvin, M. J., Winterbottom, M., Hartstone-Rose, A., Rutland, A., Burns, K. P., Butler, L., Drews, M., Fields, G. E., & Mulvey, K. L. (2021). Science and math interest and gender stereotypes: The role of educator gender in informal science learning sites. *Frontiers in Psychology, 12*, 503237. https://doi.org/10.3389/fpsyg.2021.503237

McPherson, C., Ndumbe-Eyoh, S., Betker, C., Oickle, D., & Peroff-Johnston, N. (2016). Swimming against the tide: A Canadian qualitative study examining the implementation of a province-wide public health initiative to address health equity. *International Journal for Equity in Health, 15*(1), 129. https://doi.org/10.1186/s12939-016-0419-4

Mehta, B., Jannat-Khah, D., Fontana, M. A., Moezinia, C. J., Mancuso, C. A., Bass, A. R., Antao, V. C., Gibofsky, A., Goodman, S. M., & Ibrahim, S. (2020). Impact of COVID-19 on vulnerable patients with rheumatic disease: results of a worldwide survey. *RMD Open, 6*(3), e001378. https://doi.org/10.1136/rmdopen-2020-001378

Meyer, H. M., Mocarski, R., Holt, N. R., Hope, D. A., King, R. E., & Woodruff, N. (2020). Unmet expectations in health care settings: Experiences of transgender and gender diverse adults in the Central Great Plains. *Qualitative Health Research, 30*(3), 409–422. https://doi.org/10.1177/1049732319860265

Mishori, R. (2019). The social determinants of health? Time to focus on the political determinants of health! *Medical Care, 57*(7), 491–493. https://doi.org/10.1097/mlr.0000000000001131

Misiak, B. (2020). Stress, allostatic load, and psychosis: One step forward in research but where to go next? *Frontiers in Psychiatry, 10*, 937. https://doi.org/10.3389/fpsyt.2019.00937

Morrison, V., Gagnon, F., Morestin, F., & Keeling, M. (2014). *Keywords in healthy public policy.* National Collaborating Centre for Healthy Public Policy.

Muller, J., & Raphael, D. (2023). Does unionization and working under collective agreements promote health? *Health Promotion International, 38*(4), daab181. https://doi.org/10.1093/heapro/daab181

Mulligan, C. J. (2021). Systemic racism can get under our skin and into our genes. *American Journal of Physical Anthropology, 175*(2), 399–405. https://doi.org/10.1002/ajpa.24290

Nash, R., Hudson, A., & Luttrell, C. (2006). *Mapping political context: A toolkit for civil society organizations.* Overseas Development Institute. https://odi.org/en/publications/mapping-political-context-a-toolkit-for-civil-society-organisations/

National Center for Health Statistics. (2020). *Healthy people 2020.* Centers for Disease Control and Prevention. https://www.cdc.gov/nchs/healthy_people/hp2020.htm

Olkin, R., Hayward, H. S., Abbene, M. S., & VanHeel, G. (2019). The experiences of microaggressions against women with visible and invisible disabilities. *Journal of Social Issues, 75*(3), 757–785. https://doi.org/10.1111/josi.12342

Organisation for Economic Co-operation and Development (OECD). (2019). *Health for everyone? Social inequalities in health and health systems.* OECD Publishing. https://doi.org/10.1787/3c8385d0-en

Palmen, R. (2021). *ACT on intersectionality.* Zenodo. https://doi.org/10.5281/zenodo.5602859

Park, J. E., Kim, S. Y., Kim, S. H., Jeoung, E. J., & Park, J. H. (2020). Household food insecurity: Comparison between families with and without members with disabilities. *International Journal of Environmental Research and Public Health, 17*(17), 6149. https://doi.org/10.3390%2Fijerph17176149

Raghupathi, V., & Raghupathi, W. (2020). The influence of education on health: An empirical assessment of OECD countries for the period 1995–2015. *Archives of Public Health, 78*(1), 20. https://doi.org/10.1186/s13690-020-00402-5

Raphael, D. (2021). Raising the volume on the social determinants of health in Canada and elsewhere. In E. McGibbon (Ed.), *Oppression: A social determinant of health* (2nd ed.). Fernwood Publishing.

Raphael, D., & Bryant, T. (2023). Socialism as the way forward: Updating a discourse analysis of the social determinants of health. *Critical Public Health, 33*(4), 387–394. https://doi.org/10.1080/09581596.2023.2178387

Raphael, D., Bryant, T., & Curry-Stevens, A. (2004). Toronto charter outlines future health policy directions for Canada and elsewhere. *Health Promotion International, 19*(2), 269–273. https://doi.org/10.1093/heapro/dah214

Raphael, D., T., Bryant, J., Mikkonen, J., & Raphael, A. (2020). *Social determinants of health: The Canadian facts* (2nd ed.). Ontario Tech University Faculty of Health Sciences and York University School of Health Policy and Management. https://thecanadianfacts.org/

Ratima, M., Martin, D., Castleden, H., & Delormier, T. (2019). Indigenous voices and knowledge systems—Promoting planetary health, health equity, and sustainable development now and for future generations. *Global Health Promotion, 26*(suppl. 3), 3–5. https://doi.org/10.1177/1757975919838487

Ridley, M., Rao, G., Schilbach, F., & Patel, V. (2020). Poverty, depression, and anxiety: Causal evidence and mechanisms. *Science, 370*(6522), eaay0214. https://doi.org/10.1126/science.aay0214

Rossman, K., Salamanca, P., & Macapagal, K. (2017). A qualitative study examining young adults' experiences of disclosure and nondisclosure of LGBTQ identity to health care providers. *Journal of Homosexuality, 64*(10), 1390–1410. https://doi.org/10.1080/00918369.2017.1321379

Sacks, R. M., Greene, J., Burke, R., & Owen, E. C. (2015). Mental health care among low-income pregnant women with depressive symptoms: Facilitators and barriers to care access and the effectiveness of financial incentives for increasing care. *Administration and Policy in Mental Health and Mental Health Services Research, 42*(4), 484–492. https://doi.org/10.1007/s10488-014-0562-4

Sanger, T. (2019). *Time to step up for tax justice: Important international reforms to end tax-dodging and tax havens are on the horizon. Why isn't Canada doing more?* Canadian Centre for Policy Alternatives.

Schultz, A., Nguyen, T., Sinclaire, M., Fransoo, R., & McGibbon, E. (2021). Historical and continued colonial impacts on heart health of Indigenous Peoples in Canada: What's reconciliation got to do with it? *CJC Open, 3*(12), S149–S164. https://doi.org/10.1016/j.cjco.2021.09.010

Schultz, A., Sinclair, M., McGibbon, E. & Dhal, L. (2018, May 28–31). *Cardiac health disparities in First Nation Peoples: One to five year health and treatment outcomes among all Manitoba index coronary angiogram recipients.* Canadian Public Health Association Conference, Montreal, QC, Canada.

Shanks, T. R. W., & Robinson, C. (2013). Assets, economic opportunity and toxic stress: A framework for understanding child and educational outcomes. *Economics of Education Review, 33*(C), 154–170. https://doi.org/10.1016/j.econedurev.2012.11.002

Sinclaire, M., Schultz, A., Linton, J., & McGibbon, E. (2021). Etuaptmumk (Two-Eyed Seeing) and ethical space: Ways to disrupt health researchers' colonial attraction to a singular biomedical worldview. *Witness: The Canadian Journal for Critical Nursing Discourse, 3*(1). https://doi.org/10.25071/2291-5796.94

Smith, D. (1990). *Texts, facts, and femininity: Exploring the relations of ruling.* Routledge.

Statistics Canada. (2023). *Canadian survey on disability, 2017 to 2022.* The Daily. https://www150.statcan.gc.ca/n1/daily-quotidien/231201/dq231201b-eng.htm

Statistics Canada. (2024). The disability rate in Canada increased in 2022. *StatsCAN Plus.* https://www.statcan.gc.ca/o1/en/plus/5980-disability-rate-canada-increased-2022

Stevens, P. E., & Hall, J. M. (1992). Applying critical theories to nursing in communities. *Public Health Nursing, 9*(1), 2–9. https://doi.org/10.1111/j.1525-1446.1992.tb00065.x

Stone, K., Blinn, N. & Spencer, R. (2022). Mental health impacts of climate change on women: A scoping review. *Current Environmental Health Reports 9*(2), 228–243. https://doi.org/10.1007/s40572-022-00346-8

Stroumsa, D., Shires, D. A., Richardson, C. R., Jaffee, K. D., & Woodford, M. R. (2019). Transphobia rather than education predicts provider knowledge of transgender health care. *Medical Education, 53*(4), 398–407. https://doi.org/10.1111/medu.13796

Stuart, G. (2019, February 1). *4 types of power: What are power over, power with, power to and power within?* [Blog] Sustaining Community. https://sustainingcommunity.wordpress.com/2019/02/01/4-types-of-power/

Sundberg, J. (2009). Eurocentrism. In R. Kitchin & N. Thrift (Eds.), *International Encyclopedia of Human Geography*. Elsevier.

Sylliboy, J. R., Bird, N., Butler, E., Wilmot, K., & Perley, G. (2022). Two-Spirits' response to COVID-19: Survey findings in Atlantic Canada identify priorities and developing practices. *International Journal of Indigenous Health, 17*(1), 14–25. https://doi.org/10.32799/ijih.v17i1.36724

Turin, T. C., Saad, N., Jun, M., Tonelli, M., Ma, Z., Barnabe, C. C. M., Manns, B., & Hemmelgarn, B. (2016). Lifetime risk of diabetes among First Nations and non–First Nations people. *Canadian Medical Association Journal, 188*(16), 1147–1153. https://doi.org/10.1503/cmaj.150787

Turpel-Lafond, M. E., & Johnson, H. (2021). In plain sight: Addressing Indigenous-specific racism and discrimination in BC health care. *BC Studies: The British Columbian Quarterly,* (209), 7–17. https://doi.org/10.14288/bcs.vi209.195283

Tutty, L. M., Radtke, H. L., Thurston, W. E. B., Nixon, K. L., Ursel, E. J., Ateah, C. A., & Hampton, M. (2020). The mental health and well-being of Canadian Indigenous and non-Indigenous women abused by intimate partners. *Violence Against Women, 26*(12–13), 1574–1597. https://doi.org/10.1177/1077801219884123

Van Dijk, T. A. (2015). Critical discourse analysis. In D. Tannen, D. Schiffrin, & H. Hamilton (Eds.), *Handbook of discourse analysis* (2nd ed., pp. 466–485). Blackwell.

Wesley-Esquimaux, C. C., & Smolewski, M. (2004). *Historic trauma and Aboriginal healing*. Aboriginal Healing Foundation.

World Health Organization (WHO). (n.d.). *Social determinants of health*. https://www.who.int/health-topics/social-determinants-of-health

World Health Organization. (2008). *Closing the gap in a generation: Health equity through action on the social determinants of health—Final report of the commission on social determinants of health*. https://www.who.int/publications/i/item/WHO-IER-CSDH-08.1

CHAPTER 4

Ecological Determinants of Health: Threats to Earth's Life Support Systems

CHAPTER OBJECTIVES

Using as many examples as possible:

1. Describe the Anthropocene Epoch, including the politics of language in the Anthropocene(s).
2. In the context of the ecological DoH, describe what is meant by planetary health, EcoHealth, One Health, and One World.
3. Identify and describe the main ecological DoH.
4. Identify some important structural, root causes of climate emergency.
5. Compare and contrast the International Panel on Climate Change (2021) recommendations with the Club of Rome's (Dixson-Decleve et al., 2018) recommendations for achieving "Earth 4 All."

CRITICAL THINKING QUESTIONS

1. What are the differences among descriptions of concern for the environment as "climate change," "climate crisis," and "climate emergency"?
2. What are some common features of the perpetration of environmental racism across the examples provided in this chapter?

3. What is the relationship between the Haida Gwaii First Nations' fight for land sovereignty and colonialist capitalism?
4. How are each of chapter's ecological DoH related to the social DoH?
5. How is neoliberal capitalism related to the climate emergency?

INTRODUCTION

The aim of this chapter is to describe, in more detail, the ecological determinants of health (DoH). The chapter begins with a discussion of the politics of the **Anthropocene Epoch**, which is explained within anthropogenic (human induced) planetary damage. Commodification of natural resources, colonialist and imperialist dominance, and the capitalist imperative of corporate profit are emphasized, including Kathryn Yusoff's (2018) work in tracing the colour line of the Anthropocene. The constructs of planetary health, EcoHealth, One Health, and One World lay the foundation for analyzing globe-wide responses to increasing threats to Earth's life support systems. Pivotal ecological DoH are described, along with some of their important health and policy implications: pollution and ecotoxicity, including environmental racism; resource extraction and depletion; climate and atmospheric emergency; desertification, deforestation, and acidification; and biodiversity loss, species endangerment, and extinction. The chapter concludes with International Panel on Climate Change (IPCC) recommendations for policymakers regarding actions that can be taken in the near term, based on existing knowledge, to address desertification, land degradation, and food security (Mirzabaev et al., 2019). IPCC recommendations are then contrasted with the Club of Rome's (Dixson-Declève et al., 2018) responses to direct calls to climate action from citizens around the world.

THE ANTHROPOCENE: EARTH'S LIFE SUPPORT SYSTEMS IN PERIL

> [The Anthropocene] is also the story of environmental uncertainties, geo-political struggles, and social dilemmas, which create a

> paradoxical sense of worldly involvement in, and estrangement from, this tempestuous site where the human along with every other being is intimately caught within a maelstrom of erosion and disintegration. The Earth, in other words, entangles every life form, always disallowing fence-sitting, regardless of the geological epochality of a single species [humans] pretending to occupy a position outside Earth systems. (Oppermann, 2018, p. 3)

The ecological DoH now unfold within an increasingly recognized new geological epoch, the Anthropocene. This global context is a central background for naming the pervasive ecological damage that is now being acknowledged and met with mobilization for change, along with neoliberal resistance to acknowledging the global climate emergency.

Core Descriptions of the Anthropocene

Citizen-scientist Rachel Carson's book *Silent Spring* (1962) is widely recognized as the catalyst of a global consciousness about anthropogenic impacts on health. "Our heedless and destructive acts enter into the vast cycles of the Earth and in time return to bring hazard to ourselves … By acquiescing in an act that causes such suffering to a living creature, who among us is not diminished as a human being?" (Griswold, 2012). Carson described a view of nature compromised by synthetic pesticides, especially DDT. Once these pesticides entered the biosphere, Carson argued, they not only killed bugs but also made their way up the food chain to threaten bird and fish populations and could eventually sicken children.

Complex and multiple changes in Earth's natural systems such as these are captured in the term *Anthropocene Epoch*, first described by Paul Crutzen (2005), an environmental chemist and Nobel laureate, as the current geological age (Carrington, 2016). Despite ongoing debates about the naming of a new epoch, the Anthropocene is now largely accepted as a descriptor that signals the dominance of humans over the global environment. It replaces the Holocene Epoch, a period of relative climatic stability lasting about 11,500 years, during which humanity moved from being hunter-gatherers to agriculturalists to today's predominantly urban global population (Carrington, 2016). The on-the-ground meaning of the Anthropocene involves synergistic impacts on **Earth systems**, including the ecological DoH described in this chapter. "Since we depend on these systems for the most fundamental determinants of our health, these human-induced changes present a profound threat to the health of the world's population in the 21st century" (Hancock et al., 2015, p. 23). There are five main Earth systems, or spheres, on Earth: the geosphere (the interior and surface of Earth, both of which are made up of rocks), the biosphere (the limited part of the planet that can support living things), the hydrosphere (areas of Earth that are covered with enormous amounts of water), the atmosphere (the envelope of gas that keeps the planet warm and provides oxygen for breathing and carbon dioxide for photosynthesis), and the cryosphere (the huge quantities of ice at the poles and elsewhere) (Huddart & Scott, 2020). All five of these enormous and complex systems interact with one another to maintain the Earth as we know it.

The decision to define a new geological epoch involves identifying a geological signal that occurs globally and will also be incorporated into deposits in Earth's future geological record (Waters et al., 2016). An example is the huge meteorite that ended the dinosaur age, where sediments of iridium, the meteorite's metal, can be found all over the globe in the Earth's geological record, or footprint (Carrington, 2016). Evidence of globe-wide signals, such as this one, are the measures used to define the beginning or the end of a geological epoch—in this case the end of the dinosaur age. Since these signals are relatively abrupt in the context of Earth's history, they are referred to as golden spikes. "For the Anthropocene, the best candidate for such a golden spike are radioactive elements from nuclear bomb tests, which were blown into the stratosphere before settling down to Earth... although there are an array of other signals, including plastic pollution, soot from power stations, concrete, and even the bones left by the global proliferation of the domestic chicken" (Carrington, 2016). This chapter is about on-the-ground meanings of the Anthropocene, as well as the politics of the Anthropocenes.

The Politics of Health in the Anthropocenes

There are many variations in how the Anthropocene is described, when it started, what it should be named, and its impacts on Earth systems—each of these possibilities creating its own distinct framing of the Anthropocene (Chakrabarty, 2018). The term itself is highly political, in part because its meanings vary across different ideological spectrums. Some variations concentrate on the geological and other scientific considerations, with the near exclusion of the political, sociological, historical, and anthropological contexts, to name a few. These perspectives also lack an examination of differential impacts across the social DoH, and across the northern and southern hemispheres. Some variations analyze the socially constructed notion that the Anthropocene can be siloed or separated into discrete, relatively recent time periods, and that impacts do not need to be disaggregated across social class and race, to name a few (Chakrabarty, 2018; Moore, 2017; Yusoff, 2018). In these perspectives, the politics of planetary health, such as the impacts of historical and current capitalist enterprises, tend to be absent. Concepts of the Anthropocene have also been critiqued due to the ostensibly equal blame attributed to all of humanity (Malin, 2021). Anthropogenic damage in the Anthropocene is largely collapsed into collective "human" impacts, thus supporting a persistent masking of deeply inequitable impacts across the social DoH.

A concurrent assumption is that the Anthropocene Epoch began with the Industrial Revolution (1760–1830). However, this assumption is inconsistent with the historical trajectory of capitalism, which began in the era of Christopher Columbus with first contact of European settlers and the beginning of global resource extraction and depletion. Alternative namings of the current geological epoch include "the **Capitalocene**," so that the blame is laid squarely on the root causes of this new geological epoch—capitalism, or the global economic system (Chakrabarty, 2018). The Capitalocene (Age of Capital) reflects the history of capitalism and the central political, cultural, and economic role it played in the reshaping of global ecosystems for centuries before the advent of coal and steam engines (Moore, 2017).

Dominant discourses of the Anthropocene have also been critiqued due to the erasure of historical contributions of working-class labourers, including women, as well as the Black and Brown bodies upon which early capitalism was constructed (McGibbon, in press). European colonization, and its early forms of capitalism in the Americas, caused the death of at least 56 million people by 1600, including 90 percent of the Indigenous Peoples in these territories (Moore, 2017). The Anthropocene's origins in early capitalism explain the roots of some of the main historical inequities in the social DoH. These inequities are embodied across many generations, along with concurrent deprivations of the material goods necessary for establishing and sustaining health and well-being. It is crucial to note that current impacts of the Anthropocene are built upon centuries-old, deeply disproportionate impacts across the social DoH, causing an acceleration of injustice in this new era of anthropogenic damage (McGibbon, in press). These impacts have always been political, due to their linkages with public policy: rather than being a neutral phenomenon, the Anthropocene is entrenched with financial, legal, political, and governance systems "that must be radically realigned to recognize the connectivity among social, ecological, and technological domains of urban systems in order to deliver more just, equitable, sustainable, and resilient futures" (McPhearson et al., 2021, p. 1).

Earth scientist Kathryn Yusoff's (2018) groundbreaking book, *A Billion Black Anthropocenes or None*, traces the colour line of the Anthropocene, examining how the grammar and language of geology is foundational to establishing the extractive economies of subjective life and the Earth under colonialism and slavery (Ivry, 2022). This assumption is grounded in the principles of positivism, where objectivity and facts are assumed to be value-free and apolitical, despite evidence that resource extraction across the Earth disproportionately, by far, impacts racialized peoples. The Black Anthropocene, in the singular, represents

> … an inhuman proximity organized by historical geographies of extraction, grammars of geology, imperial global geographies, and

> contemporary environmental racism. It is predicated on the presumed absorbent qualities of black and brown bodies to take up the body burdens of exposure to toxicities and to buffer the violence of the Earth. (Ivry, 2022, p. 11)

Yusoff (2018) argues that the field of geology itself is assumed to be without a subject, "thinglike and inert." This objectification allows geology to operate with impunity, distancing itself from the on-the-ground extraction and depletion impacts of mining, pipeline construction, and water commodification, all of which heavily rely on colonialist histories and public policies and the commodification of the subaltern (Yusoff, 2018). In describing these subaltern spaces, Dutta (2014) refers to erasures of the "other" from "dominant discursive sites in civil society, academic and policy spaces" (p. 70). For Yusoff, geology operates through a racist prism where the organization of geological matter and human subjects produced the idea of a standing stock of gold, energy, and slaves, all part of the bill of sale, transforming humans into things (Ivry, 2022): "Blackness is rendered as an empty signifier, like gold, silver, and other precious minerals, where the valuation of exchange is established through descriptive markers, and subjects are considered as a set of properties" (p. 78), reflecting Marx's description of humans as "bits of capital" (Marx, 1867/2019, p. 446) Yusoff underscores how geology is implicated in assaults on Earth, and life on Earth, that led to the creation of the signifiers of the Anthropocene Epoch in the first place.

Importantly, anthropogenic processes were, and are, largely predicated on whiteness as the colour of universality (Yusoff, 2018), where Black bodies become dehumanized in the chains of violent commodification and planetary damage of the Anthropocene. Yusoff argues that there are a multiplicity of Anthropocenes that take Blackness as their foundation (Ivry, 2022). How one understands, or chooses to define, the Anthropocene is closely linked to notions of its ecosystem impacts and, hence, strategies to tackle anthropogenic damage. The ecological DoH provide a framework for naming and addressing the impacts of human-induced climate emergency, and resulting debates about what "counts" as an ecodeterminant are important; however, the politics of causation, and hence solution-making, must be the overarching consideration.

ECOLOGICAL DETERMINANTS OF HEALTH IN THE ANTHROPOCENES

Ecological DoH encompass human health and the health of the whole natural world. The Earth is itself a life-support system that is the ultimate determinant of human health and that of all other species (Hancock et al., 2015). Ecodeterminants involve impacts and assaults on Earth's natural systems, including pollution and ecotoxicity, environmental racism, resource extraction and depletion, climate and atmospheric emergency, desertification and deforestation, soil erosion, and species extinction and biodiversity loss. Although these impacts are described separately in this discussion, they are synergistic. For example, deforestation contributes significantly to greenhouse gas emissions, which then contribute to global heating and its resulting species extinction. Fossil fuel industries and the burning of fossil fuels create substantive air, water, and ground pollution, which also contributes to Earth systems damage and causes global heating and hence climate emergency.

Important Existing Models of Ecological Health

Activists and scholars, including Indigenous Peoples and people of African descent, public health practitioners, civil society organizations, and others have sounded the alarm for many decades. However, the ecological DoH are in the relative beginning of entering public consciousness about human and planet health. In 1986, the Ottawa Charter, an international agreement signed at the First International Conference on Health Promotion organized by the World Health Organization, pointed to the crucial role of a stable ecosystem and sustainable resources as fundamental conditions and resources for health (WHO, 1986). Hancock's (1985) Mandala Model of the human ecosystem rejected a positivist, reductionist, medical model of human health and explained that the health of individuals "is intimately bound up with their physical and social environments and that actions within the community and a broader culture are important determinants of health" (p. 4). The 2015 report of the international Working Group on the Ecological Determinants of Health (Hancock et al., 2015) stated, "Earth's natural systems provide key ecosystem goods and services (e.g., oxygen, water, food, waste decomposition and recycling, climate stability) that are fundamental determinants of the health of humans and other species. We call these the ecological determinants of health" (p. 11).

As discussed in Chapter 1, the Dahlgren-Whitehead Rainbow Model (Dahlgren & Whitehead, 1991) of the DoH depicted socio-economic, cultural, and environmental conditions as important health determinants. Environmental conditions included water and sanitation, and agriculture and food production. More recently, characterizations of the ecodeterminants have included food, the ecological systems that support food production, and systems that provide fuel and resources that support the processing and distribution of foodstuffs (Elton, 2021). According to Elton, in areas such as public health, nutrition, and food and food systems studies, the social DoH have historically gained prominence over the ecological DoH, despite the fact that human well-being is produced at every step in the food system, from soil, to plate, to waste.

The ecological DoH "provide the language and the theoretical concept that makes explicit how these systems—be they agroecological, organic, biodynamic, and so on—are human-health supporting (Elton, 2021, p. 15). Here, human health is framed as something that involves interspecies relationships and dependencies, inseparably connecting human well-being and non-human nature (Elton, 2021). As recently as 2023, researchers and practitioners noted the near-absence of the ecological DoH in mainstream population and public health, with some notable exceptions, such as the work of Hancock (1985), Hancock et al. (2015), and Buse et al. (2023). In the following section, recent models and frameworks related to the ecological DoH are described, highlighting their similarities and differences. The term *ecological DoH* emerged from decades of scholarship in subfields such as Planetary Health, Eco-Health, One Health (Zinsstag, 2012), and One World (Calistri et al., 2013). These terms and their descriptions, although distinct in many of their components and approaches, have similarities that encompass the overarching term ***planetary health***. Planetary health is inseparably bonded to human health (Prescott et al., 2018). It refers to

> ... the interdependent vitality of all natural and anthropogenic ecosystems; this vitality includes the biologically defined ecosystems (at micro, meso and macro scales) that favor biodiversity; it includes the more broadly defined human-constructed social, political, and economic ecosystems that favor health equity and the opportunity to strive for high-level wellness; this definition also includes the business ecosystems that influence sustainable and health-promoting local and global commerce. (p. 3)

EcoHealth

EcoHealth involves understanding how social, economic, and ecological factors impact the condition and sustainability of **ecosystems** (Mi et al., 2016). These processes are supported by transdisciplinary action research, encouraging problem solving that draws upon a broad scope of knowledge from the natural, social, and health sciences and the humanities (Zinsstag, 2012). The aim of EcoHealth is to understand "how social, economic, and ecological factors and their interactions affect ecosystem health, including the condition and sustainability of ecosystems" (Mi et al., 2016, p. 12). EcoHealth's ecosystems approach arose from the merging of ecological approaches to public health with ecosystem health from the field of environmental management (Forget & Lebel, 2001). EcoHealth involves consideration of the global atmosphere, climate emergency, stratospheric ozone depletion, transcontinental air pollution and dust clouds, and the sustainability of civilization (Butler, 2000).

In response to an emphasis on the interconnections among human health and the environment, Lisitza and Wolbring (2018) developed an EcoHealth model (Figure 4.1) that includes the social DoH (SDH), the ecological DoH (EDH), the environmental DoH (EnDH), the political DoH (PDH), and the cultural DoH (CDH). These authors also described debates about distinguishing the ecological DoH and the environmental DoH, stating that "irrespective of whether the two are distinct conceptually, it would be beneficial for the field to use

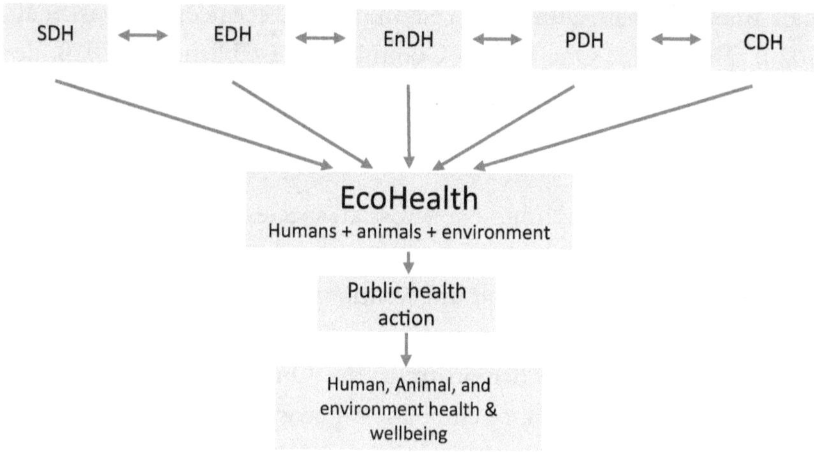

Figure 4.1: A New Analytic Framework on the Determinants of Health and EcoHealth

Source: Adapted from Lisitza & Wolbring, 2018.

consistent language to establish a more concrete way of understanding and addressing these determinants" (p. 11). Their conclusion supports the arguments in this book that the social DoH, ecological DoH, and structural DoH are theoretically and practically converging. The Eco-Health framework demonstrates this convergence, with synthesis of ecological and environmental DoH impacts on the social DoH, both of which are inseparably linked to the political DoH.

One Health

One Health is a concept that supports the recognition that the health of humans, animals, and our broader environment are interconnected (Okello, 2020). It emerged through the need for interdisciplinary responses to prevent and control zoonoses (infectious diseases that cross the animal-human species barrier), including bacteria and viruses such as COVID-19, severe acute respiratory syndrome (SARS), and Highly Pathogenic Avian Influenza (HPAI) (Okello, 2020). The One Health movement eventually included not only physicians and veterinarians but also wildlife specialists, environmentalists, anthropologists, economists, and sociologists, among others (Gibbs, 2014). One Health emphasizes the synergistic advantage of dismantling disciplinary and professional silos among human, animal, and environmental sciences (Amuasi et al., 2020). The Lancet One Health Commission, established in 2020, described three distinct but interrelated dimensions (see Figure 4.2) of One Health:

1. The shared environment across all species
2. Safe food and food systems
3. Shared medicines and interventions (Amuasi et al., 2020)

As Figure 4.2 may demonstrate, the One Health approach has been critiqued for its lack of emphasis on ecosystem health (Mi et al.,

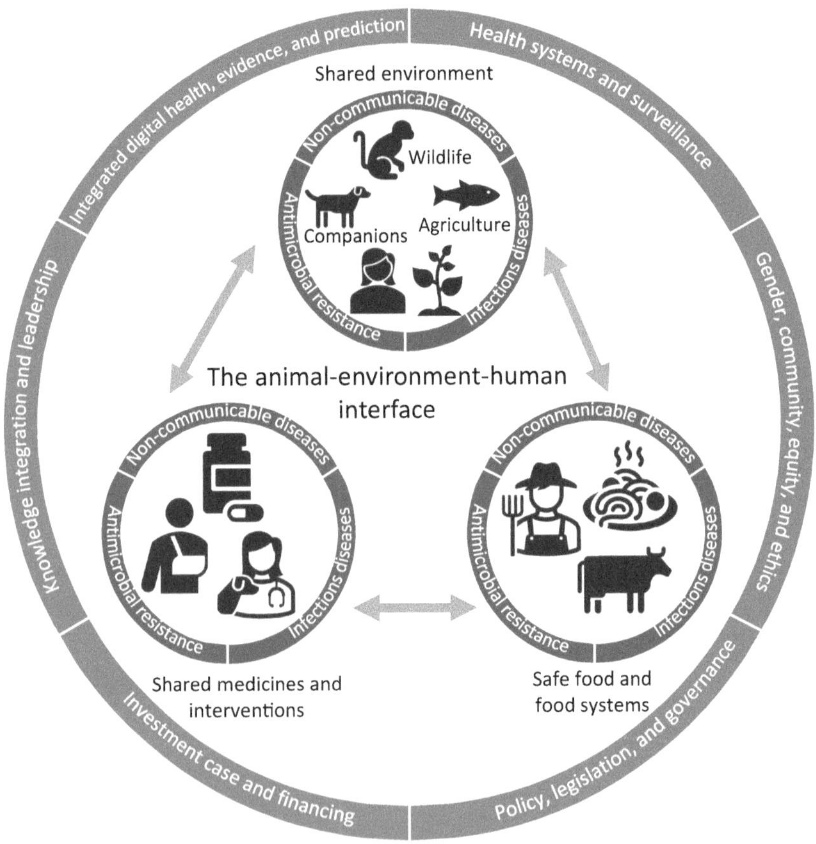

Figure 4.2: Approach of the Lancet One Health Commission

Source: Adapted from Amuasi et al., 2020.

2016). However, One Health has historically developed from a tightly defined view of zoonotic disease mitigation to an approach that can address much broader socioeconomic, environmental, human health, and livelihood challenges (Häsler et al., 2014). Both One Health and Eco-Health are evolving towards the concept of "health in socio-ecological systems, and these systems generate social and ecological determinants of human, animal, and planet health" (p. 14). Authors such as Zinsstag (2012) have described how the two concepts are converging, with the goals of exploring common ground and integrating the unique attributes of each concept. The COVID-19 crisis has intensified calls for One Health approaches, although there is neither coordinated global support nor systematic allocation of resources towards integrated, cross-sectoral policies and programs (Häsler et al., 2014; Okello, 2020). The importance of transdisciplinary research and global scientific and civil society collaboration was strongly accentuated during the COVID-19 response across the globe. The pandemic increased public awareness of the interconnectedness of humans, animals, and the environment, and it reinforced the importance of understanding these complex links—providing a wake-up call to action for improving the capacity for integrating research with public policy (Centre on Climate Change and Planetary Health, 2020).

One World–One Health

The One World approach is relatively new and for some authors it has evolved to be described as a One World–One Health approach:

> The recognitions of these relationships amongst humans, domestic animals, wildlife, ecosystem services and climate, as in the One Health concept under ecosphere and zoosphere of this One World system, are therefore being formulated. (Zeng & Li, 2021, p. 280)

The One World–One Health approach was first used in 2004 at the *One World, One Health: Building Interdisciplinary Bridges to Health in a Globalized World* workshop hosted by the Wildlife Conservation Society and Rockefeller University (Wild Conservation Society & Rockefeller University, 2004). A One World–One Health approach takes into consideration four main components: 1) effects of globalization of trade in animals and animal products and the need for a supranational approach (the geographical component, for example, trade in chickens); 2) the role of wildlife and environmental factors in the spread of infections (the ecological component, for example, avian flu); 3) the importance of integration between veterinary and human medicine into a "one medicine" strategy and the imperative to adopt a multidisciplinary approach (the human activities component); and 4) the need for a "farm to fork" approach, across the food production chain (the food-agricultural component, for example, sustainable healthy diets, food production, food consumption; food security and sovereignty; and reducing loss and waste) (Calistri et al., 2013).

Indigenous Knowledges and Environmental Health

Despite living in diverse contexts, Indigenous Peoples face common challenges within the threats of climate change (Jones, 2019). These threats are disproportionate due to many factors, including unique relationships with the natural environment and interconnectivity with the land (Ratima et al., 2019). Other central considerations are socioeconomic deprivation; a greater existing burden of disease; less access to, and quality of, health care; and political marginalization, including threats to Indigenous Peoples' rights (Ratima et al., 2019). Land defending and instilling stewardship and sustainability have flourished despite the prevailing forces of capitalism, settler colonialism, globalization, and intellectual imperialism that silences Indigenous knowledge systems (Ratima et al., 2019). Box 4.1 provides an overview of the meaning of Indigenous knowledges, quoted from the National Collaborating Centre for Indigenous Health (2022a).

Box 4.1: Indigenous Knowledges

"Indigenous knowledge, traditional ecological knowledge (TEK), traditional knowledge (TK), and Inuit knowledge or Inuit Qaujimajatuqangit are all dynamic and living concepts that denote the understanding, interdependence, and relationality between Indigenous Peoples and the lands they call home, including all Creation and beings (animate and inanimate) within that land (McGregor, 2014). [...]

Indigenous knowledges are embedded within Indigenous languages and transmitted to younger generations through community knowledge (Task Force on Aboriginal Languages and Cultures, 2005; Battiste, 2010; Tagali, 2010; Wilder et al., 2016). This includes observations about the land, plants, insects, forests, waterways, sea, sea ice, soil, weather conditions, and migratory patterns of animals (Tagalik, 2010; McGregor, 2014; Sandoval et al., 2016; Windchief & Ryan, 2018). Cosmological, medicinal, pharmacological, agricultural, and botanical knowledges, for example, are shared through direct observation and participation in them, as well as through storytelling, prayers, dance, art, protocols, teachings, and ceremonies (Neeganagwedgin, 2013; Kulnieks et al., 2016; Reo et al., 2017).

Indigenous knowledges inform ethical, social, political, legal, governance and moral practices, and are pivotal for community survival and continuity, as well as resource management and sustainability (Alexander et al., 2011; McGregor, 2012; Windchief & Ryan, 2018)."

Source: Quoted from National Collaborating Centre for Indigenous Health (NCCIH), 2022a, p. 38.

The relationships between climate change and Indigenous Peoples' health is substantial and measurable (National Collaborating Centre for Indigenous Health [NCCIH], 2022b). Although climate change impacts all Canadians' health and well-being, the distribution and health risks disproportionately impact Indigenous Peoples due to their close relationship with the land, waters, animals, plants, and natural resources, and their already-proven burden of health inequities as a result of current and historical impacts of colonial histories. Existing inequities in the social and ecological DoH are further deepened, including food and water insecurity, air quality, infrastructure, personal safety, mental well-being, land and sea-based livelihoods, and increased exposure to disease-causing organisms (NCCIH, 2022b). Indigenous knowledge systems are increasingly recognized in Canada and globally as a central foundation of informing climate change policy. "Preparing for the health impacts of climate change requires that Indigenous Peoples' rights and responsibilities over their lands, natural resources, and ways of life are respected, protected, and advanced through distinctions-based, Indigenous-led, climate change adaptation, policy, and research" (NCCIH, 2022b, pp. 1–2).

Consciousness about ecological and Earth systems, and their synergy with human health and the health of all life on Earth, has the appearance of being a relatively new phenomenon. However, Indigenous Peoples across the globe, in each of their distinctive ancestries, languages, and cultures, have acknowledged and lived for centuries within the intimate relationships of land, water and wind patterns, and sustaining life. "Indigenous Peoples possess worldviews and traditional knowledge systems that are critical to climate mitigation and adaptation, yet, paradoxically, these are devalued and marginalized and have yet to be recognized as essential foundations of public health" (Lewis et al., 2020, p. 897). The current epoch of anthropogenic climate crisis is also an epoch of intensified colonialism that presents complex challenges for Indigenous Peoples across the globe, including those in wealthier nation states (Lewis et al., 2020).

Key Ecological Determinants of Health

Knowledge about the ecological DoH includes very broad and substantive fields of knowledge, including contributions from civil society organizations as well as Indigenous and academic contributions. The following discussion highlights the main ecological DoH, emphasizing that they form complex systems that are all constantly interacting. Structural DoH, described in detail in Chapter 5, are highlighted here to underscore how structural, root causes are the drivers of threats to the ecological DoH. *Global Health Watch 6* (Bloomsbury Publishing,

2022) states that global neoliberalism is the overarching root cause of the current polycrisis, including global climate emergency. Implications for the social DoH are integrated throughout this chapter.

Pollution and Ecotoxicity

Anthropogenic activities (e.g., mining, domestic activities, dispersion of nanomaterials in personal care products, industrial effluents and air pollution, fossil fuel combustion, and pesticide use) contribute vastly to a higher pollution index across all Earth systems, polluting the global water cycle and hindering the availability of a sustainable water supply (Tijani et al., 2016). As described in Chapter 5, these anthropogenic activities are driven by structural DoH, such as political-economic DoH and the ongoing colonialism of land destruction and resource extraction and depletion. Air pollution, especially particulate matter (PM) emissions from industry, power generation, transportation, and domestic burning considerably exceed the WHO's health-based air-quality guidelines. Particulate matter is the general term used for a mixture of solid particles and liquid droplets in the air. Fine PM (2.5 microns in diameter and less) is especially known to be health damaging for living organisms, including humans. There are statistically significant associations between exposure to dangerous PM air pollution and adverse health outcomes (Jbaily et al., 2022). Exposure sources include aerosols, smoke, fumes, dust, ash, and pollen. In the United States, not only are racial and ethnic minorities (Black, Asian, Hispanic, Latinx people) and people of low socioeconomic status exposed to higher levels of dangerous fine PM air pollution than other groups, they are at a higher risk of death due to exposure (Jbaily et al., 2022).

It is estimated that hundreds of thousands of lung cancer deaths annually worldwide are attributable to PM air pollution (Turner et al., 2020). After lung cancer, female breast cancer (11.6%), prostate cancer (7.1%), and colorectal cancer (6.1%) are the next leading cancers related to air pollution (Bray et al., 2018; Turner et al., 2020). Furthermore, workers exposed to indoor air pollution, such as asbestos, polycyclic aromatic hydrocarbons (PAHs), and toxic metals are also likely to develop lung cancer (Xue et al., 2022). In a systematic review of studies investigating the associations between long-term exposure to air pollution and the risk of kidney cancer and bladder cancer, results suggested positive associations between air pollution exposure, kidney cancer incidence, and death due to bladder cancer (Sakhvidi et al., 2020). Infants and children are uniquely sensitive to air pollution, because their organs are still developing and they have higher air intake per body weight than that of adults (Brumberg et al., 2021). Air pollution impacts for children are serious, including the worsening of respiratory diseases, such as asthma, and reduced lung function development; premature birth; low birth weight; neurodevelopmental disorders; IQ loss; pediatric cancers; and increased risks for adult chronic diseases (Brumberg et al., 2021).

Major causes of air pollution also include coal-fired power plants, hydraulic fracturing (fracking), agricultural production, and forest fires, all of which cause many other forms of pollution. Fracking is a primary example of a multi-polluting process that cuts across many forms of pollution, including local and global air pollution, soil pollution, and watershed pollution (Black et al., 2021). Fracking involves the fracturing of formations of bedrock through blasting a mixture of water, chemicals, and sand into a well to break apart the rock formations and extract previously inaccessible oil and natural gas deposits. Fracking creates cracks in the deep-rock formations through which natural gas, petroleum, and brine will flow more freely (Minkow, 2017). The following combinations of activities and factors are more likely than others to result in more frequent or more severe impacts (United States Environmental Protection Agency [USEPA], 2016):

1. Depletion of water availability caused by water withdrawals for hydraulic fracturing, particularly in areas with limited or declining groundwater resources (USEPA, 2016). In British Columbia, the average frack uses between 5 million and 10 million litres of water, often requiring more than 2,000 truck trips to deliver water, which becomes contaminated after the fracking process and must be disposed of by creating toxic tailing ponds or by being injected deep underground (Minkow, 2017).
2. Contamination of large watershed areas (groundwater resources), caused by spills during the management of hydraulic

fracturing fluids and chemicals that result in large volumes or high concentrations of chemicals reaching groundwater resources; injection of hydraulic fracturing fluids into wells with inadequate mechanical integrity, allowing gases or liquids to move to groundwater resources; disposal or storage of hydraulic fracturing waste water in unlined pits, resulting in contamination of groundwater resources; injection of hydraulic fracturing fluids directly into groundwater resources; and disposal or storage of hydraulic fracturing waste water in unlined pits, resulting in contamination of groundwater resources (USEPA, 2016).

3. Discharge of inadequately treated hydraulic fracturing wastewater to surface water (USEPA, 2016).

Fracking raises significant social and ecological justice concerns related to the rights of Indigenous Peoples, public health, air and water contamination, groundwater depletion, greenhouse gas emissions, and the triggering of seismic activity (Behn, 2023):

> Fracking projects have been initiated on the traditional territories of Indigenous Peoples in New Brunswick, British Columbia and in other jurisdictions often without their free, prior and informed consent as required by the UN Declaration on the Rights of Indigenous Peoples and Section 35 of the Canadian Constitution. In considering the economic, social and environmental costs, some jurisdictions in Canada, including Quebec, Nova Scotia, and New Brunswick have instituted bans or moratoria on fracking. (para. 2)

The human health impacts of fracking are serious and ongoing. Denziel et al. (2020) conducted a scoping review of studies up to August 15, 2019, focusing on health outcomes related to fracking. They found 29 epidemiological studies of community exposure to fracking. Twenty-five of the 29 studies reported at least one statistically significant association between fracking exposure and an adverse health outcome. Adverse birth outcomes were most commonly studied, particularly preterm deliveries, low birth weight, and birth defects.

Soil pollution research has indicated that heavy metals are the main pollutants in European soils and groundwater (Panagos et al., 2013). Because heavy metals are not degradable, bioaccumulation (gradual accumulation of substances in an organism) occurs throughout all levels of the food chain, which is particularly important for humans as they are positioned at the top of their food chain, causing different diseases and poisonings across the lifecourse (Vareda et al., 2019; WHO, 2017). All of these ecological DoH heavily impact the social DoH, compounding everyday stresses, struggle, and deprivation. Susceptibility to accumulation of multiple non-communicable diseases, such as the ones described above, is rooted in social, economic, and cultural contexts, with significant inequities in the burden of disease, disease patterns and outcomes, and determinants of multimorbidity (Craig et al., 2021). Multimorbidity occurs when non-communicable diseases are synergistic with poverty-created or colonialism-created health problems, such as heart disease, diabetes, and depression (Craig et al., 2021).

In Chapter 1, ecotoxicity was introduced with the example of endocrine-disrupting chemicals (EDCs), describing how ecotoxicology is the science of studying how toxic substances are dispersed and taken up in Earth systems. EDCs, found in food, industrial byproducts, plastics and plasticizers, and consumer products, to name a few, are ubiquitous in aquatic and terrestrial environments and they interfere with hormone biosynthesis and metabolism (Vareda et al., 2019). The result is a deviation from normal control over human, animal, and aquatic species reproduction across the globe (Diamanti-Kandarakis et al., 2009). EDCs are also widely found in vertebrates, where physiological impacts include abnormalities in growth and reproductive development. Aquatic vertebrates, such as fish, are among the first organisms to be affected by waterborne EDCs, an attribute that has justified their widespread use as a sentinel species—a first alarm bell that predicts subsequent wide-spread ecotoxicity across human and animal species (Celino-Brady et al., 2021). Since 1950, studies have demonstrated that persistent organic EDC pollutants, such as polychlorinated biphenyls (PCBs), flame retardants, dioxins, and pesticides interfere with invertebrate, fish, amphibian, reptile, mammal, and human reproduction (Marlatt et al., 2022). Authors have also discussed the relationships among environmental toxicity, racial inequity, and reproductive justice, and their connection to capitalism (Grossman & Dennings, 2020), with market capitalist systems that are predicated on models of infinite industrial and financial growth. These negative reproductive impacts expose the connections between fossil fuel extraction, plastic products, industrial agriculture, and climate change (Grossman & Dennings, 2020).

The ecotoxicity of microplastics is a massive Earth systems threat. Microplastics are small plastic pieces (1 micron to 5 millimeters in diameter) that are water-soluble (Brown et al., 2023). Vast global microplastic proliferation is related to approximately 360 million tons of plastic that is produced every year (Thacharodi et al., 2024). Single use plastic accounts for approximately 40 percent of all production (Geddie et al., 2022). Microplastics, a result of the degradation of plastic products, are globally ubiquitous in the water columns and sediments of lakes and rivers and the number and mass of microplastic particles in rivers can exceed those of living organisms, such as zooplankton and fish larvae (D'Avignon et al., 2022).

Concentrations of microplastics in freshwater reach the same magnitude as in the world's most contaminated marine sediments and they act as vectors or carriers of ecotoxic substances to invertebrates, fishes, amphibians and reptiles, and waterfowl (D'Avignon et al., 2022). Microplastics have also been found throughout human tissues, such as lungs, veins, placentas, and breast milk (D'Avignon et al., 2022) and in freshly fallen snow in Antarctica (Aves et al., 2022). Microplastic pollution is seen as a worldwide problem that has a detrimental impact on every aspect of the freshwater environment, acting as carriers for various toxic components, such as additives and other hazardous substances from industrial and urbanized areas (Thacharodi et al., 2024). Global plastic production, an industry valued at US $522.6 billion, increased from 2 million tons in 1950 to 348 million tons in 2017, and it is expected to double by 2040 (Geddie et al., 2022).

> The problem of plastic encapsulates everything that is wrong with whatever international order exists today. We miscalculate its balance

> sheet of utility because we don't account properly for harms that cannot be easily measured in money. Decisions that look cheap on the surface look a lot different if we used a longer time horizon or stopped assuming that the planet has an infinite capacity to absorb human excess. Regions that are the most responsible for causing the problem are working hard to reallocate its consequences to other parts of the world. (Nyabola, 2023, para. 4)

A global explosion of disposable plastic, which is a product of megacorporation oil and gas extraction and profits, is increasing carbon emissions, damaging the world's oceans, harming wildlife, and contaminating the food chain (Geddie et al., 2022). Plastics are mainly manufactured in China, and the United States and Europe are the biggest global plastic consumers. Until recently, most plastic waste was sold to countries in Asia, allegedly to be recycled (Nyabola, 2023). However, in 2017, China banned plastic waste imports from Europe because they were rarely sorted properly and most of what could not be used ended up in China's rivers and landfills (Nyabola, 2023). For years, countries such as Madagascar and Kenya became more attractive places to offload waste material, such as plastics, because poor people physically sort through the waste instead of machines, which are less able to distinguish different types of plastic (Nyabola, 2023). However, the continent of Africa now leads the world in plastics bans, and in Kenya, a plastic bag ban remains in place and is widely seen as a success (Lerner, 2020). Since the plastics ban bill's passage in 2017, plastic bags that had previously blown around in the streets, clogged streams, and hung from trees have largely disappeared (Lerner, 2020).

The plastic crisis is built into the economic model of capitalism because waste is an inevitable consequence of a system that values the profits of consumption, while refusing to acknowledge massive amounts of waste that are the inevitable result (Lerner, 2020). This model reinforces to us that without consumption, there is no economic growth, and that consumption symbolizes progress. Fixing the proliferation of global plastic requires a fundamental shift in the way we live our lives. Despite widely believed claims of comprehensive plastic recycling programs, only 7 percent of globally produced plastics are recycled and no environmental field survey that has searched for microplastics has failed to detect their presence (D'Avignon et al., 2022). The current situation is palliative and is only a half-finished version of recycling that distorts the size and scale of the problem while diverting people's attention with individual action while industrial disasters grow.

The recycling system inspires people to take personal responsibility, but it misleads people about the value of those actions—there is no doubt that individual use is a part of the problem (Lerner, 2020); however, root causes are the massive oil and gas industry profits of plastic production. Without legislation and systematic accountability, it is impossible to tackle the plastics crisis. Initially, plastics production industries (e.g., Exxon, Chevron, Dow, DuPont) informed the public that plastics could be readily accommodated by landfills or burned in garbage incinerators; however, in the 1980s, as municipalities began considering bans on grocery bags and other plastic products, the industry began promoting a new solution—recycling (Noor, 2024)—and now spends tens of billions of dollars to foster the illusion that plastic can be recycled, though most of it cannot (Sullivan, 2020). Recycling itself has been found to release substantive microplastics into the surrounding environment. A study investigating microplastic pollution from a mixed-plastics recycling facility in the United Kingdom found that between 59 and 1184 tons of microplastics were potentially discharged annually from the facility (Brown et al., 2023). The global plastics crisis is an excellent case example of the results of global neoliberal capitalism (described further in Chapter 5).

Other ecotoxins, such as firefighting foams, cosmetics, and food packaging that contains cancer-causing "forever chemicals" (per- and polyfluorinated alkyl substances [PFAS]), are gaining increasing policy attention to achieve the slowing and halting of their manufacture (The Canadian Press, 2023). Examples include more than 4,700 different combinations of synthetic chemicals used in dozens of products that have become pervasive across the entire environment, including in the bloodstreams of people and animals. In Canada, these chemicals have the potential to be limited, or outright banned, following a 2023 federal government risk assessment of the products (The Canadian

Press, 2023). Multiple studies have found that forever chemicals pose health risks to humans and wildlife, including higher risks of certain types of cancers (Nelson & Kaminsky, 2021) and thyroid damage (Vertefeuille, 2022).

Discouragingly, despite copious studies about the pervasive and significant harms of PFAS (Panieri et al., 2022), Environment Canada limited its willingness to act by stating that it is considering regulating the use of products containing PFAS, but will wait until a 60-day comment period is over on the draft assessment before considering action (The Canadian Press, 2023). As of 2021, the Government of Canada (2021) officially cited 163 substances on its toxic substances list and also listed 46 petroleum and refinery gases, for a total of 209 substances. On April 23, 2021, Canada's Administrator in Council ordered that "plastic manufactured items" immediately be added to the list as a toxic substance (Gordner et al., 2021). The order arose from growing concerns about the amount of plastic that is not recycled, noting that of the estimated 3,268 kilotons of plastic generated in Canada in 2016, only 305 kilotons, or 9 percent, was recycled.

Environmental Racism

Environmental racism is a core substrate of the Anthropocenes, where, as Yusoff (2018) explains, Black and Brown bodies have been commodified all along the historical pathways of colonial (white) and capitalist wealth accumulation. Numerous environmental justice studies have confirmed the relationships among population characteristics, such as low-income or racialized status, and the location of environmental health hazards (Kershaw et al., 2013). The following examples of environmental racism demonstrate some of the pathways of policy-created environmental harm perpetrated on racialized communities.

The Sydney Tar Ponds in Mi'kmaq territory hunting and fishing grounds on Cape Breton Island, Nova Scotia, sparked some of the first public concerns about environmental injustice in Canada. For 87 years (1901–1988), Sydney Steel Corporation's steel mill operated in the area and there were no legislated pollution controls in place. Over a million tons of particulate matter and several thousand tons of coal tar were released into the nearby estuary, including chemicals known to cause cancer (Furimsky, 2002). In 1999, five years before site rehabilitation efforts, Sydney area residents experienced a local cancer rate 45 percent higher than the Nova Scotia average and the highest rate in Canada at the time (Nickerson, 1999). Concerns were officially raised by community members in 1980; however, it took almost 35 years for the Nova Scotia government to commit $400 million over the next 10 years (2004–2014) to rehabilitate the Sydney Tar Ponds site to reduce the ecological and human health risks to the environment (Walker & MacAskill, 2014).

The Alberta Tar Sands, further discussed in Chapter 6, is the largest industrial project on the Earth (Leahy, 2019) and is referred to as "a slow industrial genocide" of Indigenous Peoples in Treaty 8 Territory (Huseman & Short, 2012). One of the three largest tar sands in Alberta is the Athabaska Tar Sands deposit, the largest known reservoir of crude bitumen in the world (McLachlan, 2014a). The Athabasca Chipewyan First Nation and the Mikisew Cree First Nation, in collaboration with researchers from the University of Manitoba, released a 2014 report, *Environmental and Human Health Implications of the Athabasca Oil Sands for the Mikisew Cree First Nation and Athabasca Chipewyan First Nation in Northern Alberta* (McLachlan, 2014a). In his comments after the release of the report, Manitoba First Nations Mikisew Cree Chief Steve Courtoreille stated, "The Joint Oil Sands Monitoring Program has released data about the increases in these contaminants, but fails to address and monitor impacts to First Nations traditional foods. We are greatly alarmed and demand further research and studies are done to expand on the findings of this report" (Linnitt, 2014).

Results from this research demonstrated high concentrations of carcinogenic PAHs (polycyclic aromatic hydrocarbons), and the heavy metals arsenic, mercury, cadmium, and selenium in kidney and liver samples from moose, ducks, muskrats, and beavers harvested by community members (McLaghlan, 2014). These contaminants are a result of bitumen oil extraction from oil sands (McLaghlan, 2014). According to the report, contaminants in wildlife, as well as limited access due to declining water levels, have nearly eliminated the consumption of some traditional foods (McLaghlan, 2014). Fish caught in Lake Athabasca and the Athabasca River are no longer trusted, while muskrat populations have seriously declined. Compounding the impacts of environmental racism, existing health care services lack the capacity to address related declines in Indigenous health (McLaughlin, 2014), especially from a cultural safety perspective. The result is embodied racism, where more recent findings reflect this germinal 2014 study. Although these health impacts are important to expose, there is an overarching dearth of Indigenous-led perspectives and research on the tar sands (Westman & Joly, 2019). There is also a significant lack of social science integration about the health, social, and cultural impacts on Indigenous Peoples and communities who "face worrying health risks and evident pollution as they lose access to special places and preferred sources of food and water, entailing loss of cultural, spiritual, and familial connections" (Westman & Joly, 2019, p. 233).

Cancer Alley is an area in the United States along the Mississippi River from Baton Rouge to New Orleans, Louisiana, housing over 150 petrochemical plants and refineries that mainly produce plastic, the most common petrochemical product. Louisiana has one of the largest concentrations of oil and natural gas in the Western Hemisphere, and hence the most petrochemical facilities (Castellón, 2021). There are many reasons, including the Jim Crow Laws, why Cancer Alley exists and why communities of colour are disproportionately affected by pollution when compared with white communities (Castellón, 2021). "Jim Crow" was a derisive slang term for a Black man. In place until the 1960s, Jim Crow laws, based on the ideology of **white supremacy**, were state and local laws introduced in the Southern United States in the late 19th and early 20th centuries, establishing different rules for Black people and white people and enforcing racial segregation (Castellón, 2021; Teach Democracy, n.d.). White supremacy refers to the myriad conditions, practices, and ideologies that underscore the hegemony of whiteness and white political, social, cultural, and economic domination, where the interests and perceptions of white people are continually placed centre stage and assumed to be "normal" (Alang et al., 2021).

The Jim Crow laws set the legal and policy-based stage for racist zoning laws and siting processes and the US Environmental Protection

Agency's (USEPA) unequal enforcement of federal environmental laws based on the race of the population impacted (Mizutani, 2018). In her doctoral dissertation entitled *The "Disposable Others": Settler colonial processes of industrial pollution in Cancer Alley, Louisiana, 1964–2023*, Martin (2023) researched ongoing colonialist processes and policies, such as the EPA refusing to uphold its own recommendations regarding carcinogen-causing chemicals such as chloroprene, found in high concentrations in Cancer Alley. Nationally, Black people die of cancer at an average rate of 174 per 100,000 people, while in Louisiana it is up to 219 per 100,000 people (National Cancer Institute, 2021).

Chemical Valley is an area near Sarnia, Canada, that is polluted by over 60 industrial facilities, such as oil refineries, power-generating stations, and landfills. The Aamjiwnaang First Nation near Sarnia have had ongoing historical concerns about Chemical Valley air pollution. Approximately 40 percent of Canada's chemical industry is clustered in this region, which has become one of the most polluted hotspots in Canada (MacDonald & Rang, 2007; Riahi & McSorley, 2013). Researchers have found suspected respiratory toxicants, known reproductive and developmental toxicants, and known endocrine-disrupting chemicals, all considered toxic under Canada's Environmental Protection Act (MacDonald & Rang, 2007). A higher statistical risk of cancer, including rare cancers, has been found to exist among the Aamjiwnaang First Nation (Graf, 2020). The Chemical Valley crisis continues to be highlighted locally and nationally in efforts to mitigate and halt its human and planet impacts. The Chemical Valley Project is an award-winning blend of documentary theatre, innovative projection design, charismatic script writing, and playful solo-performances that engage and implicate audiences in difficult conversations about Canadian environmental policy, Treaty Rights, and Indigenous relations, and the current nature of Canadian identity and values (Wong & Howman, n.d.).

Africville was an African Nova Scotian community that originated when Black slaves escaped the United States. Zarah Tootonsab (2021) studied environmental racism in selected sites across Canada, including Africville, interviewing numerous people: "In my interview with Afro-Métis singer/songwriter, Shelley Hamilton, she describes Africville based on her Africville lineage in Africville, Nova Scotia, as a community of [B]lack slaves [who] settled in Canada when they escaped from the south in the 1820s and 1850s during the Underground Railroad" (p. 30). The City of Halifax initiated an "urban renewal" campaign in 1947 that eventually led to the destruction of Africville in 1965 because it was deemed unfit for habitation. Residents were allotted meagre relocation sums, and their community was torn down and completely destroyed, an act now widely recognized as racist dislocation (Dotto, 2021). Residents were subjected to a number of environmental hazards, including a fertilizer plant, a slaughterhouse, a tar factory, a stone and coal crushing plant, a cotton factory, a prison, two infectious disease hospitals, and three systems of railway tracks. In the 1950s, the city built an open-pit dump in Africville, which many considered to be a health menace (Nelson, 2000). Before and during the demolition of Africville property, raw sewage was discharged into the basin for roughly two centuries (Loo, 2010). One resident, 24-year-old Eddie Carvery, returned to the site of Africville in 1970 and pitched a tent in protest. Demanding a public inquiry and individual compensation for community residents, he then actively occupied the site on and off for over five decades, one of the longest civil rights protests in Canada (Bernard, 2021; Chiu, 2019). The province officially apologized in 2010, but they have not yet engaged in reparations and compensation (Bernard, 2021; Chiu, 2019). There is now a small memorial park in Africville, which still sits on one of the most expensive real estate sites in the city of Halifax. In her book *A Love Letter to Africville*, Amanda Carvery-Taylor (2021) described how Africville is so much more than just the pain. She deepened the historical narrative by emphasizing the beautiful and positive aspects of Africville with captivating stories and stunning photography that express the love, importance, and flourishing culture of Africville (Dotto, 2021).

Resource Extraction and Depletion

Resource extraction and depletion (e.g., water, oil, natural gas, fossil fuels, phosphorus, rare Earth elements) is a significant ecological DoH. Natural resource commodification has caused vast natural resource depletion, along with irreversible changes in Earth's ecosystems.

Extraction of resources such as natural gas and petroleum through fracking, described earlier in the chapter, causes significant and widespread Earth system damage. Evidence demonstrates that ecosystems, and their contributions to sustaining life on Earth, are in continuous decline, with 70 percent loss of global natural wetlands over the last century, resulting in profound impacts on economic development and social and environmental stability (UN, 2023).

Global, transnational corporations with enormous profit margins are largely responsible for massive, globe-wide extraction and depletion. As described in Chapter 6, oil extraction and processing in Canada has globe-wide impacts. As of 2023, the top five corporations in terms of market capitalization (total value of a publicly traded company's outstanding common shares owned by stockholders in US dollars) are: Saudi Aramco Base Oil Company ($1.8 trillion), Exxon Mobil Corporation ($455 billion), Chevron Corporation ($341 billion), Royal Dutch Shell plc ($201 billion), and NextEra Energy, Inc. ($166.23 billion) (Saleem, 2023). As Box 4.2 demonstrates, in the face of globe-wide evidence of the impacts of resource extraction and depletion, there is significant, and at times successful, pushback, such as "naming and shaming" fossil fuel corporations.

Box 4.2: Holding Fossil Fuel Corporations Accountable: "Naming and Shaming"

Fossil fuel corporations have come under significantly increased scrutiny, including how they access capital, what sorts of subsidies they get from the government, and the ecological damage their activities pose to local communities. McGuire et al. (2022) emphasize the importance of "naming and shaming" fossil fuel firms, along with their supply infrastructures, such as banks, and cloud computing companies such as Amazon—this process is an integral part of the advocacy tool kit of climate groups (McGuire et al., 2022).

Exxon Valdez: The 1989 Exxon Valdez disaster undermined the offshore industry's claim about their state-of-the-art safe transportation technologies. In addition to lawsuits seeking financial damages from Exxon, this

(continued)

incident motivated the enactment of the Oil Pollution Act of 1990 (McGuire et al., 2022). The Act enforced removal of spilled oil and assigned liability for the cost of cleanup and damage. A responsible party under the Oil Pollution Act is one who is found accountable for the discharge or substantial threat of discharge of oil from a vessel or facility into navigable waters (USEPA, 2023). Although this is an effective start, there is no systematic analysis of the incidence and rate of actual removals of spilled oil.

Deepwater Horizon: On April 20, 2010, BP's Gulf of Mexico Deepwater Horizon offshore oil rig exploded and sank, causing 11 deaths and the largest marine oil spill in US history. McGuire et al. (2022) examined how this accident affected the corporate reputation and the stock market return of Deepwater's operating firm, BP (formerly, British Petroleum), and found no statistically significant decline in their stock market returns either in the mid-term (1–2 years) or the long term (2–7 years) and no evidence of reputational damage.

Three Mile Island and Fukushima: Industrial nuclear accidents can inflict lasting reputational and financial damage on firms. The 1979 Three Mile Island accident brought a halt to the construction of new nuclear plants in the United States. In the wake of the 2011 Fukushima accident in Japan, most nations using nuclear power programs as their main energy source reexamined their national energy and electricity plans and policies (Jang & Park, 2020).

Thus, by strategically leveraging both the reputational and financial harms of offshore accidents, the climate movement can exert additional pressure on fossil fuel firms to forgo offshore oil drilling and production, as well as pressure financial institutions not to fund such activities.

Source: McGuire et al., 2022.

Globally, over two billion people (26% of the global population) live in countries experiencing high climate emergency stress, including an absence of safe drinking water. Access to water and improved water and wastewater management in human settlements is one of the United Nations' Sustainable Development Goals (Carlsen & Bruggemann, 2022), and water resources are embedded in all forms of development—for example, food security, health promotion, and poverty reduction; sustaining economic growth in agriculture, industry, and energy generation; and in maintaining healthy ecosystems (UN, 2023). Lack of access to safely managed sanitation is experienced by 3.6 billion (46% of the population) people. It is estimated that by 2040, one in four of the world's children under 18 years of age (600 million) will be living in areas of extremely high water stress (United Nations Educational, Scientific and Cultural Organization [UNESCO], 2023) and 700 million people worldwide could be displaced by intense water scarcity by 2030 (United Nations Environmental Programme [UNEP], 2015). UNEP has described innovative technological and policy instruments and opportunities to accelerate decoupling of economic growth from water consumption (halting water privatization), a process that the panel states is crucial to water sustainability across the planet.

Global water availability and access is also highly gendered—of the almost three-quarters of households around the globe without access to drinking water on the premises, women and girls have the primary responsibility for collecting water. In some countries, the proportion is more than 90 percent (UNICEF, 2011). The United Nations 2030 agenda for sustainable development reported that women and girls are disproportionately affected by inadequate access to water, sanitation, and hygiene services: 1 billion women lack access to safely managed drinking water, 1.7 billion lack access to safely managed sanitation, and, every year, over 800,000 women lose their lives due to insufficient access to safe water (UN, 2023). As of 2015, over 380 million women live in some of the most water-stressed countries on the globe. Gender inequalities limit their access to land and water resources, thereby increasing their vulnerability to the global water crisis (UN, 2023).

According to the UN (2018), global water governance structures are weak and fragmented, with inadequate political, institutional, and administrative policies and practices in many countries, particularly those where pressures on water resources are greatest. Earth's current water governance model is privatization (Warner, 2021). de Feyter (2005) defines **economic globalization** as the breaking down of states' borders to allow the free flow of finance, trade, production, and labour.

He argues that human rights and social justice must be considered in the age of the market, where existing state human rights obligations must be rethought because state action is enhanced, or fettered, by the global market and multinational economic institutions. In the case of water, for example, a state may jeopardize citizens' access to water by privatizing its water supply through agreements with a transnational water company, despite being bound by human rights covenants and treaties to provide a safe supply of water (de Feyter, 2005). These institutions include General Agreement on Tariffs and Trade (GATT) and its successor, the World Trade Organization (WTO); the International Monetary Fund (IMF); the World Bank; and transnational companies such as those that have an increasing control over global water supplies. For example, in 1993, during the year of its inception, the World Bank adopted the Water Resources Management policy paper, which noted the unwillingness of poor countries to pay for their water services and stated that water should be treated as an economic commodity, with an emphasis on efficiency, financial discipline, and full-cost recovery (Barlow, 2007).

The depletion of rare Earth elements (rarely found in nature) is also a significant consequence of unconstrained resource extraction by multinational mega-corporations. Rare Earth elements, typically soft, silvery metals with similar characteristics, are known as critical metals due to their high economic importance across the globe, combined with a high risk of supply disruption (Pell et al., 2019). These elements are commonly used in the manufacturing of smart phones, digital cameras, fluorescent and light-emitting-diode (LED) lights, computer monitors, and flat screen televisions. A crucial aspect of rare Earth element depletion is the interconnected process of e-waste recycling and worker safety. Although the rare Earth elements recycling industry is expected to increase worldwide in high tech industries, regulations for worker safety have yet to be established (Shin et al., 2019). Recycling processes involve worker exposure to hazardous substances, such as rare Earth elements containing dust, metals, and chemicals, along with the risk of ignition and explosion. Skin irritation and toxicities for respiratory, hepatic (liver), nervous, and cardiovascular systems have also been found (Shin et al., 2019). Exposure to polybrominated diphenyl ethers (PBDEs), which are a group of chemical fire retardants commonly associated with the disposal of electronic waste, is likely to cause thyroid problems, neurodevelopmental deficits, and cancer (Campbell, 2022). Health-damaging impacts of massive resource extraction are disproportionately distributed across the globe. For example, people in mainland China and the Global South suffer the brunt of emissions of toxic chemicals from consumer goods used in more-developed countries—core regions in Europe, North America, and parts of Asia continue to offload PBDE emissions to countries in the Global South (Campbell, 2022).

Climate and Atmospheric Emergency

Global heating is an emergency indicator of global changes in the ecological DoH. The recently published sixth assessment of the Intergovernmental Panel on Climate Change asserts that anthropogenic greenhouse gas emissions are responsible for an increase in yearly average temperatures across the world, estimated at 1.2°C over pre-industrial temperature levels; without mitigation, global temperatures are predicted to increase by 1.5°C by 2030 (IPCC, 2021). However, there is clear evidence that this process is accelerating. In fact, as of November 2023, data demonstrated that globally, the temperature was already 1.43°C above the pre-industrial average (Niranjan, 2023). Observable planetary changes due to global heating include glaciers melting, water levels rising, prolonged heat waves, floods, and droughts, all of which have accelerated from 2020–2022. For example, there are uncontrolled wild fires on the west coast of North America and in parts of Australia and southern Europe, and unprecedented flooding in China and central Europe (Arpin et al., 2021).

Greenhouse gas emission is a primary cause of global heating. In the latest World Meteorological Organization (WMO, 2023) report, researchers stated that atmospheric levels of the three main greenhouse gases—carbon dioxide (CO2), methane, and nitrous oxide all reached new record highs in 2021 and were a main contributor to global heating. Agriculture made up about 11 percent of greenhouse gas emissions, and deforestation was responsible for approximately 25 percent. Transportation accounts for nearly one-quarter of all energy-related emissions, with the process of generating electricity and heat by burning fossil fuels contributing significantly to global greenhouse gas emissions (WMO, 2023). Another significant impact of global heating is rising sea levels, with a persistent acceleration in global mean sea level since the 1960s. Approximately 76 percent of this acceleration was associated with sea-level changes in the Indo-Pacific and South Atlantic (Dangendorf et al., 2019).

Globally, there were 74 excess deaths per 100,000 people—over five million deaths were associated with non-optimal temperatures per year and cold-related deaths occurred over 10 times more than heat-related deaths (Zhao et al., 2021). Heat and cold-related threats are forms of structural violence intertwined with housing, heat energy poverty, and related social DoH (Hamstead, 2023). Heat islands and food deserts are measurable, visible evidence of the ruling relations of global capitalism and its inequitable distribution across ecological DoH (McGibbon, in press). Urban heat islands are characterized by urban canyons (streets flanked by tall buildings on both sides), increased impervious land cover (pavement and the like), and reduced sky visibility (Equere et al., 2020). Areas occupied by people of low socioeconomic status or minority groups have been consistently found to disproportionately experience extreme heat and corresponding impacts on health and quality of life (Hong et al., 2019; Saverino et al., 2021). From 2004 to 2018, there were 10,527 deaths related to heat islands in the United States (702/year) (USEPA, 2023). Worldwide, 356,000 deaths were linked to extreme heat in 2019 (The Lancet, 2021). An association has also been found between geographies of extreme heat and historical marginalization and racialization in demographic, socioeconomic, and land-use factors, where historical policies and municipal planning decisions solidified segregation and ghettoization as precursors to current geospatial inequities (Saverino et al., 2021).

Food deserts, food swamps, and underlying food apartheid—all pivotal spatial social DoH—are rooted in strangulation of material, cultural, social, and spatial asset flows. Food deserts occur in low-income census tracts where a large percentage of people have low or no access to a grocery store or a healthy and affordable retail food outlet (Fitzpatrick et al., 2019). The term *food swamps* refers to low-income urban communities that have an excess of fast-food restaurants and convenience stores that sell unhealthy food, in the near absence of healthy food access options (Yang et al., 2020). In a 2020 review of food insecurity literature, the two major causes of food insecurity in advanced capitalist nations were found to be economic inequality and neoliberalism: "throughout the international capitalist economy, food is a commodity first, and something to eat, relieve hunger, and provide nourishment second" (Long et al., 2020, p. 7).

Land zoning by-law policymakers have supported or perhaps "looked the other way" to create urban landscapes where Big Box food corporations have eliminated food-access in large swaths of urban spaces. Although food access is a central problem, a large US study with people living in food deserts found that the core or root concern for people living in food deserts is not so much what they eat but where they live: "They weren't asking for help to improve what they ate, they were asking for help to improve where they lived… to be an equal member of American society is to have equal ability to shop at the same venues and for the same goods as everyone else" (Kolb, 2021, p. 2). The term *food apartheid*, first coined by Karen Washington, is increasingly being used to describe spatial inequities in food access because it analyzes the root causes of unequal and unjust food systems on the basis of race, class, and geography (Robeson, 2019).

In 2019, the Lancet Commission on Climate Change determined that climate change is the biggest global health threat of the 21st century. Health impacts occur via direct exposures (e.g., heat waves, extreme weather events) and also by significantly impacting basic social DoH, such as food and housing insecurity. Populations most under threat for adverse climate change impacts include the elderly, children, individuals with underlying health conditions, and populations in low- and middle-income countries (Watts et al., 2019). Across the globe, underlying chronic health conditions are already most prominent for marginalized and racialized communities (Etowa & McGibbon, 2021).

Research has demonstrated that there is a serious and disproportionate distribution of climate emergency impacts, including within country inequality, between country inequality, geographic inequality, and intergenerational inequality (Arpin et al., 2021).

As described in Chapter 1 and Chapter 3, hierarchies related to the isms substantively impact access to resources and various forms of capital—a major determinant of equitable distribution of socioeconomic opportunities for individuals and population groups. As a direct extension, these opportunities in turn determine access to socioeconomic opportunities that are critical to support coping with, and recovering from, climate change impacts (Abimbola et al., 2021). Atmospheric changes lead to stratospheric ozone layer depletion, which causes increasing UV radiation and hence skin cancer. In a systematic review of socioeconomic status (SES) and melanoma (skin cancer) incidence in Canada, researchers found that people with a lower SES and those living within certain health care regions had increased risks of advanced melanoma at diagnosis, when compared to people with high SES (Li et al., 2021). The review also highlighted the potential for inequities in access to care across SES, even within countries that have a universal health care system. Financial resources to buy sunscreen and living in areas with shade and green space are crucial in decreasing skin cancers; however, these benefits are also known to be distributed along social class and racialized lines (Rigolon et al., 2021).

In a meta-review, Arpin et al. (2021) examined 520 articles to assess the current state of knowledge on the impact of climate change and its consequences on child health inequalities. Figure 4.3 explains findings from this study. Researchers found that explanatory mechanisms (determinants) of the production of child inequalities related to climate change included 1) inequities in financial and social resources that determine decreased access to protective factors within countries; 2) inadequate sanitation and infrastructure and weak economies resulting from inadequate political leadership determine inequalities within countries; 3) a double burden of high exposure to extreme weather events and low mitigation capacity determines inequalities between countries; and 4) direct effects compound already existing inequalities

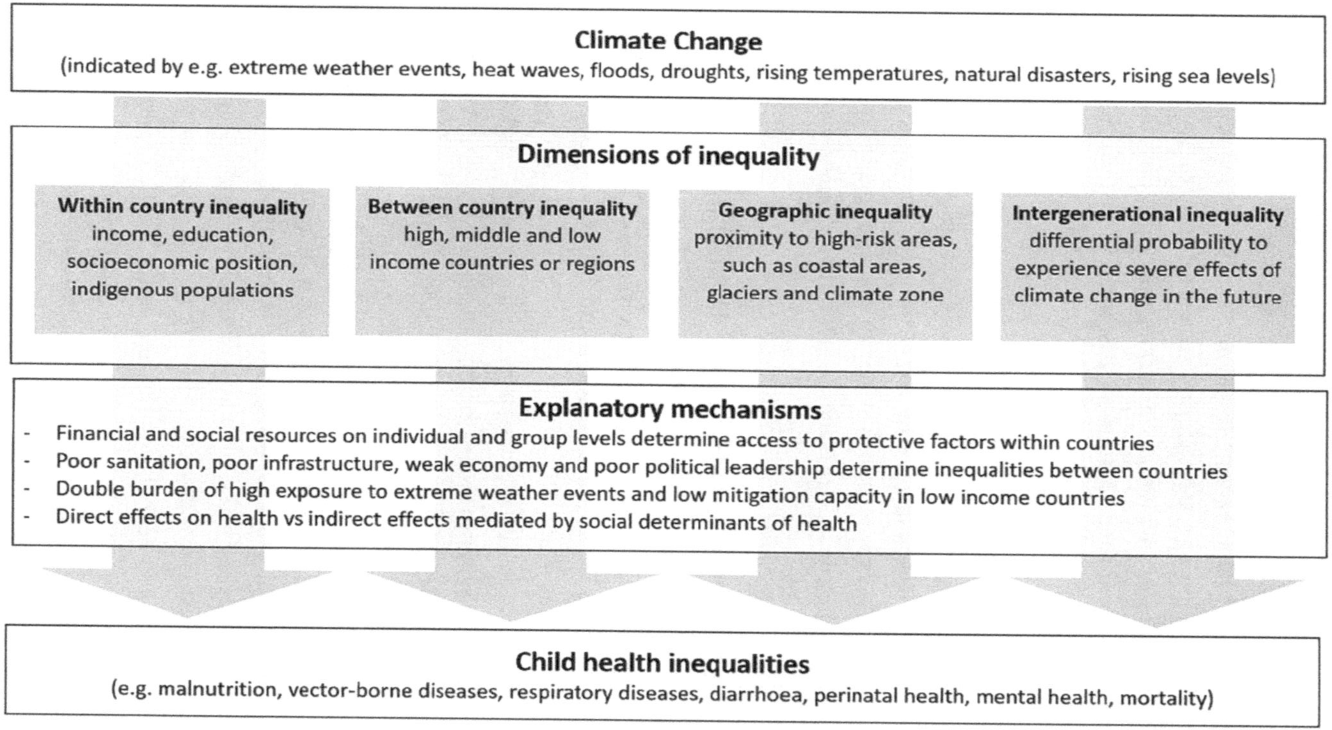

Figure 4.3: Relationship between Climate Change and Child Health Inequalities.

Source: Arpin et al., 2021.

in the social DoH. The authors pointed to the fact that health inequities are mediated or deepened by already-existing inequities in the social DoH (Arpin et al., 2021). There is also substantive evidence that differential impacts of global heating fall along income, racial, and gender lines, as well as having a greatly disproportionate impact on low-income countries. Root causes include colonization, genocide, and the racism and slavery that paved the way towards historical industrialization and massive land-use changes (Abimbola et al., 2021; Yusoff, 2018).

> Such long-standing hierarchies between White/BIPoC, men/women, and culture/nature, which have been institutionalized globally since the colonial era, also explain why BIPoC women and non-binary people continue to experience heightened vulnerability generally, and in relation to the climate crisis more specifically. (Abimbola et al., 2021, pp. 6–7)

Desertification, Deforestation, and Acidification

Interlinked and central ecological DoH include desertification, deforestation, and acidification. These DoH each involve substantive fields of knowledge. Introductory explanations and important examples are provided for all three areas.

Desertification is land degradation in arid, semi-arid, and dry subhumid areas resulting from many factors, including climatic variations and human activities (Mirzabaev et al., 2019; United Nations [UN], 1994). Drylands currently cover about 46.2 percent of the global land area, and desertification hotspots (areas with decline in vegetation productivity) affected about 500 million people in 2015, largely in South and East Asia, the Sahara regions of North Africa, and the Middle East (Mirzabaev et al., 2019). Human activities, such as pollution, the exploitation of natural land for agriculture, and overgrazing are the main factors triggering desertification and land degradation (Huang et al., 2020). The assessment of global scale desertification vulnerability to climate change and human activity is important to help policy and other decision makers formulate the best strategies for land rehabilitation and to combat global desertification in sensitive areas (Huang et al., 2020). The Intergovernmental Panel on Climate Change (IPCC, 2019) concluded that policy frameworks promoting the adoption of sustainable land management would also support poverty eradication and food security among dryland populations.

Deforestation contributes substantively to climate emergency outcomes. Over the decade since 2010, the net loss in forests globally was 4.7 million hectares per year (UN News, 2020). However, deforestation rates were significantly higher. The United Nations Food and Agriculture Organization (UNFAO) estimates that 10 million hectares of forest were cut down each year (UN News, 2020). Furthermore, an estimated one-quarter of total anthropogenic greenhouse gas emissions arise mainly from deforestation, ruminant livestock, and fertilizer application. A lack of formal (legal) ownership has often led to the loss of access rights to land, where these rights were also not formally enshrined in law, a situation that especially impacts Indigenous communities—for example, deforestation in the Amazon basin (Arneth et al., 2019). Old-growth tree logging in the Haida Gwaii territory is an urgent example of deforestation in Canada. The territory was taken when British colonial authorities formally annexed Haida Gwaii in 1853 by establishing the Colony of the Queen Charlotte Islands. For centuries, the Haida sustainably used their forests to hunt and to harvest medicinal plants and centuries-old cedar trees to create totem poles that honour their ancestors. Ongoing settler deforestation in Haida territory, such as clear-cut logging of ancient cedars, many worth upwards of $20,000 as lumber, are being cut down at an alarming rate, where more than 2,000 hectares of Haida territory forests are clear cut each year (Bertz, 2022).

After decades of protest, the fight to protect cedars was boosted by an affidavit filed with the British Columbia Supreme Court by Robert Davidson, an acclaimed Haida carver who is responsible for carving the first totem pole on the island in 100 years (Wilson, 2020). As a result, the allowable annual cut was reduced to 804,000 cubic meters in 2020, down from 929,000 in 2012. One cubic meter of timber is equivalent to about one telephone pole's worth of wood. If that many poles were spaced an average distance apart, as in most city streets, "you could run 930,000 poles from Vancouver to Halifax and back and then do it all over again" (Parfitt, 2019). Although reduction in the annual cut is movement towards truth and reconciliation, it is widely recognized by Indigenous Peoples that Indigenous forest sovereignty is the only process that can save the cedars (Zucco, 2022). "The removal of Indigenous people from forestry decision-making processes, and the lack of legislative power used to uplift Indigenous ecological knowledge, illustrate the global impacts of settler colonialism and its threat to our collective future" (Zucco, 2022, pp. 4–5). Box 4.3 details some of the contexts and successful actions of Haida Gwaii First Nations resistance to industrial logging in their territories.

Box 4.3: Haida Gwaii First Nations Resistance to Industrial Logging

Haida resistance to industrial logging in Haida Gwaii over the past four decades has transformed the political and environmental map of Canada:

- Since the mid-1970s, industrial logging on Haida Gwaii, an archipelago of over one hundred islands off the northwest coast of British Columbia, has been contested by the Haida Nation and their supporters. Haida Gwaii is home to the world's best remaining stands of cedar, hemlock, and Sitka spruce. Many waves of blockades, popular mobilizations, court battles, and intergovernmental negotiations have led to significant wins. Forests have been protected, new forms of co-management have been forged and Indigenous rights have been strengthened. Haida resistance has helped bring about treaty recognition for First Nations in Canada.
- Conflicts have been sparked again and again over industrial logging, especially of old-growth cedar trees. Communities are opposing the flow of logging revenue accruing away from local communities and concerned about impacts to rivers and salmon. The conflict also involves logging companies repeatedly violating existing agreements and quotas. "From at least the mid-1970's, the Haida have pursued a number of strategies, from participation

in cooperative management processes to illegal roadblocks, in order to reclaim control over the forests and waters of Haida Gwaii. Throughout this period the Haida continued to draw links between their opposition to the environmental damage wrought by resource extraction industries and the nature of colonialism in BC" (Dean, 2009, p. 3). Environmentalists helped raise awareness for this Haida-led struggle (Pynn, 2010).

- Haida resistance led to the creation of the Gwaii Haanas National Park in 1993, which they co-manage with the federal government. This was the first national park to be co-managed by the Government of Canada and an Indigenous nation (Dean, 2009). Fifty-two percent of Haida Gwaii is now in protected areas, while another 18.5 percent is protected through the Haida Gwaii Land-Use Objectives Order (Hudson, 2018). Logging companies continue to violate agreements and new blockades and waves of resistance have arisen as recently as 2018. The BC government is still "pursuing profit over culture and community" by selling logging rights on Haida Gwaii without Haida permission (Kurjata, 2017).
- Logging corporation names can be found at Environmental Justice Atlas (2019), Haida Gwaii Forestry Conflicts. Juridical relevant texts related to the conflict can be found in *Haida Nation v British Columbia (Minister of Forests)*, [2004] 3 S.C.R. 51.

Acidification of water and soil continues to be a major contributor to negative Earth system health outcomes. Between a quarter to a third of the CO2 emitted into the atmosphere from the burning of fossil fuels, cement manufacturing, and land-use changes has been absorbed by the ocean (Ciais et al., 2013). Research has shown that the rate at which CO2 is currently being absorbed into the ocean is too rapid to be buffered sufficiently for the prevention of substantial decreases in ocean pH, referred to as ocean acidification (Findlay & Turley, 2021). Soil acidification, caused by anthropogenic activities, such as mass application of ammonium-based and other fertilizers on agricultural land, is also of central concern (Bolan et al., 2023). Impacts of soil acidification include increases in the impacts of toxic elements, such as heavy metals (Uchimiya et al., 2020), and decreased plant production and water use (Yadav et al., 2020). If soil acidification is not treated, it can impact agricultural productivity and sustainable farming systems, and it can also spread or filter into sub-soil layers underneath agricultural areas, posing serious problems for plant root development and remedial action (Agriculture Victoria, 2024).

Biodiversity Loss, Species Endangerment, and Extinction

Biodiversity loss is related to each of the key ecological DoH described in this chapter. Due to the synergistic nature of these DoH, it is not possible to point to any one root cause. Biodiversity loss refers to the reduction of any aspect of biological diversity, such as diversity loss at the genetic level, species and individual organisms within a given species, and ecosystem levels within a defined geographic area. It includes the number and population size of wild species, the number of local varieties of domesticated species, the distinctness of ecological communities, and the extent and integrity of many terrestrial and aquatic ecosystems (Díaz et al., 2019). Loss occurs through death, including extinction; destruction or manual removal from an area, as well as air, soil, and water pollution, as described in previous sections; habitat loss; invasive species; and natural and anthropogenic catastrophes such as volcanos, wildfires, floods, hurricanes, droughts, epidemics, and tsunamis.

Biodiversity loss happens on many scales, from the smallest ecosystem to global population extinctions (Intergovernmental Science-Policy Platform on Biodiversity and Ecosystem Services [IPBES], n.d.). Anthropogenic actions now threaten more species with global extinction. An average of about 25 percent of species in assessed animal and plant groups are threatened. This data points to the likelihood that about one million species already face extinction, many within decades, unless action is taken to reduce the intensity of drivers of biodiversity loss. Without such action, there will be a further acceleration in the global rate of species extinction, which is already at least tens to hundreds of times higher than it has averaged over the past ten million years (Brondizio et al., 2019). Figure 4.4 depicts five threats to

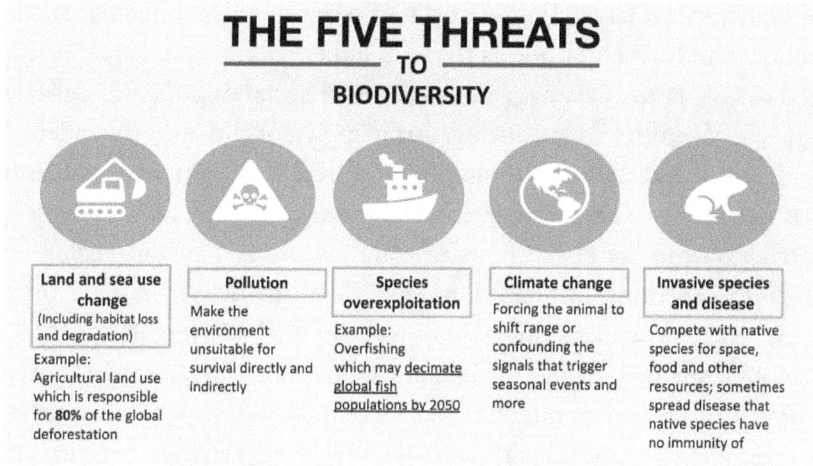

Figure 4.4: Five Threats to Biodiversity

Source: World Wildlife Fund, 2020.

biodiversity on Earth: land and sea use change, pollution, species overexploitation, climate change, and invasive species and disease.

However, these five threats or direct drivers of biodiversity loss are distal or downstream causes. The upstream or root causes (causes-of-the-causes) are grounded in neoliberal global capitalism, further described below.

> … action at the level of direct drivers of nature decline, although necessary, is not sufficient to prevent further deterioration of the fabric of life on Earth. Reversal of recent declines—and a sustainable global future—are only possible with urgent transformative change that tackles the root causes: the interconnected economic, sociocultural, demographic, political, institutional, and technological indirect drivers behind the direct drivers. (Díaz et al., 2019, p. 1)

Climate Emergency Denial and Neoliberal Global Capitalism

The shift from describing ecological damage as "climate change" to "climate crisis" to "climate emergency" in the public sphere has happened very recently amidst alarming verification of the nature and scope of planetary damage. These latter two terms are also a marker of the political and structural forces that can either continue to deny massive globe-wide climate damage or mobilize for sustaining Earth's delicate balance of health and well-being. The mapping of climate change denial with neoliberal political economies and **neoliberal global capitalism** has a relatively recent history. It refers to the phase of capitalism where restrictions on the global flows of commodities and capital, including capital in the form of finance, have been substantially removed. Since such removal happens under pressure from globally mobile (or international) finance capital, neoliberal capitalism is characterized by the dominating power of international finance capital, which ensures that a common set of neoliberal policy and global governance policies are pursued by all countries across the globe (Patnaik, 2017).

Although neoliberal global capitalism has been demonstrated to be the driver of climate emergency, its role in disrupting public knowledge about climate change is much less known. Neubauer (2011) traced these connections and provided an analysis of some of the mechanisms that play a part in this role. He first referred to the Elite Policy and Information Infrastructure (EPII) in the United States as a "decentralized yet interlocked network of conservative intellectuals, activists, think tanks, corporations, foundations, and advocacy organizations, EPII has emerged as a central force within a hegemonic neoliberal project" (Neubauer, 2011, p. 66). Despite irrefutable evidence of anthropogenic climate damage, and the naming of the Anthropocene Epoch, there remain significant numbers of people who deny climate change, including those in elected governance positions. Neubauer traced how conservative think tanks in the United States create and sustain a parallel global movement to reify climate skeptics as experts, regardless of any proven expertise or accreditation in the field of climate science—and, importantly, as described by Neubauer as early as 2011, help to sustain entry points into the media, where their expert authority is legitimized in the public sphere.

These structures have their foundations and their ongoing sustenance within neoliberal political economies, described in Chapter 2. The primacy of the market, and resulting corporate profit, are legitimized through climate denial "science" and taken up at formal policy governance levels in local to national jurisdictions. In a 2022, 31-country IPSOS survey of 23,577 adults aged 16–74, researchers found that climate change is a regular concern for fewer Canadians than citizens of most other countries (34% worry a great deal/a fair amount when compared to 48% across all other countries surveyed, and only 30% of Canadians are aware of the government's plan to tackle climate change, placing Canada in the bottom five in the list of 30 countries surveyed) (IPSOS, 2022). Although there may be other factors contributing to Canadian citizens' overall lower concern about climate change, further research is needed to determine the nature and structure of climate denial in Canada and how these processes may be contributing to IPSOS findings. This context is an important foreground for describing the ecological DoH—just as the ecological DoH form a complex adaptive system (systems-within-systems), so does the international climate skeptic infrastructure that continues to support public policy denial of the urgent need for responsible and accountable climate policy and governance. Responsible means exercising the mandate to effectively address climate emergency and accountable means publicly demonstrating measurable and consistent progress in mitigating and halting climate emergency.

WHAT'S TO BE DONE?

The IPCC (2019) recommends that actions can be taken in the near term, based on existing knowledge, to address desertification, land degradation, and food security. At the same time, it is important to support longer-term responses that enable adaptation and mitigation of climate change, as described in Box 4.4. These include actions to build individual and institutional capacity, accelerate knowledge transfer, enhance technology transfer and deployment, enable financial mechanisms, implement early warning systems, undertake risk management, and address gaps in implementation and upscaling.

Box 4.4: International Panel on Climate Change Recommendations for Policymakers: Climate Actions That Can Be Taken in the Near Term

Near-term capacity-building, technology transfer and deployment, and enabling financial mechanisms can strengthen adaptation and mitigation in the land sector. Knowledge and technology transfer can help enhance the sustainable use of natural resources for food security under a changing climate.

Measuring and monitoring land-use change, including land degradation and desertification, is supported by the expanded use of new information and communication technologies (cellphone-based applications, cloud-based services, ground sensors, drone imagery), use of climate services, and remotely sensed land and climate information on land resources (medium-term).

Early warning systems for extreme weather and climate events are critical for protecting lives and property and enhancing disaster risk reduction and management.

Upfront investment, actions to ensure sustainable land management can improve crop yields and the economic value of pasture. Land restoration and rehabilitation measures improve livelihood systems and provide both short-term positive economic returns and longer-term benefits in terms of climate change adaptation and mitigation, biodiversity, and enhanced ecosystem functions and services.

Government support and improved access to credit can help overcome barriers to adoption, especially those faced by poor smallholder farmers.

Prompt action on climate mitigation and adaptation aligned with sustainable land management and sustainable development, depending on the region, could reduce the risk to millions of people from climate extremes, desertification, land degradation, and food and livelihood insecurity.

Deferral of greenhouse gas emissions reductions from all sectors must be examined and mitigated. Deferral implies trade-offs, including irreversible loss in land ecosystem functions and services required for food, health, habitable settlements, and production, leading to increasingly significant economic impacts on many countries in many regions of the world.

Source: Mirzabaev et al., 2019.

However, each of these IPCC recommendations is dependent on a seismic shift in policy and politics across all countries—one that targets the root, structural causes of climate emergency. Building on its groundbreaking 1972 report, *The Limits to Growth* (Meadows et al., 1972), the Club of Rome produced an emergency paper with the goal of "responding to direct calls for action from citizens around the world, and to formulate a plan that will meet suitably ambitious reduction targets and ensure climate stability" (Dixson-Declève et al., 2018, p. 3). The Club of Rome is a platform of diverse thought leaders who identify solutions to complex global issues and promote policy initiatives and action to enable humanity to emerge from multiple planetary emergencies (Dixson-Declève et al., 2018). Transforming Earth's energy systems is a key area in the Club of Rome's calls to action, specifically calling for a halt in fossil fuel expansion and fossil fuel subsidies by 2020, which has not been met as of early 2024, and a total phase-out of the existing fossil fuel industry by 2050.

In tandem with fossil fuel phase-out, the Club calls for continuing to double wind and solar capacity every four years and triple annual investments in renewable energy, energy efficiency, and low-carbon technologies for high-emitting sectors before 2025, while giving priority to "developing" countries to avoid locked-into-carbon economies.

According to OECD (2023), "gross domestic product (GDP) is the standard measure of the value added created through the production of goods and services in a country during a certain period." OECD also states that although GDP is the most important indicator that will capture economic growth and/or activity, it does not provide an appropriate measure of people's material well-being and alternative indicators may be more appropriate. The Club of Rome mandate also calls for alternative indicators, such as the genuine progress indicator. Figure 4.5

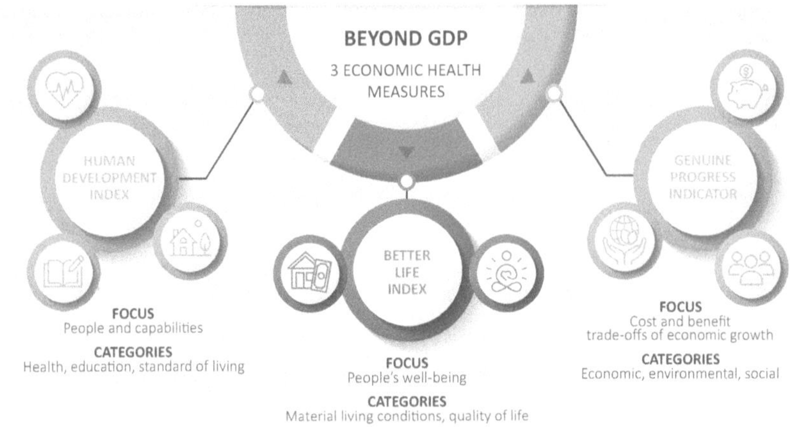

Figure 4.5: Beyond GDP: Three Alternative Indicators of a Country's Well-Being

Source: © 2023 Federal Reserve Bank of St. Louis. All rights reserved. Reproduced with permission of Federal Reserve Bank of St. Louis. https://www.stlouisfed.org/

illustrates three of these alternatives, their overall focus, and related measurement categories: the Human Development Index (United Nations Development Program [UNDP], n.d.) which measures areas such as life expectancy, education, and standard of living; the Better Life Index (Altintas, 2022), which measures areas such as material living conditions, civic engagement, quality of life, and environment; and the Genuine Progress Indicator, which measures areas such as economic, environmental, and social progress. The latter two explicitly target environmental measures, such as the ecological determinants of health described in this chapter (e.g., air and water pollution, climate change, and non-renewable resource depletion). A central Club of Rome call to action is the provision for a just transition in all affected communities, recognizing that "the degree of social change needed to make a successful transformation to a sustainable future will extend throughout society, requiring fundamental shifts in behaviour and rethinking of national and community support and care systems" (Dixson-Declève et al., 2018, p. 5). Alternative indicators and alternative political economies are further discussed in Chapter 7.

CONCLUSION

The ecological DoH illustrate how all three DoH (social, ecological, structural) are inseparable. Hence, the difficulty in creating "separate" spaces to map the intricacies of damage to ecosystems and other Earth systems. This chapter pulls together many of the ideas in the book—ecological determinants are the "bell weather signal" of the health of all living beings, including the planet. The ecodeterminants also precisely illustrate how the disciplines, sectors, civil society organizations, and first-voice expertise, such as Indigenous knowledges, Afrocentric knowledges, and local, community-driven understandings are all indispensable for intervening in what seems to be a futile effort to halt or even mitigate climate emergency. Nonetheless, this is the task at hand and synergies among all the DoH also mean that progress in one area will inevitably have ripple effects that improve progress in many other systems. The overall goal is to mitigate, stall, or halt what is now known as the age of extinction.

FURTHER READINGS

Butler, C. D. (2000) Inequality, global change, and the sustainability of civilisation. *Global Change and Human Health, 1*(2), 156–172. https://doi.org/10.1023/A:1010029222095

Campbell, R. A. (2002). A narrative analysis of success and failure in environmental remediation: The case of incineration at the Sydney tar ponds. *Organization and Environment, 15*(3), 259–277. https://doi.org/10.1177/1086026602153002

Centre on Climate Change and Planetary Health (2020, November 13). *One Health, EcoHealth and planetary health: Bridging disciplines for a post-COVID 19 world.* London School of Hygiene and Tropical Medicine. https://www.lshtm.ac.uk/newsevents/events/one-health-ecohealth-and-planetary-health-bridging-disciplines-post-COVID-19

Elton, S. (2021). Is the "obesity crisis" really the health crisis of the food system? The ecological determinants of health for food system change. *Canadian Food Studies/La Revue Canadienne des Etudes sur l'Alimentation, 8*(1). https://doi.org/10.15353/cfs-rcea.v8i1.447

Hancock, T. (2020). *Ecological economics and public health: An interview with Dr. Trevor Hancock.* National Collaborating Centre for Healthy Public Policy. http://www.ncchpp.ca/docs/2020-policy-and-climate-change-ethics-ecological-economics-and-public-health.pdf

WEBSITES OF INTEREST

The Anthropocene Project—https://theanthropocene.org/

This website presents a multidisciplinary body of work from world-renowned collaborators Nicholas de Pencier, Edward Burtynsky and Jennifer Baichwal. Combining art, film, virtual reality, augmented reality, and scientific research, the project investigates human influence on the state, dynamic and future of the Earth.

The Black Environmental Initiative (BEI)—https://beinitiative.com/

"BEI's mission is to create more opportunities for Black communities and individuals to participate in environmental action. Our objective is to increase access to green jobs, green entrepreneurship opportunities and environmental protection engagement in Black communities. We also work to ensure that Black communities have decent access to environmental benefits and we promote environmental protection and equity for all. Finally, we fight against racism and we promote better relations between all races, mostly through shared environmental values."

Community of Practice in Ecosystems Approach to Health Canada (CoPEH-Canada)—https://copeh-canada.org/en/teaching-manual/complexity.html

Access research and educational resources compiled by a dynamic group of interdisciplinary scholars and practitioners from universities across Canada. Click "Teaching Resources" to explore recorded lectures and learning modules.

The ENRiCH Project—https://www.enrichproject.org/

"The mission of the Environmental Noxiousness, Racial Inequities and Community Health Project is to examine and address the social, environmental, political, and health effects of environmental racism and climate change in Indigenous, Black, and other marginalized communities across Canada through community-based research, publications, multidisciplinary and multisectoral partnerships, student training and mentorship, advocacy, community engagement, mobilizing and capacity building in affected communities, government consultations, policy analysis and legislation, public education, multimedia, and knowledge sharing and communications."

Environmental Justice Atlas—https://ejatlas.org/

The EJ Atlas documents and catalogues social conflict around environmental issues and collects stories of communities struggling for environmental justice from around the world. The EJ Atlas aims to make these mobilizations more visible, highlight claims and testimonies, and to make the case for true corporate and state accountability for the injustices inflicted through their activities. It also attempts to serve as a virtual space for those working on EJ issues to get information, find other groups working on related issues, and increase the visibility of environmental conflicts.

UNESCO Designated Sites: A Climate Change Observatory—https://www.unesco.org/en/climate-change/unesco-sites-climate-change-observatory

This website explores the iconic UNESCO-designated World Heritage sites, Biosphere Reserves, and UNESCO Global Geoparks, which provide useful platforms to apply and test climate monitoring, mitigation and adaptation, and to raise awareness on climate change impacts on human societies, cultural diversity, biodiversity, ecosystem services, and the world's natural and cultural heritage. Spread across different regions, climates and ecosystems around the world, climate change is already being felt in many UNESCO-designated sites. Communities there are working on innovative ways to address climate change.

GLOSSARY

Anthropocene Epoch: Complex and multiple changes in Earth's natural systems such as these are captured in the term *Anthropocene Epoch*, first described by Paul Crutzen (2005). The Anthropocene signals the dominance of humans over the global environment. The on-the-ground meaning of the Anthropocene involves synergistic impacts on Earth systems, including ecological DoH (e.g., pollution and ecotoxicity, including environmental racism; resource extraction and depletion; climate and atmospheric emergency; desertification, deforestation, and acidification; and biodiversity loss, species endangerment, and extinction).

Capitalocene: Refers to the Age of Capital, reflecting the history of capitalism, and the central political, cultural, and economic role it played in the reshaping of global ecosystems for centuries before the advent of coal and steam engines (Moore, 2017). The Capitalocene is sometimes used as an alternative term for the Anthropocene.

Earth Systems: There are five main Earth systems, or spheres, on Earth: the geosphere (interior and surface of Earth, both of which are made up of rocks), the biosphere (limited part of the planet that can support living things), the hydrosphere (areas of Earth that are covered with enormous amounts of water), the atmosphere (envelope of gas that keeps the planet warm and provides oxygen for breathing and carbon dioxide for photosynthesis), and the cryosphere (the huge quantities of ice at the poles and elsewhere). All five of these enormous and complex systems interact with one another to maintain the Earth as we know it (National Geographic, 2023).

EcoHealth: Refers to the process of striving for the sustainable health of people, animals, and ecosystems. These processes are supported by transdisciplinary action research, encouraging problem solving that draws upon a broad scope of knowledge from the natural, social, and health sciences, and the humanities (Zinsstag, 2012). The aim is to understand "how social, economic, and ecological factors and their interactions affect ecosystem health, including the condition and sustainability of ecosystems" (Mi et al., 2016, p. 12).

Economic Globalization: Refers to the breaking down of states' borders to allow the free flow of finance, trade, production, and labour. Human rights and social justice must be considered in the age of the market, where existing state human rights obligations must be rethought because state action is enhanced, or fettered, by the global market and multinational economic institutions and mega-corporations (de Feyter, 2005).

Ecosystems: Refers to a collection of communities of both living and non-living things that are synergistically connected. The biotic elements in an ecosystem include living things, such as plants and animals. The abiotic elements include non-living things, such as land forms or climate. Terrestrial ecosystems are found on land and include vegetation, ecosystems, soil, terrain, and wildlife habitat. Aquatic ecosystems are found in bodies of water, such as streams, lakes, oceans, marshes, and watersheds (Province of British Columbia, 2018).

Neoliberal Global Capitalism: Refers to the phase of capitalism where restrictions on the global flows of commodities and capital, including capital in the form of finance, have been substantially removed. Since such removal happens under pressure from globally mobile (or international) finance capital, neoliberal capitalism is characterized by the hegemony of international finance capital, which ensures that a common set of neoliberal policy and global governance policies are pursued by all countries across the globe (Patnaik, 2017).

One Health: Refers to a concept that supports the recognition that the health of humans, animals, and our broader environment are interconnected (Okello, 2020). It emerged through the need for interdisciplinary responses to prevent and control zoonoses (infectious diseases that cross the animal-human species barrier), including bacteria and viruses such as COVID-19 and SARS (Okello, 2020). The One Health movement eventually included not only physicians and veterinarians but also wildlife specialists, environmentalists, anthropologists, economists, and sociologists, among others (Gibbs, 2014).

Planetary Health: Refers to "... the interdependent vitality of all natural and anthropogenic ecosystems; this vitality includes the biologically defined ecosystems (at micro, meso and macro scales) that favor biodiversity; it includes the more broadly defined human-constructed social, political, and economic ecosystems that favor health equity and the opportunity to strive for high-level wellness; this definition also includes the business ecosystems that influence sustainable and health-promoting local and global commerce" (Prescott et al., 2018, p. 3).

White Supremacy: Refers to the myriad conditions, practices, and ideologies that underscore the hegemony of whiteness and white political, social, cultural, and economic domination, where the interests and perceptions of white people are continually placed centre stage and assumed to be "normal" (Alang et al., 2021).

REFERENCES

Abimbola, O., Aikins, J. K., Makhesi-Wilkinson, T., & Roberts, E. (2021). *Racism and climate (in)justice: How racism and colonialism shape the climate crisis and climate action*. Heinrich Böll-Stiftung.

Agriculture Victoria. (2024). *Soil acidity*. https://agriculture.vic.gov.au/farm-management/soil/soil-acidity

Alang, S., Hardeman, R., Karbeah, J., Akosionu, O., McGuire, C., Abdi, H., & McAlpine, D. (2021). White supremacy and the core functions of public health. *American Journal of Public Health, 111*(5), 815–819. https://doi.org/10.2105%2FAJPH.2020.306137

Alexander, C., Bynum, N., Johnson, E., King, U., Mustonen, T., Neofotis, P., Oettlé, N., Rosenzweig, C., Sakakibara, C., Shadrin, V., Vicarelli, M., Waterhouse, J., & Weeks, B. (2011). Linking Indigenous and scientific knowledge of climate change. *BioScience, 61*(6), 477–485. https://doi.org/10.1525/bio.2011.61.6.10

Altintas, T. (2022). Grouping OECD countries according to Better Life Index indicators by multidimensional scaling analysis. *Cognizance Journal of Multidisciplinary Studies, 2*(12), 18–22. https://doi.org/10.47760/cognizance.2022.v02i12.003

Amuasi, J. H., Lucas, T., Horton, R., & Winkler, A. S. (2020). Reconnecting for our future: The Lancet One Health Commission. *The Lancet, 395*(10235), 1469–1471. https://doi.org/10.1016/s0140-6736(20)31027-8

Arneth, A., Denton, F., Agus, F., Elbehri, A., Erb, K., Osman Elasha, B., Rahimi, M., Rounsevell, M., & Spence, R. (2019). Framing and context. In P. R. Shukla, J. Skea, E. Calvo Buendia, V. Masson-Delmotte, H.-O. Pörtner, D. C. Roberts, P. Zhai, R. Slade, S. Connors, R. van Diemen, M. Ferrat, E. Haughey, S. Luz, S. Neogi, M. Pathak, J. Petzold, J. Portugal Pereira, P. Vyas, E. Huntley, … J Malley (Eds.), *Climate change and land: An IPCC special report on climate change, desertification, land degradation, sustainable land management, food security, and greenhouse gas fluxes in terrestrial ecosystems* (pp. 77–130). Cambridge University Press.

Arpin, E., Gauffin, K., Kerr, M., Hjern, A., Mashford-Pringle, A., Barros, A., Rajmil, L., Choonara, I., & Spencer, N. (2021). Climate change and child health inequality: A review of reviews. *International Journal of Environmental Research and Public Health, 18*(20), 10896. https://doi.org/10.3390/ijerph182010896

Aves, A. R., Revell, L. E., Gaw, S., Ruffell, H., Schuddeboom, A., Wotherspoon, N. E., LaRue, M., & McDonald, A. J. (2022). First evidence of microplastics in Antarctic snow. *The Cryosphere, 16*(6), 2127–2145. https://doi.org/10.5194/tc-16-2127-2022

Barlow, M. (2007). *Blue covenant: The global water crisis and the coming battle for the right to water.* McClelland and Stewart.

Behn, C. (2023). *Ecological justice: Fracking.* Kairos. https://www.kairoscanada.org/what-we-do/ecological-justice/fracking

Bernard, W. T. (2021). *Eddie Carvery.* The Progressive Senate Group. https://theprogressives.ca/in-the-senate/statements/eddie-carvery/

Bertz, K. L. (2022, September 30). The Haida's fight to save their centuries-old "trees of life." *Toronto Star.* https://www.thestar.com/news/canada/2022/09/30/the-haida-gwaiis-fight-to-save-centuries-old-trees-of-life.html

Black, K. J., Boslett, A. J., Hill, E. L., Ma, L., & McCoy, S. J. (2021). Economic, environmental, and health impacts of the fracking boom. *Annual Review of Resource Economics, 13*, 311–334. https://doi.org/10.1146/annurev-resource-110320-092648

Bloomsbury Publishing. (2022). *Global Health Watch 6: In the shadow of the pandemic.*

Bolan, N., Sarmah, A. K., Bordoloi, S., Bolan, S., Padhye, L. P., Van Zwieten, L., Sooriyakumar, P., Ahmed Khan, B. A., Ahmad, M., Solaiman, Z. M., Rinklebe, J., Wang, H., Singh, B. P., & Siddique, K. H. (2023). Soil acidification and the liming potential of biochar. *Environmental Pollution, 317*, 120632. https://doi.org/10.1016/j.envpol.2022.120632

Bray, F., Ferlay, J., Soerjomataram, I., Siegel, R. L., Torre, L. A., & Jemal, A. (2018). Global cancer statistics 2018: GLOBOCAN estimates of incidence and mortality worldwide for 36 cancers in 185 countries. *CA: A Cancer Journal for Clinicians, 68*(6), 394–424. https://doi.org/10.3322/caac.21492

Brondizio, E. S. Settele, J. Díaz, S., & Ngo, H. T. (Eds.). (2019). *Global assessment report on biodiversity and ecosystem services of the Intergovernmental Science-Policy Platform on Biodiversity and Ecosystem Services.* IPBES Secretariat.

Brown, E., MacDonald, A., Allen, S., & Allen, D. (2023). The potential for a plastic recycling facility to release microplastic pollution and possible filtration remediation effectiveness. *Journal of Hazardous Materials Advances, 10*, 100309. https://doi.org/10.1016/j.hazadv.2023.100309

Brumberg, H. L., Karr, C. J., Bole, A., Ahdoot, S., Balk, S. J., Bernstein, A. S., Byron, L. G., Landrigan, P. J., Marcus, S. M., Nerlinger, A. L., Pacheco, S. E., Woolf, A. D., Zajac, L., Baum, C. R., Campbell, C. C., Sample, J. A., Spanier, A. J., Trasande, L., & Council on Environmental Health. (2021). Ambient air pollution: health hazards to children. *Pediatrics, 147*(6), e2021051484. https://doi.org/10.1542/peds.2021-051484

Buse, C. G., Hancock, T., Allison, S., Astle, B., Cole, D., Fumerton, R., Gislason, M., Takaro, T., Howard, C., Kling, R., Maruti, S., McLaren, L., Newhouse, E., Parkes, M. W., Pollock, S., Rainham, D., Webb, J., & Woollard, R.

(2023). Where are the ecological determinants of health? *Canadian Journal of Public Health, 114*(1), 152–153. https://doi.org/10.17269%2Fs41997-022-00720-x

Butler, C. D. (2000). Inequality, global change, and the sustainability of civilisation. *Global Change and Human Health, 1*(2), 156–172.

Calistri, P., Iannetti, S., L. Danzetta, M., Narcisi, V., Cito, F., Di Sabatino, D., Bruno, R., Sauro, F., Atzeni, M., Carvelli, A., & Giovannini, A. (2013). The components of "one world—one health" approach. *Transboundary and Emerging Diseases, 60*(Suppl 2), 4–13. https://doi.org/10.1111/tbed.12145

Campbell, D. (2022, April 13). *More developed countries dumping toxic e-waste in Global South, U of T researchers find.* University of Toronto News. https://www.utoronto.ca/news/more-developed-countries-dumping-toxic-e-waste-global-south-u-t-researchers-find

The Canadian Press. (2023, May 19). *Firefighting foam ban possible as Canada looks at risks of "forever chemicals."* CTV News. https://www.ctvnews.ca/climate-and-environment/firefighting-foam-ban-possible-as-canada-looks-at-risks-of-forever-chemicals-1.6406412

Carlsen, L., & Bruggemann, R. (2022). The 17 United Nations' sustainable development goals: A status by 2020. *International Journal of Sustainable Development & World Ecology, 29*(3), 219–229. https://doi.org/10.1080/13504509.2021.1948456

Carrington, D. (2016, August 29). The Anthropocene Epoch: Scientists declare dawn of human-influenced age. *The Guardian.* https://www.theguardian.com/environment/2016/aug/29/declare-anthropocene-epoch-experts-urge-geological-congress-human-impact-earth

Carson, R. (1962). *Silent spring.* Houghton Mifflin.

Carvery-Taylor, A. (2021). *A love letter to Africville.* Fernwood Publishing.

Castellón, I. G. (2021). Cancer Alley and the fight against environmental racism. *Villanova Environmental Law Journal, 32*(1), 15–43. https://digitalcommons.law.villanova.edu/elj/vol32/iss1/2

Celino-Brady, F. T., Lerner, D. T., & Seale, A. P. (2021). Experimental approaches for characterizing the endocrine-disrupting effects of environmental chemicals in fish. *Frontiers in Endocrinology, 11*, 619361.

Centre on Climate Change and Planetary Health. (2020, November 13). *One Health, EcoHealth and planetary health: Bridging disciplines for a post-COVID 19 world.* London School of Hygiene and Tropical Medicine. https://www.lshtm.ac.uk/newsevents/events/one-health-ecohealth-and-planetary-health-bridging-disciplines-post-COVID-19

Chakrabarty, D. (2018). Anthropocene time. *History and Theory, 57*(1), 5–32. https://doi.org/10.1111/hith.12044

Chiu, E. (2019). *After 5 decades, Eddie Carvery says his Africville protest is "back at square one."* CBC News. https://www.cbc.ca/news/canada/nova-scotia/eddie-carvery-africville-protest-trailers-destroyed-1.5360104

Ciais, P., Sabine, C., Bala, G., Bopp, L., Brovkin, V., Canadell, J., Chhabra, R., DeFries, J., Galloway, M., Heimann, C., Jones, C., Le Quéré, R. B., Myneni, S. P., & Thornton, P. (2013). Carbon and other biogeochemical cycles. In T. F. Stocker, D. Qin, G.-K. Plattner, M. Tignor, S. K. Allen, J. Boschung, A. Nauels, Y. Xia, V. Bex & P. M. Midgley (Eds.), *Climate change 2013: The physical science basis. Contribution of Working Group I to the fifth assessment report of the Intergovernmental Panel on Climate Change* (pp. 465–570). Cambridge University Press.

Club of Rome. (n.d.). *About us.* https://www.clubofrome.org/about-us/

Craig, L. S., Cunningham-Myrie, C. A., Hotchkiss, D. R., Hernandez, J. H., Gustat, J., & Theall, K. P. (2021). Social determinants of multimorbidity in Jamaica: Application of latent class analysis in a cross-sectional study. *BMC Public Health, 21*(1), 1–15.

Crutzen, P. J. (2005). Human impact on climate has made this the "Anthropocene age." *New Perspectives Quarterly, 22*(2), 14–16.

Dahlgren, G., & Whitehead, M. (1991). *Policies and strategies to promote social equity in health.* Institute for Futures Studies.

Dangendorf, S., Hay, C., Calafat, F. M., Marcos, M., Piecuch, C. G., Berk, K., & Jensen, J. (2019). Persistent acceleration in global sea-level rise since the 1960s. *Nature Climate Change, 9*(9), 705–710. https://doi.org/10.1038/s41558-019-0531-8

D'Avignon, G., Gregory-Eaves, I., & Ricciardi, A. (2022). Microplastics in lakes and rivers: An issue of emerging significance to limnology. *Environmental Reviews, 30*(2), 228–244. https://doi.org/10.1139/er-2021-0048

de Feyter, K. (2005). *Human rights: Social justice in the age of the market.* Fernwood Publishing.

Dean, M. (2009). *What they are doing to the land they are doing to us: Environmental politics on Haida Gwaii* [Master's thesis]. University of British Columbia.

Deziel, N. C., Brokovich, E., Grotto, I., Clark, C. J., Barnett-Itzhaki, Z., Broday, D., & Agay-Shay, K. (2020). Unconventional oil and gas development and health outcomes: A scoping review of the epidemiological research. *Environmental Research, 182*, 109124. https://doi.org/10.1016/j.envres.2020.109124

Diamanti-Kandarakis, E., Bourguinon. J.-P., Giudice, L. C., Hauser, R., Prins, G. S., Soto, A. M., Zoeller, R. T., & Gore, A. C. (2009). Endocrine-disrupting chemicals: An Endocrine Society statement. *Endocrine Reviews, 30*(4), 293–342. https://doi.org/10.1210%2Fer.2009-0002

Díaz, S., Settele, J., Brondízio, E. S., Ngo, H. T., Agard, J., Arneth, A., Balvanera, P., Brauman, K. A., Butchart, S. H. M., Chan, K. M. A., Garibaldi, L. A., Ichii, K., Liu, J., Subramanian, S. M., Midgley, G. F., Miloslavich, P., Molnár, Z., Obura, D., Pfaff, A., ... Zayas, C. N. (2019). Pervasive human-driven decline of life on Earth points to the need for transformative change. *Science, 366*(6471), eaax3100. https://doi.org/10.1126/science.aax3100

Dixson-Declève, S., Dunlop, I., & Wijkman, A. (2018). *The Club of Rome climate emergency plan: A collaborate call for climate action*. Club of Rome. https://clubofrome.org/wp-content/uploads/2018/10/COR_Climate-Emergency-Plan-.pdf

Dotto, S. (2021). A love letter to Africville by Amanda Carvery-Taylor. *Canadian Journal of History, 56*(3), 403–405. https://doi.org/10.3138/cjh.56-3-br02

Dutta, M. J. (2014). A culture-centered approach to listening: Voices of social change. *International Journal of Listening, 28*(2), 67–81. https://doi.org/10.1080/10904018.2014.876266

Elton, S. (2021). Is the "obesity crisis" really the health crisis of the food system? The ecological determinants of health for food system change. *Canadian Food Studies/La Revue Canadienne des Etudes sur l'Alimentation, 8*(1). https://doi.org/10.15353/cfs-rcea.v8i1.447

Environmental Justice Atlas (EJAtlas). (2019, March 19). *Haida Gwaii forestry conflicts*. https://ejatlas.org/conflict/haida-gwai-forresty-dispute

Equere, V., Mirzaei, P. A., & Riffat, S. (2020). Definition of a new morphological parameter to improve prediction of urban heat island. *Sustainable Cities and Society, 56*, 102021. http://dx.doi.org/10.1016/j.scs.2020.102021

Etowa, J., & McGibbon, E. (2021). The racialization of oppression. In E. McGibbon (Ed.), *Oppression: A social determinant of health* (2nd ed., pp. 66–84). Fernwood Publishing.

Findlay, H. S., & Turley, C. (2021). Ocean acidification and climate change. In T. M. Letcher (Eds.), *Climate change* (pp. 251–279). Elsevier.

Fitzpatrick, K., Greenhalgh-Stanley, N., & Ver Ploeg, M. (2019). Food deserts and diet-related health outcomes of the elderly. *Food Policy, 87*, 101747. https://doi.org/10.1016/j.foodpol.2019.101747

Forget, G., & Lebel, J. (2001). An ecosystem approach to human health. *International Journal of Occupational and Environmental Health, 7*(Suppl 2), S3–S38.

Furimsky, E. (2002). Sydney tar ponds: Some problems in quantifying toxic waste. *Environmental Management, 30*, 0872–0879. https://doi.org/10.1007/s00267-002-2649-z

Geddie, J., Volcovici, V., & Brock, J. (2022, February 18). Insight: UN pact may restrict plastic production. Big Oil aims to stop it. *Reuters*. https://www.reuters.com/business/sustainable-business/un-pact-may-restrict-plastic-production-big-oil-aims-stop-it-2022-02-18/

Gibbs, E. P. J. (2014). The evolution of One Health: A decade of progress and challenges for the future. *The Veterinary Record, 174*(4), 85–91. https://doi.org/10.1136/vr.g143

Gordner, T., Loney, J., Cuervo-Lorens, & Ross, D. N. (2021, July 19). *Plan for the ban: Plastics classified as "toxic substance" under* Canadian Environmental Protection Act. McMillan. https://mcmillan.ca/insights/plan-for-the-banplastics-classified-as-toxic-substanceunder-canadian-environmental-protection-act/

Government of Canada. (2021). *Toxic substances list*. https://www.canada.ca/en/environment-climate-change/services/canadian-environmental-protection-act-registry/substances-list/toxic/schedule-1.html

Graf, C. (2020, January 13). New study in Aamjiwnaang finds residents may face higher health risks caused by toxic substance in air. *Anishinabek News*. https://anishinabeknews.ca/2020/01/13/new-study-in-aamjiwnaang-finds-residents-may-face-higher-health-risks-caused-by-toxic-substance-in-air/

Griswold, E. (2012, September 21). How "*Silent Spring*" ignited the environmental movement. *New York Times*. https://www.nytimes.com/2012/09/23/magazine/how-silent-spring-ignited-the-environmental-movement.html

Grittayaphong, P. (2023, April 19). *Beyond GDP: Three other ways to measure economic health*. Federal Reserve Bank of St. Louis. https://www.stlouisfed.org/open-vault/2023/apr/three-other-ways-to-measure-economic-health-beyond-gdp

Grossman, A., & Dennings, K. (2022). *The influence of environmental toxicity, inequity and capitalism on reproductive health*. Center for Biological Diversity. https://www.biologicaldiversity.org/programs/population_and_sustainability/pdfs/environmental_reproductive_health_report.pdf

Haida Nation v British Columbia (Minister of Forests), [2004] 3 S.C.R. 51

Hamstead, Z. A. (2023). Thermal insecurity: Violence of heat and cold in the urban climate refuge. *Urban Studies, 61*(3), 531–548. https://doi.org/10.1177/00420980231184466

Hancock, T. (1985). The mandala of health: A model of the human ecosystem. *Family & Community Health, 8*(3), 1–10. https://doi.org/10.1097/00003727-198511000-00002

Hancock, T., Spady, D. W., & Soskolne, C. L. (Eds.). (2015). *Global change and public health: Addressing the ecological determinants of health*. Canadian Public Health Association.

Häsler, B., Cornelsen, L., Bennani, H., & Rushton, J. (2014). A review of the metrics for One Health benefits. *Revue Scientifique et Technique de l'Office International des Epizooties, 33*(2), 453–464. https://doi.org/10.20506/rst.33.2.2294

Hong, J.-W., Hong, J., Kwon, E. E., & Yoon, D. K. (2019). Temporal dynamics of urban heat island correlated with the socio-economic development over the past half-century in Seoul, Korea. *Environmental Pollution, 254*(Pt A), 112934. https://doi.org/10.1016/j.envpol.2019.07.102

Huang, J., Zhang, G., Zhang, Y., Guan, X., Wei, Y., & Guo, R. (2020). Global desertification vulnerability to climate change and human activities. *Land Degradation & Development, 31*(11), 1380–1391. https://doi.org/10.1002/ldr.3556

Huddart, D., & Scott, T. A. (2020). *Earth environments* (2nd ed.). Wiley-Blackwell.

Hudson, A. (2018, March 16). Logging protest at Collison Point. *Haida Gwaii Observer.* https://www.haidagwaiiobserver.com/local-news/logging-protest-at-collison-point/

Huseman, J., & Short, D. (2012). "A slow industrial genocide": Tar sands and the Indigenous peoples of northern Alberta. *The International Journal of Human Rights, 16*(1), 216–237. https://doi.org/10.1080/13642987.2011.649593

Intergovernmental Panel on Climate Change (IPCC). (2019). *Climate change and land: An IPCC special report on climate change, desertification, land degradation, sustainable land management, food security, and greenhouse gas fluxes in terrestrial ecosystems.* Cambridge University Press.

Intergovernmental Panel on Climate Change. (2021). *Climate change 2021: The physical science basis. Contribution of Working Group I to the Sixth Assessment Report of the Intergovernmental Panel on Climate Change.* Cambridge University Press.

Intergovernmental Science-Policy Platform on Biodiversity and Ecosystem Services (IPBES). (n.d.). *Glossary: Biodiversity loss.* https://www.ipbes.net/glossary-tag/biodiversity-loss

IPSOS. (2022, April 22). *Canadians are concerned about climate change, yet demonstrate low awareness and low hope for action.* https://www.ipsos.com/en-ca/news-polls/canadians-are-concerned-about-climate-change-yet-demonstrate-low-awareness-and-low-hope-action

Ivry, H. (2022). Kathryn Yusoff, a billion Black Anthropocenes or none. *American Literary History Online Review*, Series XXIX 795. Oxford University Press.

Jang, Y., & Park, E. (2020). Social acceptance of nuclear power plants in Korea: The role of public perceptions following the Fukushima accident. *Renewable and Sustainable Energy Reviews, 128*, 109894. https://doi.org/10.1016/j.rser.2020.109894

Jbaily, A., Zhou, X., Liu, J., Lee, T.-H., Kamareddine, L., Verguet, S., & Dominici, F. (2022). Air pollution exposure disparities across US population and income groups. *Nature, 601*(7892), 228–233. https://doi.org/10.1038/s41586-021-04190-y

Jones, R. (2019). Climate change and Indigenous health promotion. *Global Health Promotion, 26*(Suppl 3), 73–81. https://doi.org/10.1177/1757975919829713

Kershaw, S., Gower, S., Rinner, C., & Campbell, M. (2013). Identifying inequitable exposure to toxic air pollution in racialized and low-income neighbourhoods to support pollution prevention. *Geospatial Health, 7*(2), 265–278. https://doi.org/10.4081/gh.2013.85

Kolb, K. H. (2021). *Retail inequality: Reframing the food desert debate*. University of California Press.

Kurjata, A. (2017, December 14). *Tension escalates in Haida Gwaii forestry dispute*. CBC News. https://www.cbc.ca/news/canada/british-columbia/forestry-haida-gwaii-cuts-1.4449770

The Lancet. (2021). Health in a world of extreme heat. *The Lancet, 398*(10301), 641. https://doi.org/10.1016/S0140-6736(21)01860-2

Leahy, S. (2019, April 11). This is the world's most destructive oil operation—and it's growing. *National Geographic*. https://www.nationalgeographic.com/environment/article/alberta-canadas-tar-sands-is-growing-but-indigenous-people-fight-back

Lerner, S. (2020, April 19). *Africa's exploding plastic nightmare: As Africa drowns in garbage, the plastics business keeps booming*. The Intercept. https://theintercept.com/2020/04/19/africa-plastic-waste-kenya-ethiopia/

Lewis, D., Williams, L., & Jones, R. (2020). A radical revision of the public health response to environmental crisis in a warming world: Contributions of Indigenous knowledges and Indigenous feminist perspectives. *Canadian Journal of Public Health, 111*(6), 897–900. https://doi.org/10.17269/s41997-020-00388-1

Li, H. O.-Y., Bailey, A. J.-M., Grose, E., McDonald, J. T., Quimby, A., Johnson-Obaseki, S., & Nessim, C. (2021). Socioeconomic status and melanoma in Canada: A systematic review. *Journal of Cutaneous Medicine and Surgery, 25*(1), 87–94. https://doi.org/10.1177/1203475420960426

Linnitt, C. (2014, July 7). *"Alarming" new study finds contaminants in animals downstream of oilsands*. The Narwhal. https://thenarwhal.ca/alarming-new-study-finds-contaminants-animals-downstream-oilsands/

Lisitza, A., & Wolbring, G. (2018). EcoHealth and the determinants of health: Perspectives of a small subset of Canadian academics in the EcoHealth community. *International Journal of Environmental Research and Public Health, 15*(8), 1688. https://doi.org/10.3390/ijerph15081688

Long, M. A., Gonçalves, L., Stretesky, P. B., & Defeyter, M. A. (2020). Food insecurity in advanced capitalist nations: A review. *Sustainability, 12*(9), 3654. https://doi.org/10.3390/su12093654

Loo, T. (2010). Africville and the dynamics of state power in postwar Canada. *Acadiensis, 39*(2), 23–47. https://www.jstor.org/stable/41803299

MacDonald, E., & Rang, S. (2007). *Exposing Canada's Chemical Valley: An investigation of cumulative air pollution emissions in the Sarnia, Ontario area*. Ecojustice. https://ecojustice.ca/wp-content/uploads/2015/09/2007-Exposing-Canadas-Chemial-Valley.pdf

Malin, S. (2021). Examining the Anthropocene: A contested term in capitalist times. In S. Ryder, K. Powlen, M. Laituri, S. Malin, J. Sbicca, & D. Stevis (Eds.), *Environmental Justice in the Anthropocene* (pp. 10–18). Routledge.

Martin, A. (2023). *The "disposable others": Settler colonial processes of industrial pollution in Cancer Alley, Louisiana, 1964–2023* (Publication No. 30484487) [Master's thesis, The University of North Carolina]. ProQuest Dissertations Publishing.

Marlatt, V. L., Bayen, S., Castaneda-Cortès, D., Delbès, G., Grigorova, P., Langlois, V. S., Martyniuk, C. J., Metcalfe, C. D., Parent, L., Rwigemera, A., Thomson, P., & Van Der Kraak, G. (2022). Impacts of endocrine disrupting chemicals on reproduction in wildlife and humans. *Environmental Research, 208*, 112584. https://doi.org/10.1016/j.envres.2021.112584

Marx, K. (2019). *Capital: Volume 1, A critique of political economy.* Dover Publications. (Original work published 1867)

McGibbon, E. (2021). Embodied oppression: The social, ecological and structural determinants of health. In W. Antony & J. Antony (Eds.), *Power and resistance: Critical thinking about Canadian social issues* (7th ed., pp. 452–492). Fernwood Publishing.

McGibbon, E. (In press). The Anthropocene: Collisions with the social determinants of health. In T. Bryant (Ed.), *Handbook of the social determinants of health.* Edward Elgar Publishing.

McGuire, W., Holtmaat, E. A., & Prakash, A. (2022). Penalties for industrial accidents: The impact of the Deepwater Horizon accident on BP's reputation and stock market returns. *PLoS ONE, 17*(6), e0268743. https://doi.org/10.1371/journal.pone.0268743

McLachlan, S. M. (2014a). *Environmental and human health implications of the Athabasca Oil Sands for the Mikisew Cree First Nation and Athabasca Chipewyan First Nation in Northern Alberta: Phase two report.* Clayton H. Riddell Faculty of Environment, Earth and Resources, University of Manitoba.

McLachlan, S. M. (2014b). *"Water is a living thing": Environmental and human health implications of the Athabasca Oil Sands for the Mikisew Cree First Nation and Athabasca Chipewyan First Nation in Northern Alberta.* Environmental Conservation Laboratory.

McPhearson, T., Raymond, C. M., Gulsrud, N., Albert, C., Coles, N., Fagerholm, N., Nagatsu, M., Olafsson, A. S., Soininen, N., & Vierikko, K. (2021). Radical changes are needed for transformations to a good Anthropocene. *npj Urban Sustainability, 1*(1), 5. https://doi.org/10.1038/s42949-021-00017-x

Meadows, D. H., Meadows, D. L., Randers, J., & Behrens III, W. W. (1972). *The limits to growth.* Club of Rome.

Mi, E., Mi, E., & Jeggo, M. (2016). Where to now for One Health and EcoHealth? *EcoHealth, 13*(1), 12–17. https://doi.org/10.1007/s10393-016-1112-1

Minkow, D. (2017, April 6). *What you need to know about fracking in Canada*. The Narwhal. https://thenarwhal.ca/what-is-fracking-in-canada/

Mirzabaev, A., Wu, J., Evans, J., García-Oliva, F., Hussein, I. A. G., Iqbal, M. M., Kimutai, J., Knowles, T., Meza, F., Nedjraoui, D., Tena, F., Türkeş, M., Vázquez, R. J., & Weltz, M. (2019). Desertification. In P. R. Shukla, J. Skea, E. Calvo Buendia, V. Masson-Delmotte, H.-O. Pörtner, D. C. Roberts, P. Zhai, R. Slade, S. Connors, R. van Diemen, M. Ferrat, E. Haughey, S. Luz, S. Neogi, M. Pathak, J. Petzold, J. Portugal Pereira, P. Vyas, E. Huntley, ... J. Malley (Eds.), *Climate change and land: International Panel on Climate Change (IPCC) special report on climate change, desertification, land degradation, sustainable land management, food security, and greenhouse gas fluxes in terrestrial ecosystems* (pp. 249–343). IPPC. https://doi.org/10.1017/9781009157988.005

Mizutani, J. (2019). In the backyard of segregated neighborhoods: an environmental justice case study of Louisiana. *Georgetown Environmental Law Review, 31*, 363–390. https://ssrn.com/abstract=4607301

Moore, J. W. (2017). The Capitalocene, Part I: On the nature and origins of our ecological crisis. *The Journal of Peasant Studies, 44*(3), 594–630. https://doi.org/10.1080/03066150.2016.1235036

National Cancer Institute. (2021). *State cancer profiles, 2016–2020*. https://statecancerprofiles.cancer.gov/map/map.withimage.php?00&state&001&001&28&0&02&0&1&5&0#results

National Collaborating Centre for Indigenous Health (NCCIH). (2022a). Climate Change and Indigenous People's health in Canada. Reprinted with permission from P. Berry & R. Schnitter (Eds.), *Health of Canadians in a changing climate: Advancing our knowledge for action* (pp. 53–113). Government of Canada.

National Collaborating Centre for Indigenous Health. (2022b). *Podcast—Voices from the field 20—Climate change and Indigenous Peoples' health in Canada* [Audio]. https://www.nccih.ca/495/Podcast_-_Voices_from_the_Field_20_-_Climate_change_and_Indigenous_Peoples%E2%80%99_Health_in_Canada.nccih?id=10369

National Geographic. (2023). *Earth's systems*. https://education.nationalgeographic.org/resource/earths-systems/

Nelson, B., & Kaminsky, D. B. (2021). A growing drive to get rid of cancer-linked "forever chemicals": As concern mounts over the health effects of a huge and ubiquitous family of persistent organic compounds, researchers are making headway on remediation strategies despite uncertainties over costs and regulations. *Cancer Cytopathology, 129*(1), 7–8. https://doi.org/10.1002/cncy.22403

Nelson, J. J. (2000). The space of Africville: Creating, regulating and remembering the urban "slum." *Canadian Journal of Law and Society/La Revue Canadienne Droit et Société, 15*(2), 163–185. https://doi.org/10.1017/S0829320100006402

Neubauer, R. (2011). Manufacturing junk: Think tanks, climate denial, and neoliberal hegemony. *Australian Journal of Communication, 38*(3), 65–88.

Nickerson, C. (1999, May 12). Hoping blight makes might: Cape Breton town seeks role as toxic waste learning site. *Boston Globe.*

Niranjan, A. (2023, November 8). 2023 on track to be the hottest year on record, say scientists. *The Guardian.* https://www.theguardian.com/environment/2023/nov/08/2023-on-track-to-be-the-hottest-year-on-record-say-scientists

Noor, D. (2024, February 15). "They lied": Plastics producers deceived public about recycling, report reveals. *The Guardian.* https://www.theguardian.com/us-news/2024/feb/15/recycling-plastics-producers-report

Nyabola, N. (2023, April 18). Nothing encapsulates the false promise of capitalism like plastic. *The Nation.* https://www.thenation.com/article/environment/plastic-recycling-capitalism/

Okello, A. (2020). One Health: A cross-sectoral, holistic approach to reduce disease risk and build resilience. In *Development Co-operation Report 2020: Learning from crises, building resilience* (pp. 175–182). OECD. https://www.oecd-ilibrary.org/sites/8913694e-en/index.html?itemId=/content/component/8913694e-en

Oppermann, S. (2018). The scale of the Anthropocene. *Mosaic: An Interdisciplinary Critical Journal, 51*(3), 1–17. https://www.jstor.org/stable/26974107

Organisation for Economic Co-operation and Development (OECD). (2023). *Gross domestic product (GDP).* https://data.oecd.org/gdp/gross-domestic-product-gdp.htm

Panagos, P., Van Liedekerke, M., Yigini, Y., & Montanarella, L. (2013). Contaminated sites in Europe: Review of the current situation based on data collected through a European network. *Journal of Environmental and Public Health, 2013*(1), 158764. https://doi.org/10.1155/2013/158764

Panieri, E., Baralic, K., Djukic-Cosic, D., Buha Djordjevic, A., & Saso, L. (2022). PFAS molecules: A major concern for the human health and the environment. *Toxics, 10*(2), 44. https://doi.org/10.3390/toxics10020044

Parfitt, B. (2019, August 14). *The battle for Haida Gwaii's cedars.* The Narwhal. https://thenarwhal.ca/battle-haida-gwaiis-cedars/

Patnaik, P. (2017). *Neo-liberal capitalism and its crisis.* International Development Economics Associates. https://www.networkideas.org/news-analysis/2017/10/neo-liberal-capitalism/

Pell, R. S., Wall, F., Yan, X., & Bailey, G. (2019). Applying and advancing the economic resource scarcity potential (ESP) method for rare earth elements. *Resources Policy, 62*(C), 472–481. https://doi.org/10.1016/j.resourpol.2018.10.003

Prescott, S. L., Logan, A. C., Albrecht, G., Campbell, D. E., Crane, J., Cunsolo, A., Holloway, J. W., Kozyrskyj, A. L., Lowry, C. A., Penders, J., Redvers, N., Renz, H., Stokholm, J., Svanes, C., Wegienka, G., & on Behalf of inVIVO Planetary Health, of the Worldwide Universities Network (WUN). (2018). The Canmore declaration: Statement of principles for planetary health. *Challenges, 9*(2), 31. https://doi.org/10.3390/challe9020031

Province of British Columbia. (2018). *Ecosystems*. https://www2.gov.bc.ca/gov/content/environment/plants-animals-ecosystems/ecosystems

Pynn, L. (2010, November 17). *Lyell Island: 25 years later.* Wilderness Committee. https://www.wildernesscommittee.org/news/lyell-island-25-years-later

Ratima, M., Martin, D., Castleden, H., & Delormier, T. (2019). Indigenous voices and knowledge systems–Promoting planetary health, health equity, and sustainable development now and for future generations. *Global Health Promotion, 26*(Suppl 3), 3–5. https://doi.org/10.1177/1757975919838487

Riahi, A., & McSorley, T. (2013). "Another layer of colonialism": Resource extraction, toxic pollution and First Nations. *The Free Library*. https://www.thefreelibrary.com/%22Another+layer+of+colonialism%22%3a+resource+extraction%2c+toxic+pollution...-a0354262781

Rigolon, A., Browning, H. E. M., McAnirlin, O., & Yoon, H. (2021). Green space and health equity: A systematic review on the potential of green space to reduce health disparities. *International Journal of Environmental Research and Public Health, 18*(5), 2563. https://doi.org/10.3390/ijerph18052563

Robeson, B. (2019). *Food deserts debunked and decentered: From deficit to relational mapping for food justice in Worcester, MA* (Publication No. 238) [Master's paper, Clark University]. International Development, Community and Environment (IDCE). https://commons.clarku.edu/idce_masters_papers/238

Sakhvidi, M. J. Z., Lequy, E., Goldberg, M., & Jacquemin, B. (2020). Air pollution exposure and kidney and urinary tract cancer risk: A systematic review. *Environmental Pollution, 267*, 115328. https://doi.org/10.1016/j.envpol.2020.115328

Saleem, F. (2023, January 12). 5 biggest natural resources companies in the world. *Insider Monkey*. https://www.insidermonkey.com/blog/5-biggest-natural-resources-companies-in-the-world-1107078

Saverino, K. C., Routman, E., Lookingbill, T. R., Eanes, A. M., Hoffman, J. S., & Bao, R. (2021). Thermal inequity in Richmond, VA: The effect of an unjust evolution of the urban landscape on urban heat islands. *Sustainability, 13*(3), 1511. https://doi.org/10.3390/su13031511

Shin, S. H., Kim, H. O., & Rim, K. T. (2019). Worker safety in the rare earth elements recycling process from the review of toxicity and issues. *Safety and Health at Work, 10*(4), 409–419. https://doi.org/10.1016/j.shaw.2019.08.005

Sullivan, L. (2020, September 11). How Big Oil misled the public into believing plastic would be recycled. *National Public Radio*. https://www.npr.org/2020/09/11/897692090/how-big-oil-misled-the-public-into-believing-plastic-would-be-recycled

Teach Democracy. (n.d.). *A brief history of Jim Crow*. https://www.crf-usa.org//black-history-month/a-brief-history-of-jim-crow

Thacharodi, A., Meenatchi, R., Hassan, S., Hussain, N., Bhat, M. A., Arockiaraj, J., Ngo, H. H., Le, Q. H., & Pugazhendhi, A. (2024). Microplastics in the environment: A critical overview on its fate, toxicity, implications, management, and bioremediation strategies. *Journal of Environmental Management, 349*, 119433. https://doi.org/10.1016/j.jenvman.2023.119433

Tijani, J. O., Fatoba, O. O., Babajide, O. O, & Petrik, L. F. (2016). Pharmaceuticals, endocrine disruptors, personal care products, nanomaterials and perfluorinated pollutants: A review. *Environmental Chemistry Letters, 14*, 27–49. https://doi.org/10.1007/s10311-015-0537-z

Tootonsab, Z. (2021). *Where water hits home: Colonial technologies of violence on IBPOC peoples and nonhuman nature in Canada* [Master's thesis]. University of Alberta. https://doi.org/10.7939/r3-kqg0-zr39

Turner, M. C., Andersen, Z. J., Baccarelli, A., Diver, W. R., Gapstur, S. M., Pope III, C. A., Prada, D., Samet, J., Thurston, G., & Cohen, A. (2020). Outdoor air pollution and cancer: An overview of the current evidence and public health recommendations. *CA: A Cancer Journal for Clinicians, 70*(6), 460–479. https://doi.org/10.3322/caac.21632

Uchimiya, M., Bannon, D., Nakanishi, H., McBride, M. B., Williams, M. A., & Yoshihara, T. (2020). Chemical speciation, plant uptake, and toxicity of heavy metals in agricultural soils. *Journal of Agricultural and Food Chemistry, 68*(46), 12856–12869. https://doi.org/10.1021/acs.jafc.0c00183

United Nations (UN). (1994). *United Nations convention to combat desertification.*

United Nations. (2018). *World water development report 2018.* https://www.unwater.org/publications/world-water-development-report-2018

United Nations. (2023). Progress towards the sustainable development goals: Towards a rescue plan for people and planet. Report of the Secretary-General (Special Edition). https://unstats.un.org/sdgs/report/2023/

United Nations Children's Fund (UNICEF). (2011). *Water, sanitation, and hygiene.* http://www.unicef.org/wash/

United Nations Development Program (UNDP). (n.d.). *Human Development Index (HDI).* Human Development Reports. https://hdr.undp.org/data-center/human-development-index#/indicies/HDI

United Nations Educational, Scientific and Cultural Organization (UNESCO). (2023, March 22). *Imminent risk of a global water crisis, warns the UN World Water Development Report 2023.* https://www.unesco.org/en/articles/imminent-risk-global-water-crisis-warns-un-world-water-development-report-2023

United Nations Environmental Programme (UNEP). (2015). *Options for decoupling economic growth from water use and water pollution: A report of the Water Working Group of the International Resource Panel.* https://www.resourcepanel.org/reports/options-decoupling-economic-growth-water-use-and-water-pollution

United Nations News. (2020, July 21). *Deforestation has slowed down but still remains a concern, new UN report reveals.* https://news.un.org/en/story/2020/07/1068761

United States Environmental Protection Agency (USEPA). (2016). *Hydraulic fracturing for oil and gas: Impacts from the hydraulic fracturing water cycle on drinking water resources in the United States*. https://cfpub.epa.gov/ncea/hfstudy/recordisplay.cfm?deid=332990

United States Environmental Protection Agency. (2023, September 6). *Summary of the Oil Pollution Act*. https://www.epa.gov/laws-regulations/summary-oil-pollution-act

Vareda, J. P., Valente, A. J. M., & Durães, L. (2019). Assessment of heavy metal pollution from anthropogenic activities and remediation strategies: A review. *Journal of Environmental Management, 246*, 101–118. https://doi.org/10.1016/j.jenvman.2019.05.126

Vertefeuille, K. (2022). *The detrimental effects of forever chemicals*. Digital Commons at Sacred Heart University. https://digitalcommons.sacredheart.edu/acadfest/2022/all/29/

Walker, T. R., & MacAskill, D. (2014). Monitoring water quality in Sydney Harbour using blue mussels during remediation of the Sydney Tar Ponds, Nova Scotia, Canada. *Environmental Monitoring and Assessment, 186*(3), 1623–1638. https://doi.org/10.1007/s10661-013-3479-6

Warner, M. E. (2021). Key issues in water privatization and remunicipalization. *Utilities Policy, 73*, 101300. https://doi.org/10.1016/j.jup.2021.101300

Waters, C. N., Zalasiewicz, J., Summerhayes, C., Barnosky, A. D., Poirier, C., Gałuszka, A., Cearreta, A., Edgeworth, M., Ellis, E. C., Ellis, M., Jeandel, C., Leinfelder, R., McNeill, J. R., Richter, D. D., Steffen, W., Syvitski, J., Vidas, D., Wagreich, M., Williams, M., … Wolfe, A. P. (2016). The Anthropocene is functionally and stratigraphically distinct from the Holocene. *Science, 351*(6269). https://doi.org/10.1126/science.aad2622

Watts, N., Amann, M., Arnell, N., Ayeb-Karlsson, S., Belesova, K., Boykoff, M., Byass, P., Cai, W., Campbell-Lendrum, D., Capstick, S., Chambers, J., Dalin, C., Daly, M., Dasandi, N., Davies, M., Drummond, P., Dubrow, R., Ebi, K. L., Eckelman, M., … Montgomery, H. (2019). The 2019 report of *The Lancet* Countdown on health and climate change: Ensuring that the health of a child born today is not defined by a changing climate. *The Lancet, 394*(10211), 1836–1878. https://doi.org/10.1016/S0140-6736(19)32596-6

Westman, C. N., & Joly, T. L. (2019). Oil sands extraction in Alberta, Canada: A review of impacts and processes concerning Indigenous peoples. *Human Ecology, 47*(2), 233–243. https://www.jstor.org/stable/45154288

Wild Conservation Society & Rockefeller University. (2004, September 29). *One world, one health: Building interdisciplinary bridges to health in a "globalized world."* Symposium, Manhattan, NY, USA. http://www.oneworldonehealth.org/sept2004/owoh_sept04.html

Wilson, L. (2020, May 13). *New Haida Nation tree cutting agreement with province protects "monumental cedars."* APTN News. https://www.aptnnews.ca/national-news/new-haida-nation-tree-cutting-agreement-with-province-protects-monumental-cedars/

Wong, K. M., & Howman, J. (Creators). (n.d.) *The chemical valley project.* Broadleaf Creative. http://www.broadleaftheatre.com/chemical-valley-project

World Health Organization (WHO). (1986). *Ottawa Charter for Health Promotion.*

World Health Organization (2017). *Guidelines for drinking-water quality* (4th ed.).

World Meteorological Organization (WMO). (2023, April 21). *WMO annual report highlights continuous advance of climate change.* https://wmo.int/news/media-centre/wmo-annual-report-highlights-continuous-advance-of-climate-change

World Wildlife Fund. (2020). Chapter one: An SOS for nature. In R. E. A. Almond, M. Grooten, & T. Petersen (Eds.), *Living Planet Report 2020: Bending the curve of biodiversity loss.*

Xue, Y., Wang, L., Zhang, Y., Zhao, Y., & Liu, Y. (2022). Air pollution: A culprit of lung cancer. *Journal of Hazardous Materials, 434*, 128937. https://doi.org/10.1016/j.jhazmat.2022.128937

Yadav, D. S., Jaiswal, B., Gautam, M., & Agrawal, M. (2020). Soil acidification and its impact on plants. In P. Singh, S. K. Singh, & S. M. Prasad (Eds.), *Plant responses to soil pollution* (pp. 1–26). Springer.

Yang, M., Wang, H., & Qiu, F. (2020). Neighbourhood food environments revisited: When food deserts meet food swamps. *Canadian Geographies/Géographies canadiennes, 64*(1), 135–154. https://doi.org/10.1111/cag.12570

Yusoff, K. (2018). *A billion black Anthropocenes or none.* University of Minnesota Press.

Zhao, Q., Guo, Y., Ye, T., Gasparrini, A., Tong, S., Overcenco, A., Urban A., Schneider, A., Entezari, A., Vicedo-Cabrera, A. M., Zanobetti, A., Analitis, A., Zeka, A., Tobias, A., Nunes, B., Alahmad, B., Armstrong, B., Forsberg, B., Pan, S.-C., ... Li, S. (2021). Global, regional, and national burden of mortality associated with non-optimal ambient temperatures from 2000 to 2019: A three-stage modelling study. *The Lancet Planetary Health, 5*(7), e415–e425. https://doi.org/10.1016/S2542-5196(21)00081-4

Zeng, X., & Li, J. (2021). Emerging anthropogenic circularity science: Principles, practices, and challenges. *iScience, 24*(3), 102237. https://doi.org/10.1016/j.isci.2021.102237

Zinsstag, J. (2012). Convergence of ecohealth and one health. *EcoHealth, 9*(4), 371–373. https://doi.org/10.1007%2Fs10393-013-0812-z

Zucco, M. (2022). *Settler colonialism and the movement towards Indigenous forest sovereignty* [Honours thesis]. University of Nebraska-Lincoln.

CHAPTER 5

Structural Determinants of Health: Root Cause Politics

CHAPTER OBJECTIVES

Using as many examples as possible:

1. Identify and describe four forms of power related to the structural DoH.
2. Identify and describe key political DoH: neoliberal epidemics, worker unionization, the commercial DoH, and the digital DoH.
3. Describe what is meant by colonialism and white supremacy as structural DoH.
4. Describe social murder and necropolitics as important forms of structural violence.
5. Describe what is meant by slow violence as an important form of structural violence.

CRITICAL THINKING QUESTIONS

1. What are some examples of how the invisible power of the structural DoH is so difficult to "see"?
2. What are some neoliberal epidemics not discussed in this chapter?
3. If unionization as a political DoH has been systematically proven to improve population health outcomes, what might be some of the reasons why unionization rates are decreasing globally?

4. How might Achille Mbembe's (2003) concept of necropolitics be a form of social murder?
5. How might slow violence be related to social murder?

INTRODUCTION

This chapter explores the societal structures and patterns that determine health. The systemic nature of structural DoH and their connections to the social and ecological DoH are explained. The aim is not to provide a definitive explanation of the structural DoH because the definitions are emergent—changing quickly as increasing emphasis is placed on how critical perspectives (e.g., in social, health, Earth, and data sciences; and the humanities) can inform our understandings of structural power, how it can threaten health, and how it can inform mobilization for change. The chapter begins with an explanation of three important forms of structural power: visible power, hidden power, and invisible power. These dimensions of power are applied to a case example of sexualized violence on university campuses, a pressing structural DoH that has profound impacts across the social DoH. Central structural DoH are then described, including the political DoH (e.g., neoliberal epidemics, worker unionization); the commercial, corporate DoH; the digital DoH; and colonialism and white supremacy as DoH. Although these DoH are described somewhat separately, they are continuously interconnected—distinct but interacting.

The second half of the chapter focuses on the inherent violence perpetrated by these structural DoH. The origins of the term *structural violence* are described, along with details of its current impacts on human and planet health. The resurgence of Engels' (2009) concept of social murder is explained with two main case examples: 1) the Grenfell Tower fire in West London and 2) the political economy of increasing infant mortality in rich countries. The structural violence of necropolitics is then described with a focus on the genocide of Indigenous (First Nations, Inuit, Métis) Peoples in Canada. The chapter concludes with an explanation of the foundational concept of slow violence and its implications for persistent environmental destruction and related injustices across the social DoH.

FORMS OF POWER AND THE STRUCTURAL DETERMINANTS OF HEALTH

The structural DoH are the systemic or root causes of health inequities and injustices across all life on Earth, and the health of Earth itself. Structural includes the political, economic, and social structures of society, including the culture that supports or justifies them (Navarro, 2007). The structural determinants involve explicit examination of the roles of systemic power processes in the creation and perpetuation of inequities in the distribution of the DoH in the current global polycrisis. More specifically, there is a focus on the ways that these determinants are framed and organized by dominant power structures, such as political and economic systems and institutions. Each of the structural determinants described in this chapter involve use and abuse of power across intersecting and synergistic networks, such as power involving public policy–caused infant death or white privilege and supremacy and related colonialism-caused modern genocide of Indigenous Peoples. Following along with the seaside wharf analogy in Chapter 1, these power structures are underneath the surface of what we can "see"—they are hidden from view. Gaventa (2006) describes how **visible power** is the conventional understanding of power that is negotiated through formal rules and structures, institutions, and procedures (e.g., institutional governing boards, elected officials, members of parliament, and so on). In contrast, **hidden power** focuses on the actual controls over decision making and the ways certain powerful people and institutions maintain their influence over the process and often exclude and devalue concerns and agendas of less powerful groups (Nash et al., 2006).

Invisible power is also known as internalized power, including lack of power. This power operates by influencing how individuals think of their place in society and explains why some are prevented from questioning existing power relations (Nash et al., 2006). Visible conflict is hidden through internalization of powerlessness or lack of awareness (e.g., internalized powerlessness in the workplace, women's internalized sexism, internalized racism for racialized peoples). Internalized power also involves the power of internalized privilege (e.g., male, white, heterosexual) that invisibly entitles the more powerful to enact power over the less powerful. Table 5.1 illustrates visible, hidden, and invisible

Table 5.1: Forms of Structural Power: Sexualized Violence on University Campuses

Form of Power	Description	Structural DoH Application
Visible Power	Involves formal laws, policies, rules, structures, institutions, and procedures of decision making and the people who ensure that the rules are kept, or not kept (e.g., police, government officials, boards of directors).	Rates of sexualized violence on university campuses are steadily increasing (Linder et al., 2020). Many universities have formal policies and procedures (e.g., searchable documents on university websites) to ensure that the "rules are kept." Certain university officials are formally designated to oversee this process.
Hidden Power	Powerful people (including those who make the laws, policies, rules) may exert their power even when they are not physically present. This may influence the behaviour of others. This process acts as a means of excluding others or maintaining privileged entry by certain people to decision making, governance, and public spaces, including those where "public participation" is ostensibly mandated.	Behind-the-scenes power to ignore the rules is a hidden form of power. It is not visible in universities' formal rules, meeting minutes, marketing images, etc. This hidden power deeply supports universities' normalization of cultures of sexualized violence. Changing these norms requires that activists find a way to claim space in university decision-making structures, where they are either formally or informally excluded.
Invisible Power	We internalize the norms, values, and culture of our society. This may lead to individuals unconsciously controlling their own behaviour to meet social and institutional expectations. This process might involve not being able to act or not feeling that it is legitimate for them to act. Internalized power also involves the power of internalized privilege (e.g., male, white, heterosexual) that invisibly entitles the powerful to enact power over the less powerful.	This process involves internalized privilege and power, causing institutional decision makers to feel entitled to ignore and/or actively dismiss the dissenting voices of those who join the decades-long protests of sexualized violence on campus. Here, power also involves the structural power of patriarchal and colonialist systems. These forms of power provide the substantive and invisibly embedded contexts for sexualized violence.

Source: Nash et al., 2006 (Form of Power and Description); Author (Structural DoH Application).

forms of structural power operating in the context of sexualized violence on university campuses. This kind of violence is an especially good illustrative example, in part because it is so normalized, and therefore difficult to "see," whether it occurs in university settings or anywhere else. Linder et al. (2020) used a power-conscious, root-cause framework to interpret findings across 540 peer-reviewed articles about sexualized violence against women. Findings indicated that 1) most scholarship focuses on victims, rather than perpetrators of sexual violence, leaving significant gaps in effectively eradicating campus sexual violence (perpetrators remain largely invisible as discursive subjects), and 2) campus sexual violence research primarily focuses on white, cisgender, heterosexual college women as victims of sexual violence (Linder et al., 2020). These findings reflect historical and current intersecting power structures of patriarchy, misogyny, and colonialism. Despite decades of resistance and gains in terms of human rights, including the rights of women, these forms of power persist and in many cases are increasing, as is the case with growing hatred and exclusion of trans people in many jurisdictions (Walters et al., 2020). They also illustrate the insidiousness of structural power and the cohesive machinery/apparatus that supports it.

These structural forms of power are embedded across the structural DoH. Visible power in areas such as the political DoH is more readily identifiable, such as elected officials in the various political parties. However, due to its hidden nature, it is much more difficult to trace or make a map of the political processes and decision making that cause the structural DoH described in the following sections.

KEY STRUCTURAL DETERMINANTS OF HEALTH

The structural DoH form the hidden scaffolding of power that determines health, including planetary health. It is important to note that each of the structural determinants discussed here is a stand-alone field of study in and of itself. There are many ways to bring them all together and the configuration chosen for this chapter is by no means conclusive. It is a starting point for explaining the distinct but interacting machinery that operates to produce human and planetary health damage.

The political DoH include 1) neoliberal epidemics, due to their measurable population-wide, serious impacts on health; 2) worker unionization, due to the power of unions to improve population health, and the power of neoliberal governance structures to disrupt or damage worker rights; 3) the commercial/corporate DoH because commodification and marketing of consumer products have significant health and economic consequences that ultimately must be tackled with policy-based, structural solutions; and 4) digital technologies, due to their impact on already-existing, policy-created health and social inequities, and their threats to democracy. Colonialism and white privilege are foundational DoH because they are the cause of historical and current political DoH that exploit Indigenous land and resources to buttress economic gain for governments, corporations, and wealthy, powerful individuals.

Political Determinants of Health

The political DoH are sometimes referred to as the political-economic DoH because politics and economics are inseparable, as described in the political economy of health discussions in Chapter 2. They involve understanding health as a political choice, which requires an analysis of how power processes, interests, and ideological positions impact health (Kickbusch, 2015). This analysis requires mapping power within political systems and cultures, and at different levels of governance. As early as 2005, Bambra et al. (2005) stated that health is political because

1. Like any other resource or commodity under a neoliberal economic system, some social groups have more of it than others;
2. Its social determinants are amenable to political interventions and are thereby dependent on political action (or more usually, inaction);
3. The right to "a standard of living adequate for health and well-being" (United Nations, 1948) is, or should be, an aspect of citizenship and a human right (p. 187).

There is growing interest in the connections between politics and health, described almost 20 years ago by Kickbusch (2005) as the political DoH.

Citing the first edition of Global Health Watch's Alternative Health Report (People's Health Movement et al., 2005), Kickbusch critiqued prevailing notions of global health and called for a new alignment with other citizens' rights movements for global social justice. "Instead, the world needs a new policy model based on entitlement, in which good health is an integral part of social, economic, and cultural rights and citizenship, and is ensured as a global public good" (Kickbusch, 2005, p. 246). Ten years later, Kickbusch (2015) emphasized the importance of politicization of health at all levels of governance—within governments, global institutions, the private sector, and through civil society organizations. In 2014, the Lancet–Oslo University Commission on Global Health (Ottersen et al., 2014) called for global political solutions to decrease health inequities, stating that "norms, policies, and practices that arise from transnational interaction should be understood as political DoH that cause and maintain health inequities" (p. 630).

> The time is right to engage in a serious joint intellectual endeavour to further explore the political DoH. It can bring together work that is being done under various headings: politics of health, global health, political epidemiology, health political science, and political economy of health. Above all it requires a willingness to bring together a public health perspective reared on causality, evidence, determinants, and interventions with a lens that deals with the nature of power, systems, wicked problems, uncertainty, and complexity. (Kickbusch, 2015, p. 2)

Political DoH are framed, organized, implemented, and redeployed by dominant systems and institutions. Emphasis is on the role of the economic organization of society in the production and distribution of disease and the burden of illness and the ways that disease and illness, and wellness itself, are framed and treated (Coburn, 2010).

Neoliberal Epidemics

In Chapter 2, two major welfare-state policy approaches were discussed: social democratic and neoliberal political economies. Based in the tenets of neoliberalism, Schrecker (2016a, 2016b) and Schrecker and Bambra

(2015) described population-wide epidemics resulting from neoliberal policy structures, such as the austerity measures that caused inequality and health damage for a whole generation of children in countries such as the United Kingdom. "Epidemics" was used to describe these phenomena because they have been transmitted so quickly across populations, and on a global scale that if they were a biological contagion they would be considered as having epidemic proportions (Schrecker & Bambra, 2015). Austerity measures put in place as a result of the 2008 global financial crisis produced, and are still producing, epidemic-scale and measurable impacts, such as significant increases in child poverty (Barnett & Bagshaw, 2020; Taylor-Robinson et al., 2019), unemployment (Barnett & Bagshaw, 2020), malnutrition, scurvy (Hill, 2023), and resurgence of Victorian era diseases such as rickets (Chanchlani et al., 2020), as described in Chapter 2. For Schrecker and Bambra (2015), reversing neoliberal epidemics demands policies supporting "a state that is more willing to challenge the values of the unfettered marketplace in order to increase and equalize opportunities for everyone to lead healthy lives" (p. 120).

Also prominent among neoliberal epidemics is neoliberalism's impact on the global food supply, including food production and distribution. In his groundbreaking book, *The Neoliberal Diet*, Otero (2018) describes how free-market governance leads to replacement of traditional agriculture and healthful diets by commodity agriculture and ultra-processed (junk) foods. The neoliberal diet results in cheaper and more convenient diets, but at high cost to health and society across the globe. The health costs include Type 2 diabetes and other chronic diseases for millions of people globally; the social costs are also devastating, resulting in loss of subsistence farms, depopulation of farming communities, rural-to-urban migration, low-wage employment, and greater economic inequity (Otero, 2018).

The neoliberal food regime is characterized by trade liberalization and other state and supra-state regulatory structures and legal frameworks that favour large corporations, such as the food processors and agribusiness multinationals that profit from the proliferation of the neoliberal diet (Big Food)—the globalization of food production means that the neoliberal diet is globally consolidated as it becomes disseminated to nations in the Global South, thus deepening its epidemic proportions (Otero et al., 2018). Importantly, the neoliberal diet cuts across class lines as people with lower socioeconomic status are significantly more likely to buy health-damaging junk food because they do not have sufficient money to buy healthier food (Otero et al., 2018). The evidence is sufficiently strong to warrant naming the neoliberal diet as a form of food oppression—structurally-induced subordination that builds on, and deepens, pre-existing social inequities along class lines (Freeman, 2007; Otero et al., 2018). The most recent *Global Health Watch Alternative Health Report, Health Watch 6* (Bloomsbury Publishing, 2022) now has the goal of targeting neoliberalism as the key driver of global health damage, thus clarifying the target of mobilization for change in current health and climate emergencies. Not surprisingly, neoliberal epidemics have also been directly linked to many of the other structural DoH described in this chapter: commercial, corporate DoH (e.g., mass promotion of products that are health-damaging), digital DoH (e.g., generation of profits by influencing patterns of health, disease, disability, and death), and social murder (e.g., increasing infant mortality).

Worker Unionization Rates

Unionization rates are an important political DoH across OECD countries. Leigh and Chakalov (2021) conducted a systematic review of studies from the United States, Europe, and Canada from 1980 to April 1, 2021. Researchers used the Healthy People 2020's five domains for the social DoH (National Center for Health Statistics, 2020) to assess the impacts of unionization rates on economic stability, education, health and health care, neighbourhood and built environment, and social and community context. Findings demonstrated that unions

1. Lower wage inequality;
2. Increase wages, especially for low-wage workers, and reduce within-firm inequality compared to non-union workplaces;
3. Increase paid sick leave;
4. Decrease dangerous safety or environmental hazards;

5. Decrease fatal injuries;
6. Increase right-to-know hazards and right-to-refuse dangerous work, and have light duty after injury;
7. Increase employer-provided health insurance; and
8. Increase vacation leave, either with or without pay. (Leigh & Chakalov, 2021)

Findings also indicated that unionized workers are 53.9 percent more likely to have employer-provided pensions, and unionized workplaces have more Occupational Health and Safety inspections. Countries with high unionization rates also act to reduce economy-wide inequality through increased wages (Leigh & Chakalov, 2021). The health impacts of unionization are significant. For example, Figure 5.1 demonstrates

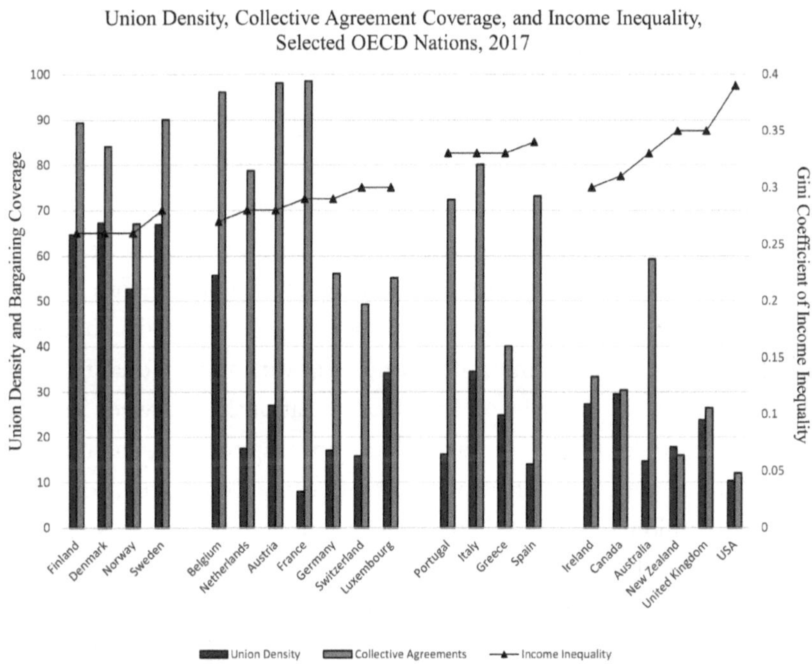

Figure 5.1: Union Density, Collective Agreement Coverage, and Income Inequality, Selected OECD Nations, 2017.

Source: OECD, 2017.

that unions are a crucial ingredient for achieving income equality (Muller & Raphael, 2023). As union density (number of employees who are union members as a proportion of the total number of employees) and collective agreements (legally binding agreements between employers and employees that specify the rights of employees) increase, so does income equality. Here, the Gini coefficient (a measure of statistical dispersion that represents income inequality within a nation or a social group) is used as a measure of income inequality. Conversely, as unionization rates decrease, income inequality increases (Muller & Raphael, 2023).

Worker advantages, and resulting health and social benefits, are closely linked to prevailing political economies and hence their prominence as political DoH. Unionization rates are a strong political DoH because social democratic political economies (e.g., Norway, Sweden, Denmark, and sometimes Finland) typically have strong unionization densities, resulting in measurable population health outcome improvements. In contrast, neoliberal political economies (e.g., Ireland, Canada, Australia, United Kingdom, United States) typically have low union densities, resulting in increased income inequality. Since income inequality is a pivotal social DoH that impacts all the other social determinants, union density is an accurate marker of health and social (in)equality. Although disaggregated statistics provide a clearer intersectional/intersectoral analysis of the impacts of unions—for example women versus men, public versus private sector (Card et al., 2020)—it is clear that a country's union density predicts income inequality (Figure 5.1). Given the established and strong relationship between income and the social DoH (e.g., access to education, employment, and housing and food security), it is not surprising that on the global scale, countries with more unionized workers consistently have better population health outcomes (Muller & Raphael, 2023).

Due to its declining unionization rates, Canada ranks 17th out of 21 OECD countries in unionization rates of employed individuals (OECD, 2017; see Figure 5.1). This decline has been linked to neoliberal governance, emphasizing the primacy of the market over workplace safety and worker rights (Muller & Raphael, 2023). Furthermore, Canada's employment insurance system was scaled back during the 1990s, so that by 1996 fewer than half of unemployed Canadian workers qualified for regular benefits, compared to an average of 75 percent during the 1980s (Stanford, 2005). One of the central functions of capitalist governance systems, including welfare states such as Canada, is to integrate the trade union movement, for better or for worse, within the capitalist state (Panitch, 1986). For Canada, this process has resulted in the steady erosion of the legislative power of unions through 1) regressive labour law changes, such as making strikes illegal through relying on changeable definitions of "essential services"; 2) privatization and contracting-out of core public services, thus weakening unions in those sectors; 3) growth in non-standard and precarious employment, such as working in the gig economy, has eroded union density and collective bargaining capacity; and 4) growth in anti-union organizations, such as the Canadian Labour Watch Association. The three pillars of labour relations are collective bargaining, union representation, and the right to strike (Smith & Stevens, 2019). Political and economic developments have also hampered these pillars of unionization through processes, such as the overt pursuit of a neoliberal policy agenda in which trade unions and collective bargaining are viewed as sources of rigidity (hampering corporate profit) within the labour market (Müller et al., 2019). Figure 5.2 demonstrates steadily declining unionization rates in Canada from 1981–2014.

However, steeply rising inflation, stagnant real wages (wages that reflect inflation rates), and an exhausted work force have revived a dormant labour movement in Canada, putting unions back at the forefront of economic discourse (Subramaniam, 2022). "A tight labor market, rising inflation, and the usual indignities of capitalist workplaces are emboldening young workers to organize, especially in private sector unions" that serve workers in areas such as the café, cinema, and grocery store industries (Vescera, 2023). The renewal of organizing workers for worker rights is, in part, the result of what is now known as the Starbucks effect, with high-profile union drives at the coffee giant's stores in the United States and now Canada (Vescera, 2023).

Worker unionization contexts are an accurate reflection of the long-term impacts of neoliberal political economies. A prominent example

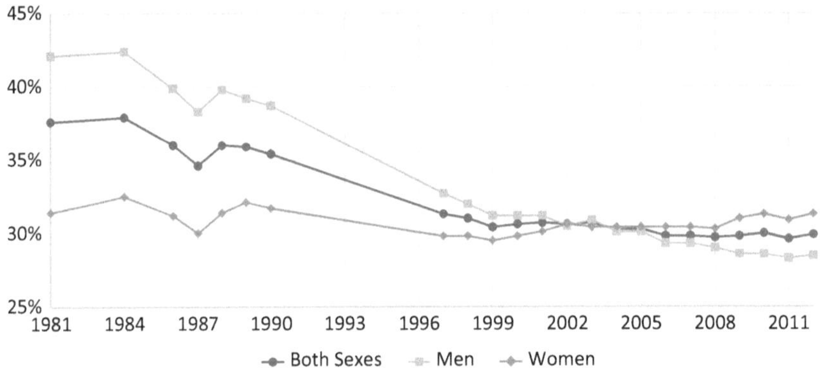

Figure 5.2: Unionization Rates of Employed Individuals, Canada, 1981–2012

Source: Adapted from Statistics Canada, 2015.

involves the 2022 strike of the Canadian Union of Public Employees (CUPE) education workers in Ontario, Canada, with over 95 percent approval from its members (83% turnout) (Hoges, 2022). The bargaining unit consisted of teachers and other school employees, such as education assistants, library workers, administrative assistants, custodians, early childhood educators, cafeteria workers, safety monitors, and social workers due to neoliberal retrenchment of wage stagnation. Some of these employees were the lowest-paid workers in the education system (Hoges, 2022). When CUPE announced its intention to strike, the Ontario provincial Conservative government responded with a fast-tracked passage of Bill 28, which would have fined striking workers $4,000 for every day on strike and penalties of $500,000 a day on a striking union. The law provoked province-wide worker mobilization for breaching workers' rights to collectively bargain, and it was seen as setting an ominous anti-union precedent in Canada's most populous province. It was deployed using a rarely used mechanism called the notwithstanding clause of the country's constitution (Cecco, 2022).

In response on the following day, nearly 55,000 CUPE education workers went on strike. Within hours of Bill 28's introduction on

October 31, 2022, the Ontario Federation of Labour (OFL) launched its "Hands Off Workers' Rights" campaign and called an emergency rally for the next day at the Ministry of Labour in downtown Toronto—the intention of a general strike was announced (Hoges, 2022). A general strike would potentially extend strike action well beyond the education workers to a much broader number of associated unions under the umbrella of CUPE, which includes 250,000 members. Just four days after the threat of a general strike, Premier Doug Ford repealed Bill 28 (Hoges, 2022). This example demonstrates the on-the-ground context of the crucial foundations of labour solidarity and the impact that solidarity can have on the strength of unions to fight for worker rights. Given the proven and strong relationship between the protection of worker rights and health outcomes, these events have the potential to reduce or even reverse current trends of worsening population health outcomes for millions of marginalized and racialized Canadians.

Commercial, Corporate Determinants of Health

The term *commercial determinants of health* (CDoH) was first introduced in the literature by West and Marteau (2013). It became popular after 2016 when defined by Kickbusch et al. (2016) as "strategies and approaches used by the private sector to promote products and choices that are detrimental to health" (p. e895). These authors explained that CDoH operate at the micro level (e.g., consumer and health behaviour, individualization, and choice) and at the macro level (e.g., the global risk society, the global consumer society, and the political economy of globalization). More recently, Lee and Freudenberg (2020) proposed a definition of the CDoH that included the social, political, and economic structures, norms, rules, and practices designed to generate profits and influence patterns of health and disease, disability, and death. This definition is consistent with Mialon's (2020) framing of the CDoH to include three areas. First, the CDoH relate to the production and systematic distribution of unhealthy commodities that are contributing to ill-health. The neoliberal diet, discussed in a prior section about neoliberal epidemics, is a central example of the CDoH.

Second, they include business, market, and political practices that are harmful to health and used to sell these commodities and secure a favourable policy environment. Finally, they include the global drivers of ill-health described in *Global Health Watch 6*, such as market-driven economies and economic globalization, that have facilitated the use of harmful practices and supporting government policies (Bloomsbury Publishing, 2022). For these reasons, the commercial DoH are also described as the corporate DoH.

These definitions illustrate the emergent nature of the CDoH because they have evolved to include key structural DoH: the political economy of globalization; social, political, and economic structures that promote market-driven practices that damage health; and the embedded process of corporations strategically manipulating public policy to ensure increasing profits. The commercial DoH act in synergy with neoliberal epidemics, for example, due to the relationships among Big Food (i.e., global food distribution market dominated by just a few mega-corporations) and the altering of planetary food consumption towards cheap foods with relatively little nutrition and high levels of "empty calories."

Digital Determinants of Health

The global impacts of digital technologies are a new subfield of the political DoH (Özdemir, 2021), termed the ***digital DoH***, which refer to digital technologies, including digital devices, systems, and resources that help create, store, and manage data, as well as other electronically produced and disseminated digital technologies that have substantial political and population health implications. These impacts include areas such as mental health outcomes related to social media engagement, online harassment, and exposure to fake news. Although there is evidence that social media use may have positive impacts on mental health (see Keles et al., 2024; Naslund et al., 2020), there are increasing indications of its harms. Some examples include a systematic review of the influence of social media use on depression, anxiety, and psychological distress in adolescents, where researchers studied the impacts of four domains of social media: time spent, activity, investment, and addiction

(Keles et al., 2020). All domains correlated with depression, anxiety, and psychological distress. In the United States, with a school-based sample of 687 adolescents (48.6% girls; 38.1% white, 29.4% Hispanic, 23.0% Black), researchers found that higher levels of depressive symptoms were associated with more frequent negative emotional responses to social media experiences (Nesi et al., 2022). Research about gender differences in social media impacts on mental health at times produces conflicting results, depending on areas such as the strengths of methodologies used (see Svensson et al., 2022). Researchers have also cautioned that research about social media's mental health impacts on youths should integrate gender identity; "directing children and adolescents to spend less time on social media may backfire for those transgender and gender non-binary youths who are intentional about creating safe spaces on social media that may not exist in their offline world" (Coyne et al., 2023, p. 1).

The term *digital capitalism* was introduced in the late 1990s to emphasize the role of digital technologies in the promotion and success of economic globalization (de Rivera, 2020). Fuchs (2022) also tackles the phenomena of digital capitalism, which has been described as a globe-wide economic system consisting of the digital mediation of property, markets (as in neoliberal capitalism), production styles, accumulation styles, and management styles. As a new epoch of cyberspace, digital capitalism now plays a central role in shaping global political economies (Schiller, 2000). Digital platforms provide the mechanisms for capitalism to thrive in digital cyberspace (market capitalization). Google, Apple, Facebook, Amazon, and Microsoft (GAFAM), are considered an internet oligopoly over public cloud services (Smyrnaios, 2016). Although a thorough discussion is beyond the scope of this book, the principles of neoliberalism, described in Chapter 2, all apply to an analysis and critique of digital capitalism: the individual is essentially "a piece of capital"—to be developed just like any other piece of capital—where digital platform-mediated commodification and thus profit is the goal and markets are normalized in the public consciousness as the natural and superior way of unifying and shaping most forms of human interaction, not just economic transactions (Schrecker, 2016b). This distinction is paramount in analyzing digital capitalism because overt wealth generation for GAFAM is accompanied by hidden processes of massive global alteration of social and cultural human interactions and processes.

Newly recognized threats of artificial intelligence (AI) are becoming central digital DoH. In the public domain, as well as in industry and academia, opinions about AI tend to focus on its capacity to be a welcome player in data management and in data applications such as ChatGPT. Although a description of the health determinant implications of AI are beyond the scope of this chapter, it is important to note their rapidly increasing relevance for the DoH. For example, researchers surveyed relevant literature about bias and discrimination in AI from an interdisciplinary perspective that embedded technical, legal, social, and ethical dimensions (Ferrer et al., 2021). One of AI's negative consequences is discrimination—the unfair or unequal treatment of individuals based on certain characteristics (Ferrer et al., 2021). As governments, companies, and people around the world grapple with the challenges of hate speech, terrorist propaganda, and disinformation online, artificial intelligence (AI) is often proposed as a key tool for identifying and filtering out problematic content (Llansó et al., 2020). However, "the use of AI technologies raises significant questions about the influence of AI on our information environment and, ultimately, on our rights to freedom of expression and access to information" (Llansó et al., 2020, p. 2).

A central aspect of digital determinants has become the potential consequences for democracy posed by generative AI (artificial intelligence capable of producing new content) (Kreps & Kriner, 2023). Generative AI "threatens three pillars of democratic governance: representation, accountability, and, ultimately, the most important currency in a political system—trust" (p. 123). Since most citizens largely lack basic political knowledge, especially levels of policy-specific knowledge, in an era of generative AI, messages sent by the balance of electronic communication about serious policy issues can create space to promote false voter sentiments. There are numerous examples where journalists and others have tracked the use of AI strategies such as bot nets, troll farms, and deep fakes to successfully alter election results, at times significantly, in various countries (see Swenson & Chan, 2024). The question is not whether AI forms can interfere with democracy. Rather, it is about determining the extent and potential mitigation of these already-existing processes.

In an internet "with democratic credentials users would be able to understand which of their own data have been used to target them and why. During elections, people would immediately understand how different campaigns target different people with different messages, who is behind campaigns, and how much they spend" (Lewandowsky & Pomerantsev, 2022, p. 6). Although online anonymity may be a basic right for reasons of safety and others, the public should have the right to know if they are being targeted by a real person (known or anonymous), a political campaign, a corporation, or a state that is pretending to be a real person (Lewandowsky & Pomerantsev, 2022). Digital DoH implications for global democracy are also highly problematic in rich countries where digital technology access cuts across social class and rural location, to name a few, and also in countries in the Global South that do not have internet infrastructure to support citizen access. The internet, through digital technologies, is literally mapping new terrains in the pathways of oppression.

According to *Global Health Watch 6*, the digital revolution and the social acceleration of the information age has widespread consequences for the structure and functioning of society, culture, politics, education, entertainment, and the economy (Bloomsbury Publishing, 2022). In their analysis of digital DoH inequities, Jahnel et al. (2022) adapted Dahlgren and Whitehead's Rainbow Model of the DoH (1991, 2021), described in Chapter 1. Given the interconnectedness of the DoH and digital technologies, these authors argued for not introducing a separate digital sphere of the DoH, but for understanding digitization as a phenomenon that permeates all levels of DoH inequities (Jahnel et al., 2022). As a result, Figure 5.3 demonstrates how digital technologies are integral in driving inequities in the DoH. For example, digital technology is increasingly a gatekeeper to health services and other social DoH, especially for those who cannot afford to pay for internet access (expensive contracts) and/or do not have stable and reliable internet services or

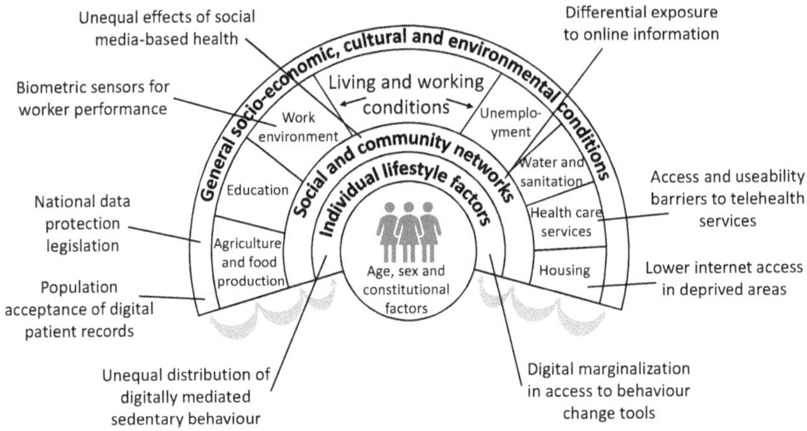

Figure 5.3: Dahlgren and Whitehead's Rainbow Model: Digital Entry Points for Inequality

Source: Adapted from Jahnel et al., 2022.

who must share internet access with one or more households—access to the housing market, job searching, health information, and telehealth are therefore all limited (Jahnel et al., 2022). Another example of the health impacts of digital DoH is labour exploitation in the relatively new processes of digital capitalism. Fuchs (2018) described new unpaid forms of labour, such as the use of Facebook or crowd-sourced labour, where the question arises: "What can we learn from studies of the relationship of exploitation and oppression that helps us to better understand unpaid digital labour?" (p. 678), where historical patterns of patriarchy, slavery, and racism are reproducing themselves within ongoing digital hierarchies of labour.

Data collection, storage, and analyses themselves are political due to implications across countless areas of everyday life, such as personal data safety in any of the new online health-provision services. The need for national data protection legislation has taken on new significance in the digital age, because trust in effective data protection is central to the success of digital interventions (Jahnel et al., 2022). An urgent example was the capacity to contact-trace during COVID-19, where inequities in digital access and related technology design significantly increased COVID-19 morbidity and mortality (Özdemir, 2021). The deeply political nature of digital technologies is increasingly being problematized, especially as they pertain to health care provision, one of the fastest growing applications of digital technology:

> The digital determinants of health are shaped by constitution and contestation of human power and values, the ends to which the new digital world is designed and deployed... to respond to digital determinants of health, we need to surface not only the technology-related dimensions but also the power-laden human and institutional relationships and long-standing politics embedded in health care. (Özdemir, 2021, p. 250)

Colonialism and White Supremacy Determinants of Health

Colonialism and white supremacy are important structural DoH (Bonilla-Silva, 2001; Wilcox, 2023). They are intimately intertwined with all the other political DoH because the very structures that politics and economics produce(d) are underpinned by colonialism and imperialism. These DoH are crucial elements in any discussion of the structural DoH due to the vast impacts of colonialism and imperialism on the social DoH (e.g., housing, food and land security, education). White supremacy, also discussed in Chapter 4, involves conditions, practices, and ideologies that support the dominance of whiteness and white political, social, cultural, and economic domination (Alang et al., 2021).

When we think of white supremacy, many people often think of disturbing and chilling historical racist contexts associated with the Ku Klux Klan in the United States. In Canada, the supremacy of whiteness is demonstrated through the racism of our history. It includes complex processes such as sustained control and power over public policy and other forms of decision making and governance, including: 1) stewardship of the land and natural resources and decisions about protecting the environment (or not); 2) design, delivery, and evaluation of health, social, legal, policing, and education systems, and their philosophical foundations, among others; 3) design and implementation of the governance and electoral processes of the nation; and 4) design and implementation of human rights instruments, along with decisions about whose rights are more legal or valid than others (e.g., human rights and treaty rights) (McGibbon, 2018). Colonialism and white supremacy are created, sustained, and redeployed through the ruling relations inherent in structural racism and racialization, recently brought into more broad public consciousness by actions such as the killing of George Floyd at the hands of police in the United States, and in Canada, the death of Joyce Echaquan, an Indigenous First Nations mother, described in Chapter 3.

White supremacy, including white privilege and colonialism, are DoH that create the systemic substrate for racialization and its health and social damage. **Racialization** is the very complex and contradictory systemic process through which groups come to be designated as being of a particular "race," and on that basis are subjected to differential and/or unequal treatment (Alberta Civil Liberties Research Centre, n.d.). Racialization involves discrimination, injustice, and, ultimately, serious harm towards racialized peoples. For example, persistent compromised health outcomes of Indigenous Peoples can best be traced to structural causes, such as the racialization that led to genocide perpetrated by white colonial imperialists, rather than to personal shortcomings or deficits in "lifestyle" (McGibbon & Etowa, 2009). White supremacy as a DoH is also evidenced by the health outcomes of Canadians of African descent, who have suffered numerous structural inequities that render them more under threat of diseases such as COVID-19 and HIV, and Black people are more likely than white people to experience household food insecurity, inequity in the criminal justice system, and discriminatory treatment in education (Husbands et al., 2019).

Racialization and white supremacy operate through many different mechanisms, such as the mass enslavement of Black people to support colonial conquests around the globe (Alang et al., 2021) and the mass incarceration of Indigenous Peoples and Black people: although Indigenous Peoples represent only 4.1% of the population in Canada, Indigenous inmates in federal institutions rose from 20% of the total inmate population in 2008–2009 to 28% in 2017–2018. During this same time period, the percentage of federally incarcerated Indigenous women rose from 32% of the female inmate population to 40% (Clark, 2019). In 2020, police-reported hate crimes, motivated by hatred of a race or ethnicity, represented 62% of all hate crimes (Statistics Canada, 2020). These crimes most frequently targeted the Black population (42% of all hate crimes). Although Black youth represent almost 4% of the combined youth population in Nova Scotia, Alberta, and British Columbia, they accounted for 10% of youth admissions to correctional services (custody and community) (Government of Canada, 2022b). These stark numbers are evidence of the nature and societal embeddedness of colonial, white supremacy as DoH in the criminal justice system Canada. Further processes of racism, colonialism, and white supremacy are described in Chapter 4 (e.g., environmental racism) and Chapter 6 (e.g., Alberta Tar Sands).

STRUCTURAL VIOLENCE

> Structural violence is silent, it does not show—it is essentially static, it *is* the tranquil waters. In a static society, personal violence will be registered, whereas structural violence may be seen as about as natural as the air around us. (Galtung, 1969, p. 173)

Structural violence is the result of historical and ongoing impacts of the structural DoH. Given the synergies among the social, ecological, and structural DoH, the importance of structural violence lies in its embeddedness within and across all the DoH. Structural violence, first described by Johan Galtung (1969) in *Violence, Peace, and Peace Research*, is distinguished from personal or direct violence, where the actor(s) may be directly identified, such as damage or death by fist, gun, or knife; whereas, in structural violence (built into, embedded in societal structures), there is no such actor. In this first description, Galtung used structural violence and social injustice interchangeably, thus linking structural violence explicitly to the concept of injustice, which inherently opens up the possibility, and even the expectation, of collective responsibility for action (McGibbon, 2021). For Galtung, "structural violence is also meaningful as a blueprint, as an abstract form without social life, used to threaten people into subordination" (1969, p. 172). Galtung makes a distinction between unavoidable death and avoidable death, the latter in keeping with current definitions of health inequalities as avoidable outcomes of inequitable social, economic and political conditions (Bambra et al., 2005; WHO, 2008). The general formula behind structural violence is inequality, with the overarching foundation of the unequal distribution of power (Galtung, 1969):

> Obviously, just as military science and related subjects would be indispensable for the understanding of personal violence, so is the science of social structure, and particularly of stratification, indispensable for the understanding of structural violence. (p. 175)

Zakrison et al. (2019) described how structural violence has its roots in structures of discrimination and alienation, leading to the "normalization of the abnormal" (p. 667). **Normalization** refers to ongoing processes that eventually make something seem more normal or regular, and thus more acceptable and therefore not open to critique or outrage. Normalization results in the framing of societal processes, such as violence against women and queer and trans people, as something that is "just part of life" and therefore does not require being taken seriously in terms of obligations to decrease or halt the occurrences of these kinds of violence. This framing of normalization reflects Said's (2005) portrayal of "the normalized quiet of unseen power." At the centre of structural violence is the social organization of power within ruling structures, such as legal, education, and health systems, and public and private policy and governance systems. These hidden ruling relations share a set of dominant ideological positions and practices that produce, reproduce, and reinstall various forms of structural violence. Social murder, necropolitics, and slow violence are constructs that have been consistently associated with structural violence (see Davies, 2022; Grover, 2019; Nixon, 2011). It is crucial to note that the beneficiaries of sustained structural violence, including public policy–created violence, are largely hidden. In the following sections, the focus is on social murder, necropolitics, and slow violence as pivotal forms of structural violence.

Social Murder: "Not by Gun or Knife, but Murder Just the Same"

> When one individual inflicts bodily injury upon another such that death results, we call the deed manslaughter; when the assailant knew in advance that the injury would be fatal, we call this deed murder. But when society places hundreds of proletarians in such a position that they inevitably meet a too early and an unnatural death, one which is quite as much a death by violence as a sword or a bullet; when it deprives thousands of the necessities of life, places them under conditions in which they cannot live—forces them, through the strong arm of the law, to remain in such conditions until that death ensues, which is the inevitable consequence—knows that these thousands of victims must perish, yet permits these conditions to remain, its deed is murder just as surely as the deed of the single individual; disguised malicious murder, murder against which none can defend himself, which does not seem what it is, because no man sees the murderer, because the death of the victim seems a natural one, since the offence is more one of omission than commission. But murder it remains. (Engels, 2009, p. 152)

Chernomas and Hudson (2007) described how public policies are designed to maximize the accumulation of profit. The authors traced how the implementation of these policies devolved the associated risks and costs on the general public. These processes are perpetuated by dominant uncritical analyses of conservative economic theory and the immense size of private corporations who are able to perpetrate social and environmental destruction with few serious consequences (Chernomas & Hudson, 2007, 2015). For example, the impacts of COVID-19 demonstrated the synergies between the pandemic and the capitalist world food system, which serves to simultaneously multiply and deepen threats to global health by creating global food insecurities and malnutrition, both of which have a well-established co-morbidity with the COVID-19 virus (Akram-Lodhi, 2020). Another strong example is the Alberta Tar Sands, further described in Chapter 6, where the unrestrained profits of Big Oil have created a "slow industrial genocide" among Indigenous Peoples (Huseman & Short, 2012).

The conservative economics of capitalism provide the building blocks for **social murder** to flourish (e.g., reduction of state interventionism in economic and social activities; deregulation of labour and financial markets; and stimulation of commerce and investments by eliminating borders/barriers for mobility of labour, financial capital, goods, and services). These building blocks represent a sanitized language that belies the brutality of social murder, a process that Birn (2009) described as the on-the-ground killing fields and factories of social injustice. Social murder refers to a term described by Engels in 1845 (2009), who defined four components: 1) individuals, usually workers, die prematurely as a result of their living and working conditions; 2) these conditions are a result of workers' exploitation under capitalism; 3) there is a class within society, the bourgeoisie, that benefits from this exploitation; and 4) since the bourgeoisie and ruling authorities are aware of these processes yet do nothing to change them, they are guilty of social murder (Medvedyuk et al., 2021). Bourgeoisie refers to the sector of society that has the most money and power and the most interest in supporting the status quo of health and social inequities (e.g., CEOs of corporations and powerful figures at various levels of government). Marx (1977) also emphasized that the bourgeoisie acquired this power as a result of the labour of ordinary people. The following sections describe two contemporary examples of social murder: the Grenfell Tower fire and increasing infant mortality in "rich" countries.

The Grenfell Tower Fire

A prominent modern-day example of social murder is the Grenfell Tower fire. Hodkinson (2020) traced the historical trajectory of public-policy action and inaction that led to "one of Britain's most deadly infernos since the Great Fire of London of 1666" (p. 1). On June 14, 2017, a high-rise fire broke out in the 24-storey Grenfell Tower block of flats in North Kensington, West London, and burned for 60 hours. Seventy people died at the scene, and nine others died later in hospital, with more than 70 injured and 223 escaping (Global Resilience Institute, 2018). Surrounded by conspicuously more affluent neighborhoods, the

Tower was located in a district that consisted mostly of social housing and was home to people of modest and lower income, working class, and racialized communities (MacLeod, 2018). Since 2013, on numerous documented occasions, the residents of Grenfell raised serious concerns about fire safety with the Kensington and Chelsea Tenant Management Organization (MacLeod, 2018).

Despite these concerns, the Tower continued to lack significantly important safety features, including fire alarms and sprinkler systems, along with having only one fire escape (Global Resilience Institute, 2018). Further worsening the fire's impact was the Arconic company's decision to use a cheaper, less fire-resistant form of cladding to cover the outside of the Tower, despite its own guidelines and brochures warning that the cladding was unsuitable for buildings above 10m tall (the Grenfell Tower was 60m tall) (Davies, 2017). The social murder of the Grenfell Tower fire—from the willful building of the Tower without adequate fire-resistant cladding and foundational, building code–required inclusion of fire alarms, sprinklers, and adequate fire escapes, all the way to the lack of action regarding residents' concerns about the lack of safety in the building—was the result of a confluence of public policy complicity in the marginalization and racialization of the Grenfell Tower residents:

> ... amid an incremental neoliberal political assault on the national welfare state, public housing across the country has become wretchedly devalued, stigmatized, and the subject of scandalous maladministration. (MacLeod, 2018)

This kind of trajectory also applies to neoliberal countries such as Canada, where people living in public housing are significantly more likely to be unemployed or to have compromised employment quality and are more likely to live in crowded, substandard housing circumstances (McGibbon, 2021). These inequities in the social DoH are not due to individual shortcomings, where the blame for substandard living conditions rests on them for "not trying hard enough," and so on. Rather, these difficulties are intimately connected to power relations in society, where class, skill, gender, race, age, and other axes of social inequality shape differential life chances (Julià et al., 2017). Although social murder is activated within complex and hidden processes, it is nonetheless put in place by actual policymakers who have the governance mandate to impact public policy to decrease health inequities (or not).

Increasing Infant Mortality in "Rich" Countries

Infant mortality rate, often regarded as a barometer for overall welfare of a country, is a well-known explanatory variable to capture the socioeconomic development of a country (Gonzalez & Gilleskie, 2017). Increasing infant mortality rates are examples of modern-day social murder because they have empirically been linked to public policies that create inequities in the social DoH, such as barriers in maternal access to health care, and household food and housing insecurity (Reno & Hyder, 2018). Decades of structural assaults, such as neoliberal retrenchment of social support policies (e.g., provision of a living wage, unemployment insurance, state-funded options for re-education/training when unemployed, housing supports) have measurably impacted maternal-child health (Garcia, 2023). Lack of access to money and resources, individually and at the societal level, contributes to compromised health, where the least wealthy experience deprivation and worse health outcomes than the more advantaged, regardless of country of origin (Garcia, 2023). For example, along with being an example of social murder, the root causes of increasing infant mortality rates in rich countries are referred to as a neoliberal epidemic:

> I argue that the analytical literature on neoliberalism, the historical record of neoliberalism's promotion and diffusion, and the empirical evidence of its health consequences support the view that "neoliberal epidemics" represent a substantial and clearly definable threat to public health and health equity. (Schrecker, 2016a, p. 477)

These inequities have been directly linked to the root causes of neoliberal public policy in countries such as Canada, which has steadily eroded universal social supports (Muller & Raphael, 2023)—such as miniscule increases in minimum wages that do not match inflation rates—and the principles of the Canada Health Act (public administration, comprehensiveness, universality, portability and accessibility) through policy decisions such as increasing health care privatization. Canada has continually slipped in the rankings of infant mortality in OECD nations: from 10th out of 24 countries in 1980, to 26th out of 34 countries in 2011, and finally to 32nd out of 38 countries in 2021 (Brend, 2023). Figure 5.4 depicts infant mortality rankings in OECD

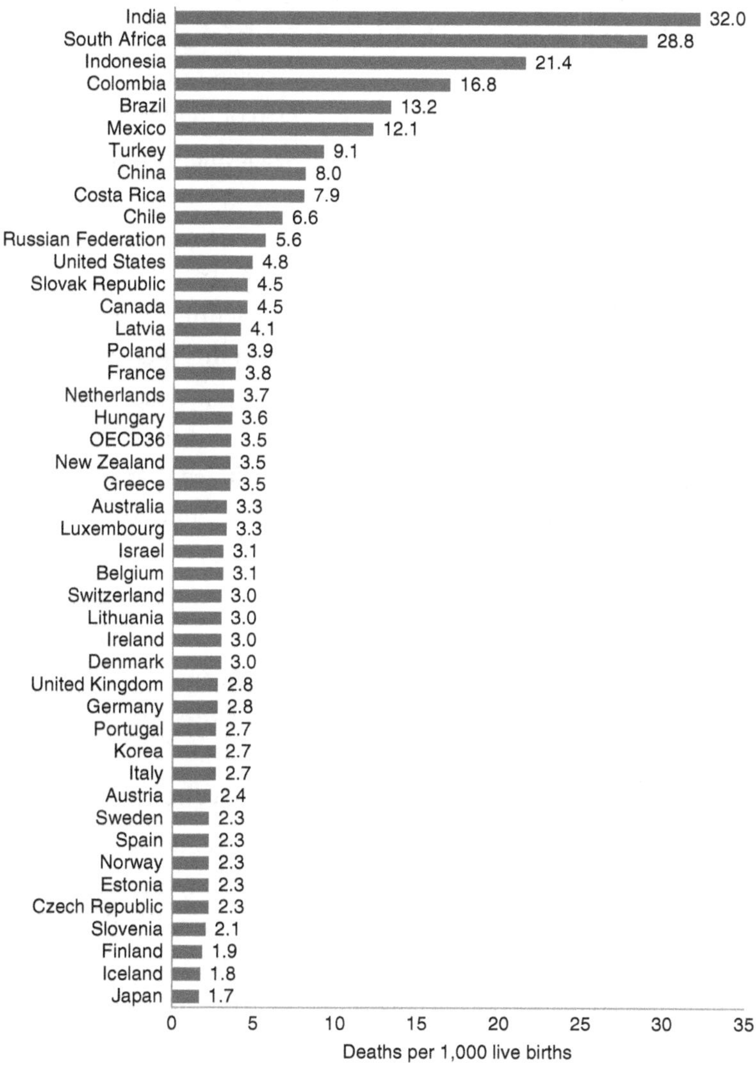

Figure 5.4: Infant Mortality Rates in OECD Countries: 2017 (or Nearest Year)

Source: Adapted from OECD, 2019.

countries in 2021 (OECD, 2023). The Indigenous infant mortality rate was more than twice that, at 9.2 deaths per 1,000 births (Hayward & Cidro, 2021). Canadian neoliberal policy and governance decision making over the past three decades (regardless of the governing political party) has resulted in a public policy–induced lock-in of implicit acceptance that baby death across racism and classism lines is unavoidable collateral damage in the neoliberal dominance of austerity measures and the primacy of the market above the survival of our most vulnerable humans. This implicit acceptance is a form of hidden power, which in the case of baby deaths, proves to be just as lethal as actual murder.

Neoliberal economic policy takes aim at the already racialized and disenfranchised, through fiscally cutting social supports that would enhance maternal-child well-being. In the United Kingdom between 2014 and 2017, the previously declining trend in infant mortality reversed, and inequalities in infant mortality increased (Taylor-Robinson et al., 2019). Researchers estimated that each 1 percent increase in child poverty was significantly associated with an extra 5.8 infant deaths per 100,000 live births. They concluded that about a third of the increases in infant mortality between 2014 and 2017 can be attributed to rising public policy–created child poverty. Infant mortality rates in affluent families remained unaffected—infant mortality rates in "rich" countries largely remain stable for those at the top-income quintiles, and other health indicators such as life expectancy continue to rise at the population health level (Aoyama et al., 2020).

Necropolitics: "Deciding Who Lives and Who Must Die"

Achille Mbembe (2003) offers a salient context to understand discrepancies in the ways that social murders, such as the social murder of newborn babies, play themselves out in the structural realm. He first described the term ***necropolitics*** as the use of social and political power to dictate how some people may live and how some must die:

> The ultimate expression of sovereignty (political power) in nations resides, to a large degree, in the power and the capacity to dictate who may live and who must die. Hence, to kill or to allow to live

> constitute the limits of sovereignty… To exercise sovereignty is to exercise control over mortality and to define life as the deployment and manifestation of power. (pp. 11–12)

Mbembe (2003) differentiates between notions of sovereignty, found in the discipline of political science, which locates sovereignty within the boundaries of the nation-state, within institutions empowered by the state, or within institutions and networks beyond the state. Mbembe's focus is not on the struggle for autonomy but the generalized instrumentalization of human existence (where humans are used as instruments to support or manipulate larger power processes such as imperialism and colonialism) and the material destruction of human bodies and populations. For Mbembe, sovereignty is expressed predominately as the right to kill, the biopower (Foucault, 1990) to "regulate the distribution of death and to make possible the murderous function of the state" (Mbembe, 2003, p. 17). Colonialism is a central example of necropolitics, where in countries such as Canada, Indigenous Peoples and peoples of African descent have been instrumentalized to build a "new" country on substrates of slavery and genocide. For example, persistent historical settler assaults on the Haida Gwaii First Nation is example of necropolitics, with settler policies and governance leading to the smallpox-induced genocide of an estimated 19,000 Haida Gwaii People on the West coast of Canada in 1862 (Parfitt, 2019).

Another instance of necropolitics in Canada involves a government-based initiative known as the Clearing of the Plains (up to and after 1870), where the government of Canada used a policy of starvation against Indigenous Peoples to clear the way for settlement. The I.G. Baker Company, hired by the Government of Canada to provide winter food rations for the Cree Nation, allowed food to rot in warehouses, while tuberculosis and other diseases ravaged an already-weakened people (Daschuk, 2013; McGibbon, 2019). To prevent the death of their families, mothers and daughters were forced into prostitution at the hands of settler officials who controlled the food supply. At the time, Sir John A. MacDonald (Prime Minister of Canada, serving from 1867–1873 and 1878–1891) had the legal authority to solve "The Indian

Problem," which was the notion that Indigenous groups presented an obstacle to land acquisition and colonial settlement. Solutions turned towards ideas of assimilation and civilization of the "savages" (Woolford, 2023). MacDonald famously stated, "We are doing all we can, by refusing food until the Indians are on the verge of starvation, to reduce the expense" (Daschuk, 2013). A related and pressing modern example is lack of policy intervention to support Indigenous community access to potable water, where 73 percent of First Nations communities in Canada have drinking water that is at medium or high risk for contamination (The Council of Canadians, n.d.). These examples explain what is meant by the structural DoH, where public policy–created, political decisions determine health and death across generations.

Necropolitics involved in the historical genocide of Indigenous Peoples in Canada can be directly linked to the criteria in Article 2 (2a to 2e) of the United Nations (UN) Convention on the Prevention and Punishment of the Crime of Genocide (UN, 1948). The Convention states that **genocide** means any of the following acts committed with intent to destroy, in whole or in part, a national, ethnical, racial, or religious group:

a. Killing members of the group;
b. Causing serious bodily or mental harm to members of the group;
c. Deliberately inflicting on the group conditions of life calculated to bring about its physical destruction in whole or in part;
d. Imposing measures intended to prevent births within the group;
e. Forcibly transferring children of the group to another group. (UN, 1948)

Box 5.1 details some of the necropolitics involved in the genocide of Indigenous Peoples in Canada, as defined in the UN Convention on Genocide.

Box 5.1: Canadian Necropolitics: Genocide of Indigenous Peoples in Canada, as per *United Nations Convention on the Prevention and Punishment of the Crime of Genocide* (UN, 1948)

Article 2, a), b), c): Clearing of the Plains (more fully described above)
Within two years of Cree negotiation of Treaty 6 in 1876, between 15,000 and 20,000 people faced starvation as a result of federal government action, with the sudden disappearance of the bison, and a way of life that endured for 10,000 years (Daschuk, 2013).

Article 2, a), b), c): The Beothuk
The Beothuk, Indigenous inhabitants of Newfoundland, were actively hunted and killed by British farmers, fishers, and trappers who settled on the bays of the Beothuk's summer camps since the island's invasion in 1497. Weakened by hunger and diseases, such as smallpox, measles, influenza, and tuberculosis, the population decreased from approximately 345 in 1768 to 72 in 1811 (Wesley-Esquimaux & Smolewski, 2004). Indigenous historian, Dan Paul (2006) stated that as early as 1506, many of the Beothuk were being sold as slaves in Europe and many were simply slaughtered. The assault caused traditional food supplies to be cut off, which led to starvation and malnutrition, causing them to die of European diseases. In time, these barbarities led to the extinction of the Beothuk Tribe.

Article 2, a), b), c): Germ Warfare, Biological Weapons
It is a matter of public record (publicly archived historical documents) that germ warfare was conducted against Indigenous Peoples in North America, such as the distribution of smallpox-infected blankets to Indigenous tribes (Paul, 2006). The UN Convention on the Prohibition of the Development, Production, and Stockpiling of Bacteriological (Biological) and Toxin Weapons, and on their Destruction, commonly known as the Biological Weapons Convention (BWC) or Biological and Toxin Weapons Convention (BTWC), was signed in 1975, officially recognizing biological agents as effective methods of warfare.

(*continued*)

Article 2 a): British Scalp Proclamation 1756

"And, we do hereby promise, by and with the advice and consent of His Majesty's Council, a reward of 30£ for every male Indian Prisoner, above the age of sixteen years, brought in alive; or for a scalp of such male Indian twenty-five pounds, and twenty-five pounds for every Indian woman or child brought in alive. Such rewards are to be paid by the Officer commanding at any of His Majesty's Forts in this Province, immediately on receiving the Prisoners or Scalps above mentioned, according to the intent and meaning of this Proclamation." The Proclamation is still legal in Nova Scotia, despite lobbying to remove it in respect for the Mi'kmaq people in the ancestral, unceded territory of Mi'kma'ki (Paul, 2006).

Article 2, a), b), c): Indian Residential Schools; Article 2, e) Relocations

Please see text analysis below.

Article 2, b), d): Coerced Sterilization of Indigenous Women

Coercive sterilization of Indigenous women occurred during the eugenics movement in the early 1900s. According to Stote (2012), evidence indicates this practice was carried out by eugenically minded doctors in Ontario and Northern Canada, where Aboriginal women were the prime targets (Stote, 2012).

Article 2, b): Medical Experiments on Indigenous Peoples, including Children in Indian Residential Schools (IRS)

Between 1942 and 1952, some of Canada's leading nutrition experts, in cooperation with various federal departments, conducted an unprecedented series of nutritional experiments and studies on Aboriginal communities and on children in IRS. The largest study was the James Bay Survey of the Attawapiskat and Rupert's House Cree First Nations (1947–1948). There were also two separate long-term controlled experiments on malnourished Indigenous Peoples in Northern Manitoba, and later in six IRS. Experiments were conducted without the "subjects'" informed consent or knowledge (McCallum, 2017).

Source: McGibbon, 2018.

Perhaps the most well-known instance of genocidal necropolitics in Canada is the Indian residential school (IRS) system. Facts, in both Indigenous and settler historical accounts, tell us that at least 150,000 children were taken from their homes, often under circumstances of abduction by Indian Agents of the Canadian government (Truth and Reconciliation Commission, 2015). Many thousands of first-voice accounts verify that Indigenous children were subjected to physical and psychological abuse, rape, and torture (e.g., electroshocked in a small, homemade electric chair; placed in bathtubs full of snakes) (Truth and Reconciliation Commission, 2015). Telling the truths of these atrocities against Indigenous Peoples' bodies is a central aspect of the Truth and Reconciliation process in Canada, one that acknowledges ongoing anti-Indigenous racism and necropolitics in the country. In 2022, Kimberly Murray was appointed as *Independent Special Interlocutor for Missing Children and Unmarked Graves and Burial Sites* associated with IRSs. She now works closely with Indigenous leaders, communities, survivors, families, and experts to accomplish two foundational processes: 1) determine measures to be used for identification of unmarked graves, and 2) recommend a new federal legal framework to ensure the respectful and culturally appropriate treatment and protection of unmarked graves and burial sites of children at former IRSs (Government of Canada, 2022a).

A massive, country-wide process has been initiated to locate these missing and murdered children, using archival data, surface examination, and excavation; historical records and community historical research and interviews, including historical research involving interviews with survivors, and oral history; ground-penetrating radar; and LiDar (laser imaging, detection, and ranging). Indigenous children were also found accidently and as a result of flooding and construction-related digging. As mass IRS graves are discovered, contributors are collating an ongoing record of news reports (largely from CBC News) on Wikipedia (2021). In High River, Alberta, at the site of the Dunbow Industrial School, 34 children's remains in caskets were exposed when the banks of the Highwood River eroded in a flood (Rollie, 2021).

In Saddle Lake Cree Nation, Alberta, at the site of the Blue Quills Indian Residential School, there was accidental discovery of child-sized skeletons wrapped in white cloth, which was incorrectly suspected to be a mass burial of typhoid victims (Parsons, 2022). In Lestock/Muskowekwan First Nation, Saskatchewan, at the site of the Muscowequan Indian Residential School, 19 graves were uncovered during water-line construction in 1992; subsequently, 10–15 potential graves were identified using ground-penetrating radar (Snowdon, 2019). As of April 20, 2023, results indicate that there were 2,614 suspected unmarked graves and 151 confirmed human remains, excluding Saddle Lake, where numerous remains were found and the counting process is still ongoing (Parsons, 2022). These atrocities signify the systematic and historically repetitive necropolitics, genocide, and social murder of Indigenous children across Canada.

Missing and murdered Indigenous women in Canada is another example of necropolitics, due to the historical persistence and lack of state-based preventive measures, as well as the absence of systematic initiatives to locate and charge perpetrators. This situation eventually led to the call for a National Inquiry into Missing and Murdered Indigenous Women and Girls (Truth and Reconciliation Commission of Canada, 2015), which was launched in 2016. The number of Indigenous women murdered in Canada is steadily increasing: in 1980, Indigenous women accounted for 9 percent (18) of female homicide victims, whereas in 2014, they accounted for 21 percent (30) of female homicide victims. In 2014, the rate of homicide of Indigenous women (3.64 per 100,000) was almost six times higher than non-Indigenous women (0.65 per 100,000) (Government of Canada, 2017). The situation is similarly urgent in the United States: Indigenous women and girls are murdered 10 times more often than all other ethnicities combined (Native Womens Wilderness, n.d.).

Slow Violence: People and Planet Under Threat

> In contrast to the static connotations of structural violence, I have sought, through the notion of slow violence, to foreground questions of time, movement, and change, however gradual. The explicitly

> temporal emphasis of slow violence allows us to keep front and center the representational challenges and imaginative dilemmas posed not just by imperceptible violence but by imperceptible change whereby violence is decoupled from its original causes by the workings of time. (Nixon, 2011, p. 11)

The term ***slow violence*** was first described in 2011 by Rob Nixon, environmentalist and literary scholar of Princeton University (Nixon, 2011). The ecological DoH, described in Chapter 4, are all examples of slow violence and their roots in capitalism and colonialism: pollution and ecotoxicity; environmental racism; resource extraction and depletion; climate and atmospheric emergency; desertification, deforestation, and soil and ocean acidification. Slow violence also includes the brutalities of over 100 million unexploded landmines from wars officially concluded decades ago, causing an annexing of vast tracts of precious agricultural land and pastures in countries such as Cambodia, Laos, and Somalia (Nixon, 2011). These agricultural losses further stress already oversubscribed resources and compound already-existing malnutrition. As discussed in this chapter and in Chapter 4, the ideological apparatus of neoliberalism remains central in critical perspectives on the structural violence that reinforces the anthropogenic damage of slow violence.

Violence often evokes powerful images such as explosions, physical and psychological confrontations, tornados, volcanos, and the like. We can readily see the shape, and at least the short-term impacts of these kinds of violence. In contrast, slow violence refers to the gradual impacts of environmental destruction, such as global capitalism's assaults on Earth systems so beautifully and paradoxically illustrated by photographer Edward Burtynsky and his team, Jennifer Baichwal and Nicholas de Pencier (Burtynsky et al., 2018). Although the trail of destruction is clear in the photographs, hidden beneath these assaults on the Earth's surface are massive and destructive impacts on millions of people. Jennifer Baichwal points out that their *Anthropocene* book is a culmination of the authors' conversations about how art can provoke change, and the merits and drawbacks of developing a project that has an experiential approach to engagement with the public: "to not preach, harangue, or blame, but to witness, and in that witnessing, to try to shift consciousness" (p. 197).

In her dialogue about the immediacy of the Anthropocene photography project, Baichwal discusses how there is some danger in this approach of engagement with the public through experiential art exhibits around the globe, due to the scale and urgency of planetary damage—she wonders if perhaps it would be better to use an approach that more stridently signals an emergency. However, she concludes by saying, "I still believe that lateral exploration, the open-ended conversation, can provoke transformation more deeply than hard argument" (Burtynsky et al., 2018, p. 197). Here, Baichwal grapples with a central puzzle in the slow violence of environmental destruction and its on-the-ground impacts on humanity and planet: despite overpowering evidence, how can transformative action continue to be a pivotal aspect of moving forward for climate action?

To confront slow violence is to take up, in all its temporal complexity, toxic geographies and the politics of the visible and the invisible (Nixon, 2011). Pushing back on framings of slow violence as invisible to the people who have ongoing, everyday experiences with the brutalities of such violence, Davies (2022) challenges these definitions of slow violence as "out of sight" and asks instead "out of sight for whom?" Slow violence urges us to expand our imaginations of the notion of harm, requiring that we take seriously the forms of slow violence that have become "unmoored" from their original causes (Davies, 2022). Rather, Nixon states that we must look beyond the incremental horrors of the climate emergencies we see all around us to the many other "slowly evolving environmental catastrophes" (Nixon, 2011, p. 2):

> As a spatial concept, slow violence invites us to include the gradual deaths, destructions, and layered deposits of uneven social brutalities within the geographic here-and-now. At the same time, by unchaining our geographical imaginations from the shackles of the present, slow violence provokes us to delve into the past to unEarth the violent structures of inequality that saturate contemporary life, and may well lay waste to the future. (p. 410)

Structural violence is sometimes referred to as the conceptual predecessor of slow violence; however, the use of slow violence as a concept does not necessarily imply its structural origins (Davies, 2022). As argued in the ecological DoH and social DoH discussions in this book, these complex concepts do not necessarily evoke analyses of their structural or root causes. Although the impacts of slow violence are quantifiable (e.g., toxic petrochemical seepage into watersheds), quantification does not overtly, or even covertly in many cases, identify the perpetrators of this violence. Structural perspectives involve identifying these perpetrators and holding them accountable for violent institutional, public, corporate, and governance policies and practices. Rob Nixon opened his 2011 book *Slow Violence and the Environmentalism of the Poor* with an analysis of the World Bank's dedication to offloading US and European toxic waste, garbage, and heavily polluting industries to African countries. The World Bank proposed more aggressive "poison-distribution" (p. 2) to avert potential economic damage at the hands of rich-nation environmentalists who were campaigning against garbage dumps and industrial effluent.

> I think the economic logic behind dumping a load of toxic waste in the lowest-wage country is impeccable and we should face up to that... I've always thought that countries in Africa are vastly under polluted; their air quality is probably vastly inefficiently low compared to Los Angeles... Just between you and me, shouldn't the World Bank be encouraging more migration of the dirty industries to the least developed countries? (Lawrence Summers, confidential World Bank memo, December 12, 1991, as cited in Nixon, 2011)

The Geopolitics of War and Conflict

The chapter would not be complete without a brief discussion of the geopolitics of war and conflict, one of the most important political DoH. Geopolitics instigates ideas of war, empire, and diplomacy, including the practice of states controlling and competing for territory (Flint, 2021). However, the geopolitics of war involves more than the competition over territory and the means of justifying such actions: geopolitics is a way of "seeing" the world (Flint, 2021). It encompasses many structural DoH, including neoliberal epidemics of profit-related "flight to arms" by global defense companies during increased global conflict (Zhang et al, 2022), Big Oil megaprofits and the "war on terror" (Lafer, 2004), and slow violence and the environmental ravages of armed conflict across urban and rural landscapes over decades (Davies, 2022). Geopolitics is grounded in the fields of political science and geography, the latter of which may include broad and diverse disciplines such as human, physical, feminist, economic, historical, and political geography.

Geographic areas heavily impacted by war and conflict in 2023, according to percent of population impacted, included Ukraine (46), Syria (61), Somalia (31), Palestine (100), and Brazil (41), resulting in vast inequities in the social DoH and capacity to survive (Armed Conflict Location & Event Data Project [ACLED], 2023). This mass displacement has had deep and global ripple effects for countries such as Canada. From 2019 to 2022 inclusive, Canada accepted 481,717 refugees (Macro Trends, n.d.). These humanitarian actions also reflect Canada's complex history of choosing which refugees are worthy of immigration to Canada and which are not (Bangarth, 2019). War and conflict deployment of Canadian military personnel, such as combat soldiers and medical personnel, also has a corresponding current and intergenerational social DoH impact on Canadian families and communities.

Salience of the geopolitics of war and conflict as a structural, political DoH lies in its massive role in determining global human and planet health. The geopolitics of war and conflict is an exceptional example of how the social DoH are inseparable from the political, structural DoH. The social DoH illustrate the pointy edges of on-the-ground family and community inequities and suffering caused by food, housing, and employment insecurity and racism, along with rural, remote, northern, and urban geographies (see Figure 3.3). At the same time, structural forces such as global neoliberal capitalism and neoliberal epidemics insidiously make their way into the lives of these same people in the form of health damage–related austerity measures that harm health for generations, to name a few. War and conflict cause significant displacement, economic instability, and disease burden and hence damaging impacts on community and individual health (Martin & Evans, 2015): "conflict is the result of inequalities realized and justice unserved" (p. 4).

CONCLUSION

This chapter illustrates how the structural DoH are embedded across and within our everyday lives. Rather than being an abstract concept, these discussions demonstrate that politics and power (or lack of power) are embedded in the politics and policymaking of the institutional structures that govern where we work, learn, buy groceries, navigate the internet, and countless other aspects of our daily lives. This chapter uncovers many things that are hard to imagine or emotionally digest, as is the case with the ecodeterminants chapter and the other chapters in this book (e.g., globe-wide austerity measures, which caused a generation of UK children to have stunted growth and nutrition-related bone deformities that were thought to have been gone since the early 1800s). These and other polycrisis results have led to the globe-wide movement and mobilization for an alternative, Earth-centred political economy, discussed in Chapter 7.

FURTHER READINGS

Burtynsky, E., Baichwal, J., & de Pencier, N. (2018). *Anthropocene*. Steidl.

Card, D., Lemieux, T., & Riddell, W. C. (2020). Unions and wage inequality: The roles of gender, skill and public sector employment. *Canadian Journal of Economics/Revue Canadienne d'Economique, 53*(1), 140–173. https://doi.org/10.1111/caje.12432

Davies, T. (2022). Slow violence and toxic geographies: "Out of sight" to whom? *Environment and Planning C: Politics and Space, 40*(2), 409–427. https://doi.org/10.1177/2399654419841063

Drescher, J. (2015). Out of DSM: Depathologizing homosexuality. *Behavioral Sciences, 5*(4), 565–575. https://doi.org/10.3390%2Fbs5040565

Labonté, R., & Stuckler, D. (2016). The rise of neoliberalism: How bad economics imperils health and what to do about it. *Journal of Epidemiology Community Health, 70*(3), 312–318. https://www.jstor.org/stable/44017712

WEBSITES OF INTEREST

The Centre for Social Justice—https://www.socialjustice.org/community/news.php

The Centre for Social Justice (CSJ) is an advocacy organization that seeks to strengthen the struggle for social justice. CSJ conducts research, education and advocacy in a bid to narrow the gap in income, wealth, and power, and enhance peace and human security; brings together people from universities and unions, faith groups and community organizations in the pursuit of greater equality and democracy; supports social movements in the struggle for social justice; offers a non-partisan perspective on political, social and economic issues; and uses creative communications to educate Canadians about public policies. See their weekly CSJ Newsletter, which includes calls to action, events, and articles.

Global Inequalities Observatory (GIO)—https://www.lse.ac.uk/International-Inequalities/Research/Global-Inequalities-Observatory

"The GIO seeks to promote rigorous research methods from a wide range of social sciences to foster a greater understanding of the levels, trends, causes, and consequences of economic inequality in multiple countries and regions. The Observatory's core values for empirical research are 1) rigour; 2) transparency for reproducibility; and 3) interdisciplinarity. It aims for broad—but not exhaustive—geographical coverage, including the Global South as well as advanced industrial countries. By working across a range of themes related to economic inequality, the GIO complements—and collaborates with—the Research Programs currently in operation at the International Inequalities Institute."

Idle No More—https://idlenomore.ca/

"From the Idle No More Hawai'i campaign to Protect Mauna Kea to the actions of Tiny House Warriors in defense of Secwepemc lands and waters—a peaceful Indigenous revolution is rising around the planet… A continent-wide network of urban and rural Indigenous Peoples working hand in hand with non-Indigenous allies, Idle No More is an Indigenous-led movement that calls on all people to join in a peaceful revolution which honours and fulfills Indigenous sovereignty and which protects the land, the water, and the sky. This website includes detailed activism campaigns and contexts for taking action for reconciliation."

National Inquiry into Missing and Murdered Indigenous Women and Girls—https://www.mmiwg-ffada.ca/

"Indigenous women and Two-Spirit people have traditionally been revered as life-givers and caregivers. This is why we say, 'our women and girls are sacred.' But Indigenous women and girls, including those who are 2SLGBTQQIA, continue to be devalued. All too many become the victims of violence. Our vision for the

National Inquiry is to build a foundation that allows Indigenous women and girls to reclaim their power and place. Because of Indigenous Peoples' rich diversity, this reclaiming will look different in different places. First Nations, Métis, and Inuit peoples each have their own distinct cultures, languages, and ways of life. Their communities have their own distinct political, legal, social, cultural, and economic systems. There can be no one-size-fits-all, pan-Indigenous approach. Solutions must instead be culturally appropriate to First Nations, Métis, and Inuit women and girls, their respective communities, and their Nations."

OECD Inequality—https://www.oecd.org/social/inequality.htm/

This OECD website focuses on measuring and mapping global inequality. It includes numerous resources to learn more about the breadth and scope of inequality across the OECD countries, including Canada: "'We have reached a tipping point. Inequality can no longer be treated as an afterthought. We need to focus the debate on how the benefits of growth are distributed. Our report "*In it Together*" and our work on *inclusive growth* have clearly shown that there doesn't have to be a trade-off between growth and equality. On the contrary, the opening up of opportunity can spur stronger economic performance and improve living standards across the board!' OECD Secretary-General."

GLOSSARY

Digital DoH: Refers to digital technologies, including digital devices, systems, and resources that help create, store, and manage data, as well as other electronically produced and disseminated digital technologies that have substantial political implications. Impacts include mental health and democracy implications for social media, online harassment, and exposure to fake news, as well as health consequences of inequities in access to digital technologies.

Genocide: For the UN Convention on the Prevention and Punishment of the Crime of Genocide (UN, 1948), genocide means any of the following acts committed with intent to destroy, in whole or in part, a national, ethnical, racial, or religious group: 1) killing members of the group, 2) causing serious bodily or mental harm to members of the group, 3) deliberately inflicting on the group conditions of life calculated to bring about its physical destruction in whole or in part, 4) imposing measures intended to prevent births within the group, and 5) forcibly transferring children of the group to another group.

Hidden Power: Refers to the actual controls over decision making and the ways certain powerful people and institutions maintain their influence over the process and often exclude and devalue concerns and agendas of less powerful groups (Nash et al., 2006).

Invisible Power: Refers to internalized power. This power operates by influencing how individuals think of their place in society and explains why some are prevented from questioning existing power relations (Nash et al., 2006). Visible conflict is hidden through internalization of powerlessness or lack of awareness (e.g., internalized powerlessness in the workplace, womens' internalized sexism, internalized racism for racialized peoples). Internalized power also involves the power of internalized privilege (e.g., male, white, heterosexual) that invisibly entitles the more powerful to enact power over the less powerful.

Necropolitics: Refers to the use of social and political power to dictate how some people may live and how some must die (Mbembe, 2003). Colonialism is a central example of necropolitics because in countries such as Canada, Indigenous Peoples and peoples of African descent have been instrumentalized to build a "new" country on substrates of slavery and genocide.

Normalization: Refers to ongoing processes that eventually make something seem more normal or regular, and thus more acceptable and therefore not open to critique or outrage. Normalization results in the framing of societal processes, such as violence against women and queer and trans people, as something that is "just part of life" and therefore does not require being taken seriously in terms of obligations to decrease or halt the occurrences of these kinds of violence.

Racialization: The very complex and contradictory systemic process through which groups come to be designated as being of a particular "race," and on that basis are subjected to differential and/or unequal treatment (Alberta Civil Liberties Research Centre, n.d.).

Slow Violence: Refers to the gradual impacts of environmental destruction, including global capitalism's assaults on Earth systems that are slowly (over decades and even centuries) resulting in devastating biodiversity loss and species extinction, deforestation, global heating, and climate emergency. Slow violence contrasts with everyday notions of violence, which often evoke powerful images such as explosions, physical and psychological confrontations, tornados, volcanos, and the like. We can readily see the shape, and at least the short-term impacts, of these kinds of violence.

Social Murder: Refers to a term first described by Engels in 1845 (2009), who described four components: 1) individuals, usually workers, die prematurely as a result of their living and working conditions; 2) these conditions are a result of workers' exploitation under capitalism; 3) there is a class within society, the bourgeoisie, that benefits from this exploitation; and 4) since the bourgeoisie and ruling authorities are aware of these processes yet do nothing to change them, they are guilty of social murder (Medvedyuk et al., 2021).

Structural Violence: Refers to violence that is built into and embedded in societal structures, such as political and economic governance systems. Some examples include systemic racism, which ultimately results in bodily damage because it is a form of embodied oppression that impacts body systems such as the cardiovascular system to produce heart disease. Structural violence is distinguished from personal or direct violence, where the actor(s) may be directly identified, such as damage or death by fist, gun or knife; whereas, in structural violence, there is no such actor (Galung, 1969).

Visible Power: Refers to the conventional understanding of power that is negotiated through formal rules and structures, institutions, and procedures (e.g., institutional governing boards, elected officials, members of parliament, and so on).

REFERENCES

Akram-Lodhi, A. H. (2021). Contemporary pathogens and the capitalist world food system. *Canadian Journal of Development Studies/Revue Canadienne d'Etudes du Dévelopement, 42*(1-2), 18–27. https://doi.org/10.1080/02255189.2020.1834361

Alang, S., Hardeman, R., Karbeah, J., Akosionu, O., McGuire, C., Abdi, H., & McAlpine, D. (2021). White supremacy and the core functions of public health. *American Journal of Public Health, 111*(5), 815–819. https://doi.org/10.2105%2FAJPH.2020.306137

Alberta Civil Liberties Research Centre. (n.d.). *Racialization.* http://www.aclrc.com/racialization

Aoyama, K., Park, A. L., Davidson, A. J., & Ray, J. G. (2020). Severe maternal morbidity and infant mortality in Canada. *Pediatrics, 146*(3), e20193870. https://doi.org/10.1542/peds.2019-3870

Armed Conflict Location & Event Data Project (ACLED). (2023). *Conflict exposure: A new measure of the impact of conflict on civilians.* https://acleddata.com/conflict-exposure/

Bambra, C., Fox, D., & Scott-Samuel, A. (2005). Towards a politics of health. *Health Promotion International, 20*(2), 187–193. https://doi.org/10.1093/heapro/dah608

Bangarth. S. (2019). Canada's complicated history of refugee reception. In D. Ross (Ed.)., *Confronting Canadian migration history* (pp. 7–14). Active History.

Barnett, P., & Bagshaw, P. (2020). Neoliberalism: What it is, how it affects health and what to do about it. *The New Zealand Medical Journal, 133*(1512), 76–84.

Birn, A.-E. (2009). Making it politic(al): Closing the gap in a generation: Health equity through action on the social determinants of health. *War & Social Medicine, 4*(3), 166–182.

Bloomsbury Publishing. (2022). *Global Health Watch 6: In the shadow of the pandemic.*

Bonilla-Silva, E. (2001). *White supremacy and racism in the post-civil rights era.* Lynne Rienner.

Brend, Y. (2023, April 2). *What Canada's slipping global ranking in infant deaths says about the overall health of society.* CBC News. https://www.cbc.ca/news/canada/infant-mortality-ranking-canada-1.6772351

Burtynsky, E., Baichwal, J., & de Pencier, N. (2018). *Anthropocene.* Steidl.

Card, D., Lemieux, T., & Riddell, W. C. (2020). Unions and wage inequality: The roles of gender, skill and public sector employment. *Canadian Journal of Economics/Revue Canadienne d'Economique, 53*(1), 140–173. https://doi.org/10.1111/caje.12432

Cecco, L. (2022, November 7). Ontario to repeal new law threatening workers' right to strike following pushback. *The Guardian.* https://www.theguardian.com/world/2022/nov/07/ontario-repeal-law-right-to-strike

Chanchlani, R., Nemer, P., Sinha, R., Nemer, L., Krishnappa, V., Sochett, E., Safadi, F., & Raina, R. (2020). An overview of rickets in children. *Kidney International Reports, 5*(7), 980–990. https://doi.org/10.1016/j.ekir.2020.03.025

Chernomas, R., & Hudson, I. (2007). *Social murder and other shortcomings of conservative economics.* Arbeiter Ring Publishing.

Chernomas, R., & Hudson, I. (2015). Social murder and conservative economics. *Criminal Justice Matters, 102*(1), 15–16. https://doi.org/10.1080/09627251.2015.1143625

Clark, S. (2019). *Overrepresentation of Indigenous people in the Canadian criminal justice system: Causes and responses.* Research and Statistics Division, Department of Justice Canada.

Coburn, D. (2010). Health and health care: A political economy perspective. In T. Bryant, D. Raphael, & M. Rioux (Eds.), *Staying alive: Critical perspectives on health, illness, and health care* (2nd ed.). Canadian Scholars.

The Council of Canadians (n.d.). *Safe water for First Nations.* https://canadians.org/fn-water/

Coyne, S. M., Weinstein, E., Sheppard, J. A., James, S., Gale, M., Van Alfen, M., Ririe, N., Monson, C., Ashby, S., Weston, A., & Banks, K. (2023). Analysis of social media use, mental health, and gender identity among US youths. *JAMA Network Open, 6*(7), e2324389. https://doi.org/10.1001/jamanetworkopen.2023.24389

Dahlgren, G., & Whitehead, M. (1991). *Policies and strategies to promote social equity in health.* Institute for Futures Studies.

Dahlgren, G., & Whitehead, M. (2021). The Dahlgren-Whitehead model of health determinants: 30 years on and still chasing rainbows. *Public Health, 199,* 20–24. https://doi.org/10.1016/j.puhe.2021.08.009

Davies, R. (2017, June 26). Grenfell Tower: Cladding material linked to fire pulled from sale worldwide. *The Guardian.* https://www.theguardian.com/uk-news/2017/jun/26/grenfell-tower-cladding-linked-to-fire-pulled-from-sale-worldwide

Davies, T. (2022). Slow violence and toxic geographies: "Out of sight" to whom? *Environment and Planning C: Politics and Space, 40*(2), 409–427. https://doi.org/10.1177/2399654419841063

Daschuk, J. (2013). *Clearing the plains: Disease, politics of starvation, and the loss of Indigenous life*. University of Regina Press.

de Rivera, J. (2020). A guide to understanding and combatting digital capitalism. *tripleC: Communication, Capitalism & Critique. Journal for a Global Sustainable Information Society, 18*(2), 725–743. https://doi.org/10.31269/triplec.v18i2.1173

Engels, F. (2009). *The condition of the working class in England in 1844*. Penguin Classics. (Original work published 1845)

Ferrer, X., van Nuenen, T., Such, J. M., Coté, M., & Criado, N. (2021). Bias and discrimination in AI: A cross-disciplinary perspective. *IEEE Technology and Society Magazine, 40*(2), 72–80. https://doi.org/10.48550/arXiv.2008.07309

Flint, C. (2021). *Introduction to geopolitics* (4th ed.). Routledge.

Foucault, M. (1990). *The history of sexuality: An introduction* (Vol. I, R. Hurley, Trans.). Vintage. (Original work published in 1976)

Freeman, A. (2007). Fast food: Oppression through poor nutrition. *California Law Review, 95*(6), 2221–2259. https://doi.org/10.15779/Z386997

Fuchs, C. (2018). Capitalism, patriarchy, slavery, and racism in the age of digital capitalism and digital labour. *Critical Sociology, 44*(4–5), 677–702. https://doi.org/10.1177/0896920517691108

Fuchs, C. (2022). *Digital capitalism: Media, communication and society* (Vol. 3). Routlegde.

Galtung, J. (1969). Violence, peace, and peace research. *Journal of Peace Research, 6*(3), 167–191. https://doi.org/10.1177/002234336900600301

Garcia, R. (2023). The social determinants of health. In G. Faye and M. Lotas (Eds.), *A population health approach to health disparities for nurses: Care for vulnerable* (pp. 107–130). Springer.

Gaventa, J. (2006). Finding the spaces for change: A power analysis. *Institute of Development Studies Bulletin, 37*(6), 23–33. https://doi.org/10.1111/j.1759-5436.2006.tb00320.x

Gaventa, J. (2017, December 18). *What have we learned from the powercube?* Institute of Development Studies. https://www.ids.ac.uk/news/what-have-we-learned-from-the-powercube/

Global Resilience Institute. (2018). *Grenfell Tower fire demonstrates the effects of cascading failures*. Resilience News. https://globalresilience.northeastern.edu/grenfell-tower-fire-information-demonstrates-effects-cascading-failures/

Gonzalez, R. M., & Gilleskie, D. (2017). Infant mortality rate as a measure of a country's health: A robust method to improve reliability and comparability. *Demography, 54*(2), 701–720. https://doi.org/10.1007/s13524-017-0553-7

Government of Canada. (2017, July 4). *Just facts: Missing and murdered Indigenous women and girls.* https://www.justice.gc.ca/eng/rp-pr/jr/jf-pf/2017/july04.html

Government of Canada. (2022a, October 27). *Independent Special Interlocutor for missing children and unmarked graves and burial sites associated with Indian residential schools.* https://www.justice.gc.ca/eng/interlocutor-interlocuteur/index.html

Government of Canada. (2022b, December 15). *Just facts: Overrepresentation of Black people in the Canadian criminal justice system.* https://www.justice.gc.ca/eng/rp-pr/jr/obpccjs-spnsjpc/index.html

Grover, C. (2019). Violent proletarianisation: Social murder, the reserve army of labour and social security "austerity" in Britain. *Critical Social Policy, 39*(3), 335–355. https://doi.org/10.1177/0261018318816932

Hayward, A., & Cidro, J. (2021). Indigenous birth as ceremony and a human right. *Health and Human Rights, 23*(1), 213–224. https://www.hhrjournal.org/2021/06/indigenous-birth-as-ceremony-and-a-human-right/

Hill, A. (2023, June 21). Children raised under UK austerity shorter than European peers, study finds. *The Guardian.* https://www.theguardian.com/business/2023/jun/21/children-raised-under-uk-austerity-shorter-than-european-peers-study

Hodkinson, S. (2020). *Safe as houses: Private greed, political negligence and housing policy after Grenfell.* Manchester University Press.

Hoges, P. (2022, November 10). *General strike threat beats Ontario's anti-worker law.* Labor Notes. https://labornotes.org/2022/11/general-strike-threat-beats-ontario-anti-worker-law

Husbands, W., Nelson, L., Owino, M., & Tharao, W. (2019, December 2). Black Canadians and HIV: How will it end? *Toronto Star.* https://www.thestar.com/opinion/contributors/black-canadians-and-hiv-how-will-it-end/article_73aa40e8-5cd4-58b5-9274-1b9e2db5e135.html

Huseman, J., & Short, D. (2012). "A slow industrial genocide": Tar sands and the Indigenous peoples of northern Alberta. *The International Journal of Human Rights, 16*(1), 216–237, https://doi.org/10.1080/13642987.2011.649593

Jahnel, T., Dassow, H. H., Gerhardus, A., & Schüz, B. (2022). The digital rainbow: Digital determinants of health inequities. *Digital Health, 8.* https://doi.org/10.1177%2F20552076221129093

Julià, M., Vanroelen, C., Bosmans, K., Van Aerden, K., & Benach, J. (2017). Precarious employment and quality of employment in relation to health and well-being in Europe. *International Journal of Health Services, 47*(3), 389–409. https://doi.org/10.1177/0020731417707491

Keles, B., Grealish, A., & Leamy, M. (2024). The beauty and the beast of social media: An interpretative phenomenological analysis of the impact of adolescents' social media experiences on their mental health during the

Covid-19 pandemic. *Current Psychology, 43*(1), 96–112. https://doi.org/10.1007/s12144-023-04271-3

Keles, B., McCrae, N., & Grealish, A. (2020). A systematic review: The influence of social media on depression, anxiety and psychological distress in adolescents. *International Journal of Adolescence and Youth, 25*(1), 79–93. https://doi.org/10.1080/02673843.2019.1590851

Kickbusch, I. (2005). Tackling the political determinants of global health. *BMJ, 331*(7511), 246–247. https://doi.org/10.1136%2Fbmj.331.7511.246

Kickbusch, I. (2015). The political determinants of health—10 years on. *BMJ, 350,* h81. https://doi.org/10.1136/bmj.h81

Kickbusch, I., Allen, L., & Franz, C. (2016). The commercial determinants of health. *The Lancet Global Health, 4*(12), e895–e896. https://doi.org/10.1016/s2214-109x(16)30217-0

Kreps, S., & Kriner, D. L. (2023). The potential impact of emerging technologies on democratic representation: Evidence from a field experiment. *New Media & Society, 0*(0). https://doi.org/10.1177/14614448231160526

Lafer, G. (2004). Neoliberalism by other means: The "war on terror" at home and abroad. *New Political Science, 26*(3), 323–346. https://doi.org/10.1080/07393140 42000251306

Lee, K., & Freudenberg, N. (2020). Addressing the commercial determinants of health begins with clearer definition and measurement. *Global Health Promotion, 27*(2), 3–5. https://doi.org/10.1177/1757975920931249

Leigh, J. P., & Chakalov, B. (2021). Labor unions and health: A literature review of pathways and outcomes in the workplace. *Preventive Medicine Report, 24,* 101502. https://doi.org/10.1016/j.pmedr.2021.101502

Lewandowsky, S., & Pomerantsev, P. (2022). Technology and democracy: A paradox wrapped in a contradiction inside an irony. In A. Hoskins & A. J. Barnier (Eds.), *Memory, Mind & Media, 1,* e5. Cambridge University Press. https://doi.org/doi:10.1017/mem.2021.7

Linder, C., Grimes, N., Williams, B. M., Lacy, M. C., & Parker, B. (2020). What do we know about campus sexual violence? A content analysis of 10 years of research. *The Review of Higher Education, 43*(4), 1017–1040. https://doi.org/10.1353/rhe.2020.0029

Llansó, E., van Hoboken, J., Leerssen, L., & Harambam, J. (2020, February 26). *Artificial intelligence, content moderation, and freedom of expression.* Policy Commons. https://policycommons.net/artifacts/8986433/untitled/9875488/

MacLeod, G. (2018). The Grenfell Tower atrocity: Exposing urban worlds of inequality, injustice, and an impaired democracy. *City: Analysis of Urban Change, Theory, Action, 22*(4), 460–489. https://doi.org/10.1080/13604813.2018.1507099

Macro Trends. (n.d.). *Refugee statistics by country*. https://www.macrotrends.net/globalmetrics/countries/ranking/refugee-statistics

Martin, L. S., & Evans, D. P. (2015). Conflict as a social determinant of health. *SM Journal of Public Health and Epidemiology, 1*(2), 1008.

Marx, K. (1977). *A contribution to the critique of political economy*. Progress Publishers. (Original work published 1859)

Mbembe, J. A. (2003). Necropolitics (L. Meintjes, Trans.). *Public Culture, 15*(1), 11–40. https://doi.org/10.1215/08992363-15-1-11

McCallum, M. J. L. (2017). Starvation, experimentation, segregation, and trauma: Words for reading Indigenous health history. *Canadian Historical Review, 98*(1), 96–113. https://doi.org/10.3138/chr.98.1.McCallum

McGibbon, E. (2018). Decolonizing health care: Reconciliation roles and responsibilities for white settlers. *Women's Health and Urban Life, 13*(2), 18–52. https://doi.org/10.51357/cs.v13i2.127

McGibbon, E. (2019). Truth and reconciliation: Healthcare organizational leadership. *Healthcare Management Forum, 32*(1), 20–24. https://doi.org/10.1177/0840470418803379

McGibbon, E. (2021). The COVID-19 pandemic: On the everyday mechanisms of social murder. *Critical Studies: An International and Interdisciplinary Journal, 16*(1), 35–42. https://doi.org/10.51357/cs.v16i1.148

McGibbon, E., & Etowa, J. (2009). *Anti-racist health care practice*. Canadian Scholars.

Medvedyuk, S., Govender, P., & Raphael, D. (2021). The reemergence of Engels' concept of social murder in response to growing social and health inequalities. *Social Science & Medicine, 289*, 114377. https://doi.org/10.1016/j.socscimed.2021.114377

Mialon, M. (2020). An overview of the commercial determinants of health. *Globalization and Health, 16*(1), 74. https://doi.org/10.1186/s12992-020-00607-x

Muller, J., & Raphael, D. (2023). Does unionization and working under collective agreements promote health? *Health Promotion International, 38*(4), daab181. https://doi.org/10.1093/heapro/daab181

Müller, T., Vandaele, K., & Waddington, J. (2019). *Collective bargaining in Europe: Towards an endgame* (Vol. 2). European Trade Union Institute (ETUI).

Nash, R., Hudson, A., & Luttrell, C. (2006). *Mapping political context: A toolkit for civil society organisations*. Overseas Development Institute.

Naslund, J. A., Bondre, A., Torous, J., & Aschbrenner, K. A. (2020). Social media and mental health: Benefits, risks, and opportunities for research and practice. *Journal of Technology in Behavioral Science, 5*(3), 245–257. https://doi.org/10.1007/s41347-020-00134-x

National Center for Health Statistics. (2020). *Healthy people 2020*. Centers for Disease Control and Prevention. https://www.cdc.gov/nchs/healthy_people/hp2020.htm

Native Womens Wilderness. (n.d.). *Murdered and missing Indigenous women*. https://www.nativewomenswilderness.org/mmiw

Navarro, V. (2007). Neoliberalism as class ideology; or, the political causes of the growth of inequalities. *International Journal of Health Services, 37*(1), 47–62. https://doi.org/10.2190/ap65-x154-4513-r520

Nesi, J., Rothenberg, W. A., Bettis, A. H., Massing-Schaffer, M., Fox, K. A., Telzer, E. H., Lindquist, K. A., & Prinstein, M. J. (2022). Emotional responses to social media experiences among adolescents: Longitudinal associations with depressive symptoms. *Journal of Clinical Child & Adolescent Psychology, 51*(6), 907–922. https://doi.org/10.1080/15374416.2021.1955370

Nixon, R. (2011). *Slow violence and the environmentalism of the poor*. Harvard University Press.

Organisation for Economic Co-operation and Development (OECD). (2017). *OECD employment outlook 2017*. https://doi.org/10.1787/empl_outlook-2017-en

Organisation for Economic Co-operation and Development (OECD). (2019). *Infant mortality rates in OECD countries: 2017 (or nearest year)*. https://www.oecd-ilibrary.org/sites/ea7e9e6a-en/index.html?itemId=/content/component/ea7e9e6a-en

Organisation for Economic Co-operation and Development (OECD). (2023). *Health at a glance 2023: OECD Indicators, infant mortality rates*. https://data.oecd.org/healthstat/infant-mortality-rates.htm

Otero, G. (2018). *The neoliberal diet: Healthy profits, unhealthy people*. University of Texas Press.

Otero, G., Gürcan, E. C., Pechlaner, G., & Liberman, G. (2018). Food security, obesity, and inequality: Measuring the risk of exposure to the neoliberal diet. *Journal of Agrarian Change, 18*(3), 536–554. https://doi.org/10.1111/joac.12252

Ottersen, O. P., Dasgupta, J., Blouin, C., Buss, P., Chongsuvivatwong, V., Frenk, J., Fukuda-Parr, S. Gawanas, B. P., Giacaman, R., Gyapong, J., Leaning, J., Marmot, M., McNeill, D., Mongella, G. I., Moyo, N., Møgedal, S., Ntsaluba, A., Ooms, G., Bjertness, E., … Scheel, I. B. (2014). The political origins of health inequity: Prospects for change. *The Lancet, 383*(9917), 630–667. https://doi.org/10.1016/s0140-6736(13)62407-1

Özdemir, V. (2021). Digital is political: Why we need a feminist conceptual lens on determinants of digital health. *OMICS: A Journal of Integrative Biology, 25*(4), 249–254. https://doi.org/10.1089/omi.2021.0020

Panitch, L. (1986). Working class politics in crisis: Essays on labour and the state. *Capital & Class, 11*(1), 125–128. https://doi.org/10.1177/030981688703100110

Parfitt, B. (2019, August 14). *The battle for Haida Gwaii's cedars*. The Narwhal. https://thenarwhal.ca/battle-haida-gwaiis-cedars/

Parsons, P. (2022, May 17). *Human remains found near Alberta residential school site likely children, First Nation says*. CBC News. https://www.cbc.ca/news/canada/edmonton/human-remains-found-near-alberta-residential-school-site-likely-children-first-nation-says-1.6457286

Paul, D. N. (2006). *We were not the savages: Collision between European and Native American civilizations.* Fernwood Publishing.
People's Health Movement, Medact, Global Equity Gauge Alliance, & University of South Africa. (2005). *Global health watch 2005–2006: An alternative world health report.* Zed Books.
Reno, R., & Hyder, A. (2018). The evidence base for social determinants of health as risk factors for infant mortality: A systematic scoping review. *Journal of Health Care for the Poor and Underserved, 29*(4), 1188–1208. https://doi.org/10.1353/hpu.2018.0091
Rollie, T. (2021, June 8). *Horrors of residential schools existed not far from Okotoks.* Western Wheel. https://www.westernwheel.ca/local-news/horrors-of-residential-schools-existed-not-far-from-okotoks-3849354
Said, E. (2005). *The public role of writers and intellectuals.* In S. Bermann & M. Wood (Eds.), Nation, language, and the ethics of translation (pp. 15–29). Princeton University Press.
Schiller, D. (2000). *Digital capitalism: Networking the global market system.* MIT Press.
Schrecker, T. (2016a). "Neoliberal epidemics" and public health: Sometimes the world is less complicated than it appears. *Critical Public Health, 26*(5), 477–480. https://doi.org/10.1080/09581596.2016.1184229
Schrecker, T. (2016b). Neoliberalism and health: The linkages and the dangers. *Sociology Compass, 10*(10), 952–971. https://doi.org/10.1111/soc4.12408
Schrecker, T., & Bambra, C. (2015). *How politics makes us sick: Neoliberal epidemics.* Springer.
Smith, C., & Stevens, A. (2019). The architecture of modern anti-unionism in Canada: Class struggle and the erosion of workers' collective freedoms. *Capital & Class, 43*(3), 459–481. https://doi.org/10.1177/0309816818815262
Smyrnaios, N. (2016). The GAFAM effect: Strategies and logics of the internet oligopoly. *Communication & Languages, 188*(2), 61–83. https://www.cairn-int.info/article-E_COMLA_188_0061-the-gafam-effect-strategies-and-logics.htm
Snowdon, W. (2019, March 8). *There was a "heaviness": Alberta anthropologists locate unmarked graves of residential schoolchildren.* CBC News. https://www.cbc.ca/news/canada/edmonton/unmarked-graves-residential-school-alberta-saskatchewan-1.5045182
Stanford, J. (2005). Revisiting the "flexibility hypothesis." *Canadian Public Policy/Analyse de Politiques, 31*(1), 109–116. https://doi.org/10.2307/3552600
Statistics Canada. (2015). *Unionization rates of employed individuals aged 17 to 64, 1981 to 2012, percentage.* https://www150.statcan.gc.ca/n1/pub/75-006-x/2013001/article/11878/c-g/desc/desc01-eng.htm
Statistics Canada. (2020). *Canadian Centre for Justice and Community Safety Statistics: Incident-based uniform crime reporting survey.*

Stote, K.-A. (2012). The coercive sterilization of Aboriginal women in Canada. *American Indian Culture and Research Journal, 36*(3), 117–150. https://api.fqpn.qc.ca/wp-content/uploads/2021/02/AICRJ_STOTE-STERILIZATION.pdf

Subramaniam, V. (2022, December 10). Inside the emboldening of Canada's unions. *The Globe and Mail.* https://www.theglobeandmail.com/business/article-canada-unions-emboldened-labour/

Svensson, R., Johnson, B., & Olsson, A. (2022). Does gender matter? The association between different digital media activities and adolescent well-being. *BMC Public Health, 22*(1), 273. https://doi.org/10.1186/s12889-022-12670-7

Swenson, A., & Chan, K. (2024, March 14). Election disinformation takes a big leap with AI being used to deceive worldwide. *Associated Press.* https://apnews.com/article/artificial-intelligence-elections-disinformation-chatgpt-bc283e7426402f0b4baa7df280a4c3fd

Taylor-Robinson, D., Lai, E. T. C., Wickham, S., Rose, T., Norman, P., Bambra, C., Whitehead, M., & Barr, B. (2019). Assessing the impact of rising child poverty on the unprecedented rise in infant mortality in England, 2000–2017: Time trend analysis. *BMJ Open, 9*(10), e029424. https://doi.org/10.1136/bmjopen-2019-029424

Truth and Reconciliation Commission of Canada. (2015). *Honouring the truth, reconciling for the future: Summary of the final report of the Truth and Reconciliation Commission of Canada.* https://ehprnh2mwo3.exactdn.com/wp-content/uploads/2021/01/Executive_Summary_English_Web.pdf

United Nations. (1948, December 9). *UN Treaty Collection: Convention on the Prevention and Punishment of the Crime of Genocide.* https://treaties.un.org/pages/ViewDetails.aspx?src=TREATY&mtdsg_no=IV-1&chapter=4

Vescera, Z. (2023, January 9). Conditions actually look good for Canadian unions in 2023. *Jacobin.* https://jacobin.com/2023/01/british-columbia-labor-organizing-union-drives-private-sector

Walters, M. A., Paterson, J., Brown, R., & McDonnell, L. (2020). Hate crimes against trans people: Assessing emotions, behaviors, and attitudes toward criminal justice agencies. *Journal of Interpersonal Violence, 35*(21–22), 4583–4613. https://doi.org/10.1177/0886260517715026

Wesley-Esquimaux, C. C., & Smolewski, M. (2004). *Historic trauma and Aboriginal healing.* Aboriginal Healing Foundation.

West, R., & Marteau, T. (2013). Commentary on Casswell (2013): The commercial determinants of health. *Addiction, 108*(4), 686–687. https://doi.org/10.1111/add.12118

Wikipedia. (2021, June 25). *Canadian Indian residential school gravesites.* Retrieved April 20, 2023, from https://en.wikipedia.org/wiki/Canadian_Indian_residential_school_gravesites#cite_note-dunbow-20

Wilcox, M. M. (2023). Oppression is not "culture": The need to center systemic and structural determinants to address anti-Black racism and racial trauma in psychotherapy. *Psychotherapy, 60*(1), 76–85. https://doi.org/10.1037/pst0000446

Woolford, A. (2023). The destruction of families Canadian Indian residential schools and the refamilialization of Indigenous children. In V. Chartrand & J. Savarese (Eds.), *Unsettling colonialism in the Canadian criminal justice system* (pp. 45–72). Athabasca University Press.

World Health Organization (WHO). (2008, August 27). *Closing the gap in a generation: Health equity through action on the social determinants of health—Final report of the commission on social determinants of health.* https://www.who.int/publications/i/item/WHO-IER-CSDH-08.1

Zakrison, T. L., Milian Valdés, D., & Muntaner, C. (2019). Social violence, structural violence, hate, and the trauma surgeon. *International Journal of Health Services, 49*(4), 665–681. https://doi.org/10.1177/0020731419859834

Zhang, Z., Bouri, E., Klein, T., & Jalkh, N. (2022). Geopolitical risk and the returns and volatility of global defense companies: A new race to arms? *International Review of Financial Analysis, 83*, 102327. https://doi.org/10.1016/j.irfa.2022.102327

CHAPTER 6

Root Determinants of Health are Complex Adaptive Systems

CHAPTER OBJECTIVES

Using as many examples as possible:

1. Identify and discuss five main characteristics of complex adaptive systems.
2. Explain how the Root Determinants of Health Framework, with social DoH, ecological DoH, and structural DoH may form a complex adaptive system.
3. Using the examples in the chapter, describe what is meant by "wicked problems."
4. Explain how the Alberta Tar Sands, a "slow industrial genocide," form a complex adaptive system.
5. Explain how the COVID-19 pandemic forms a complex adaptive system.

CRITICAL THINKING QUESTIONS

1. What are some of the public policy ways that the Canadian government has been complicit in the Alberta Tar Sands CAS?
2. What are some policy actions that the Canadian government can take to slow climate destruction in Canada?
3. What are some CAS elements of the COVID-19 pandemic that are not discussed in the chapter?

4. Applying the CAS concepts and descriptions in Table 6.1, explain how increasing university tuition in Canada is an example of a CAS.
5. How would you explain CAS to someone who is not familiar with the concept?

INTRODUCTION

This chapter synthesizes the ideas throughout the book by demonstrating how a Root Determinants of Health Framework can be applied to understand relationships among the social, ecological, and structural DoH. Each of the previous chapters included many examples of how it is impossible to separate the DoH because they form a complex adaptive system (CAS), a group of semi-autonomous, independent agents (components of the system, such as humans, animals, ecosystems) that interact in interdependent ways to produce system-wide patterns. The chapter begins with an overview of CAS thinking, including some of the main ideas in complexity science, such as their dynamic, unpredictable, and multidimensional nature. Five main CAS concepts are described and applied to urgent root-cause issues, such as some of those described throughout the book. CAS are then explored within the book's Root Determinants of Health Framework, including some of the ways that the DoH pose "**wicked problems**." Building on the complex adaptive systems (CAS) discussion in Chapter 1, two urgent examples of synergies in the DoH are analyzed through the lens of CAS: 1) the Alberta, Canada, Tar Sands, and 2) the COVID-19 pandemic. Although there are numerous possibilities of environmental and structural DoH in the chapters of this book, these two examples provide an exceptional base to describe synergies among the social, ecological, and structural DoH. The tar sands and the pandemic are especially strong examples due to their "problem wickedness" and the ways that their devastating global impacts so clearly cut across the social, ecological, and structural DoH. These insights contribute to new knowledge that can inform action to tackle the social murder, necropolitics, and slow violence that so insidiously targets and murders the already-dispossessed and poses immediate threats to Earth's very life-support systems.

ROOT DETERMINANTS: A COMPLEX ADAPTIVE SYSTEMS APPROACH

A CAS approach is an ideal way to deepen an understanding of how the Root Determinants of Health Framework may be applied to understand the complexities of the social, ecological, and structural DoH. CAS thinking is unapologetically "messy." The unpredictability and interconnectedness of CAS means that they cannot be broken down into their component parts, a strategy that is unfortunately endemic in many public systems, such as health, education, and public governance, to mention a few. Hence the seemingly impossible task of understanding and even solving wicked problems, such as the environmental and human health damage associated with the Alberta Tar Sands, and the unfolding of the COVID-19 pandemic since its official emergence in 2020.

Overview of CAS Thinking

The study of CAS evolved within the field of complexity science, which has its roots in physics, mathematics, and biology. **Complexity science** refers to the methodical investigation of emergent phenomena within systems. It continues to stretch across disciplines, from physics, mathematics, biology, and chemistry, to health and social sciences. Examples of these phenomena include ecosystems, the human brain, ant colonies, and economic networks, which are all complex systems displaying collective behaviour, or emergence, beyond the sum of their parts (Jensen, 2022). The field of CAS has numerous origins, including the work of physicist Fritjof Capra (1996, 2005; Capra & Luisi, 2014) who critiqued Cartesian, linear (positivist) approaches to understanding natural and social phenomena. He explained that insights about systems may be generated by analyzing the relationships among all the parts of the system and how these relationships contribute significantly to the character of the whole. Capra's work emphasized the web-like structure of all systems and thus the interconnectedness of all system parts.

Complexity science is not based in any unified theory—it is a collection of theories and constructs that have conceptual integrity among themselves (Begun et al., 2003). Begun et al. (2003) explained that in CAS, the "complex" portion implies diversity and a wide variety of elements. "Adaptive" denotes the capacity to change and to learn from experience, and "systems" refers to elements that are independent agents. These CAS agents are located within a densely connected, interacting web and the agents act based on local knowledge and conditions. This system aspect is not associated with the traditionally used machine metaphor (Morgan, 1998), which is of limited utility for understanding and mapping non-linear, continuously changing and deeply connected systems such as the DoH. "Given the inherent complexity of human-Earth systems, the plurality of their candidate pathways of change, and their diverse sources of uncertainty, there is a need to rethink our traditional disciplinary approaches to human-Earth systems science as well as the ways scientific knowledge is produced" (Reed et al., 2022, p. 1).

Table 6.1 describes core concepts for applying a CAS approach to understanding the DoH. Within the field of complexity science, CAS have several central characteristics: 1) they are dynamic, unpredictable, and multidimensional (e.g., COVID-19); 2) they have interconnected relationships and parts that are not possible to disentangle (e.g., structural policy intervention to increase housing security); 3) they have positive and negative **feedback loops** (e.g., operation of the Alberta Tar Sands over time); 4) they self-organize into **system-wide coherent patterns** (e.g., austerity measures after the 2008 global financial crisis); and 5) they demonstrate an overall **emergence of control**, where processes

Table 6.1: CAS Characteristics and Root Determinants of Health: Case Applications

CAS Characteristic and Description	Root Determinants of Health: Case Application for Selected Root-Cause Problems*
1) *Are dynamic, unpredictable, and multidimensional*: The large number of agents in a CAS, the connections among the agents, and the influence of external forces all combine to result in constant and discontinuous (unpredictable) change in the CAS (Begun et al., 2003).	*The COVID-19 pandemic* involves a vast number of "agents" (e.g., humans; the ecosystem; the virus itself, which is continuously mutating; and multiple levels of people engaged in public health clinical and community intervention and policymaking). External forces were, and continue to be, central (e.g., Big Pharma and vaccine access, as well as unpredictable social DoH such as barriers in health care access across the isms). (Also see Chapter 3.)

Table 6.1: CAS Characteristics and Root Determinants of Health: Case Applications (*Continued*)

CAS Characteristic and Description	**Root Determinants of Health: Case Application for Selected Root-Cause Problems***
2) *Have interconnected relationships and parts that are not possible to disentangle:* Systems parts are not linear, not separable.	*Structural policy intervention to decrease homelessness is based in increasing housing security*: If policies do not integrate interconnected relationships such as intersections of the isms as social DoH (ageism, classism, genderism, racism), the policy outcomes are not likely to increase housing access for those experiencing these isms (also see Chapter 3).
3) *Have feedback loops, positive and negative*: What is happening in one part of the system impacts the other parts of the system, forming a feedback loop that can either enhance solutions to complex problems or increase these problems (also see emergence of control).	*Alberta Tar Sands Feedback Loop*: 1) Capitalist, colonialist governance systems create and sustain Big Oil tar sands as a root cause of unchecked human-planet toxin proliferation in Treaty 8 Territories; 2) Big Oil creates severe ecological damage in Treaty 8 Territories and whole-planet impacts (e.g., greenhouse gas emission, loss of Boreal forests as global carbon sink, vital habitat destruction, pollution, eco-toxicity, biodiversity loss...); 3) Tar sands damage Indigenous Peoples' health, a "slow industrial genocide." Social DoH are already deeply and negatively impacted by colonial, capitalist supra-systems (food, housing insecurity, access barriers to culturally safe health care...). (See Figure 6.2.)
4) *Are self-organizing into system-wide, coherent patterns*: There is no individual leader, no overall plan or collective intention devised together among the players. Nevertheless, the rules, operating individually and at a local level, broadly defined (e.g., community, individual, nation), are sufficient to produce globally coherent patterns that look as if someone, or at any rate something, is directing them (Paley, 2007).	*Austerity measures* after the 2008 financial crisis quickly self-organized across global neoliberal political economies in rich countries (e.g., United Kingdom, United States, Canada), resulting in a relatively cohesive global pattern of measurable and persistent increases in health and social inequities (also see Chapter 2).

(*continued*)

Table 6.1: CAS Characteristics and Root Determinants of Health: Case Applications (*Continued*)

CAS Characteristic and Description	**Root Determinants of Health: Case Application for Selected Root-Cause Problems***
5) *Demonstrate the emergence of control*: Processes occurring at the fine scale bring about emergent higher-level regimes (ways of organizing a system, prevailing patterns over time) that in turn feed back to regulate what occurs at the fine scale, leading to the emergence of control—interactions in the system create and maintain a regime that reinforces the system state, a phenomenon known as lock-in (Centre for Complex Systems Studies, n.d.).	*Fossil fuel* energy provision is a sociotechnical regime in the structural DoH realm, developing over a long period of time (e.g., liquid fuel for transportation; oil, gas for heating houses; coal, natural gas for conversion into electricity). This regime also includes oil drilling, refining, coal mining, gas exploration and transportation, research and development in coal, oil and gas, rules and regulations, international treaties, financial markets, and stock exchanges (Vergragt et al., 2011). The regime involves powerful economic and political actors, with success in fighting off challenges related to renewable energy sources and energy conservation—fossil fuel energy provision thus represents a mature sociotechnical regime with a high degree of technological lock-in (Vergragt et al., 2011).

*Each of these case applications has been described more fully elsewhere in this book.

occurring at the fine scale produce prevailing whole-system patterns over time (e.g., fossil fuel lock-in).

The DoH themselves are also operating as a CAS. The gradual emergence of globally coherent patterns of organization, such as neoliberal epidemics, is reflected in the ways that definitions, frameworks, and descriptions of the DoH are converging. Meanings within each of the three DoH areas largely began with somewhat distinct definitions. As described in Chapters 1 and 3, over the past 20 years, conceptualization of the social, ecological, and structural DoH have continued to theoretically converge: social DoH increasingly include structural DoH, such as globalization and racism, and ecological DoH, such as pollution and land dispossession. Ecological DoH increasingly include structural DoH, such as neoliberal globalization and resulting corporate profit on the scale of trillions of dollars. The emergent complexity of the DoH is shaped by contested perspectives, evolving and continuously changing synergies, and the pressing uncertainties that influence their development over space and time. This is why it is not possible or fruitful to craft static definitions of the three DoH.

The Root Determinants of Health Framework as a CAS

The science of CAS is increasingly recognized as a major advancement for understanding human and planet health, especially in the field of environmental sciences. For example, Nayak and Waterson (2019) applied a CAS model to study global food safety and the food supply chain, from subsistence farmers to multinational food companies. They analyzed how these processes can be viewed as a multifaceted structure with multiple interactions, including the globalization of the food industry and the impact of globalization on food safety. CAS have also been applied to study climate risks and vulnerabilities, with empirical evidence to demonstrate the importance of factors such as modulation (connectedness), feedback mechanisms, redundancy, and the susceptibility to change of individual components within a climate system (Naylor et al., 2020). CAS thinking has contributed to the development of ecosystem research methodologies, exploring methodological challenges such as how to set study boundaries for ecosystems and their structures and relationships, and how to explain the temporal dynamics of co-evolution (how ecosystems change over time) (Phillips & Ritala, 2019).

Phillipps et al. (2022) applied an intersectionality-based policy analysis framework to examine complexities in access to wild game and fish for urban Indigenous (First Nations, Inuit, Métis) women. Researchers linked "colonial control over wildlife and the Western food safety discourse, with infringements on Indigenous food sovereignty, experiences of racism in food settings and on the land, as well as broad control over Indigenous sovereignty in Ontario" (p. 1). In CAS applications within the social DoH, health services and health systems have been emphasized, for example, in the study of health care organizations as CAS (Begun et al., 2003), in health care itself as a CAS (Rouse, 2008), and in understanding health systems reform as a CAS (Sturmberg et al., 2012). Researchers have also studied systems thinking, systems mapping, and organizational change in education, specifically in the teaching and learning process (Cabrera & Cabrera, 2019). Importantly, although the uptake of CAS thinking is increasing across areas such as the social, ecological, and structural DoH, discussions and real-world applications do not necessarily apply an equity or justice-focused analysis, thereby limiting the criticality of analysis, and in some cases, their utility to contribute to justice-oriented public policy and governance change to mitigate or halt inequities across the DoH.

The Root Determinants of Health Framework illustrates the **permeable boundaries** among the social, ecological, and structural DoH. Permeable boundaries refers to processes whereby the boundaries or limits of CAS, such as the social, ecological, and structural DoH, also have common building blocks or ideas that they share across these boundaries. For example, although each of the DoH areas have distinct definitions and properties (boundaries) in and of themselves, ideas such as the DoH impacts of neoliberal public policy cut across all three areas. Due to their practical (on-the-ground, everyday) and theoretical synergies, these three areas of investigation and action may be best understood as a complex adaptive system (or systems)—evolving, emergent, and unpredictable. As demonstrated in this chapter, when examined from the lens of multiple critical perspectives, each of the three broad DoH areas are in and of themselves also inter-webbed, living, changing systems that are not possible to disentangle. These systems contain numerous positive and negative feedback loops—what is happening in one part of the system impacts the other parts of the system, forming a feedback loop that can either enhance solutions to complex problems or make them worse. CAS applications are useful in gaining a better understanding of how social, ecological, and structural DoH come together and how we may find entry points to provoke public policy change (McGibbon & McPherson, 2011); spur collective social action across civil society, academic, and community mobilization; and gain valuable insights for transforming our understanding of the benefits, risks, and resilience of complex adaptive human-Earth systems (Reed et al., 2022). "Confronting human-Earth systems complexity requires a diverse, transdisciplinary workforce and community-level open science" (p. 1).

Examples of CAS Synergies among Social, Ecological, and Structural Determinants of Health

The social, ecological, and structural DoH are not distinct constructs, as illustrated in Figure 6.1 (repeated here from Chapter 1 for clarity).

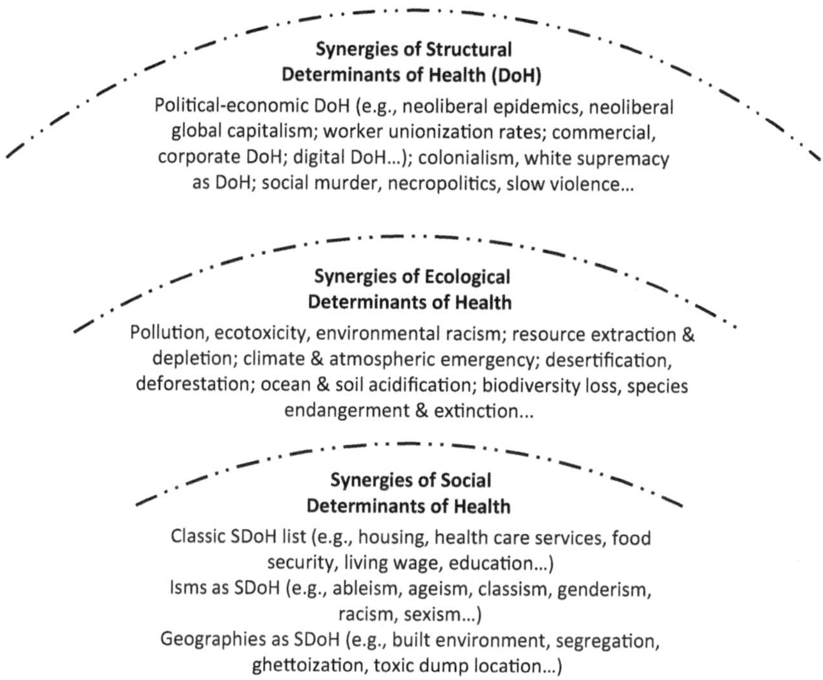

Figure 6.1: Snapshot: Synergies of Social, Ecological, and Structural Determinants of Health (Repeated here from Chapter 1, Figure 1.3, for clarity)

Source: Created by author.

Rather, they operate in tandem with each other and are always related and interacting. Social DoH, such as inequitable income distribution across class and racialization barriers, are directly connected to the structural DoH. Neoliberal political economies, a central structural DoH, have the aim of supporting market-driven management of economic matters in a country. This approach results in bolstering key market players, such as mega-corporations, in part through laws and strategies that decrease, and in some cases eliminate, corporate taxation (Sanger, 2019). To make up the loss of taxation revenue, one of the strategies is austerity measures, which have devastating impacts on a population's health and well-being because these measures target social supports, such as income supplements, minimum wages, and health and social programs, such as universal, not-for-profit health care.

Ecological DoH permeate the social and structural DoH. An example involves living in crowded indoor spaces due to deprivation and poverty. These living conditions are caused by structural DoH, such as lack of equitable access to resources needed to ensure equity across social DoH such as housing security, including equitable access to educational opportunities, and hence, stable employment. Living in crowded indoor spaces is known to cause significant increases in infectious diseases, such as tuberculosis and other respiratory infections, as evidenced during the pandemic, where people living in crowded homes were also found to have significant increases in COVID-19 infections (Azuma et al., 2020). At the same time, it is known that the pandemic was caused by unprecedented increases in global zoonoses (viruses and bacteria that cross the human-animal barrier), such as the COVID-19 virus (Okello, 2020). Increasing incidence of zoonotic disease emergence is well documented to be caused by major changes in land use, increasing urbanization, global connectedness, and climate change (Holmes, 2022).

Furthermore, global heating results in changing geographic distributions of wildlife as appropriate habitats are destroyed by resource extraction and depletion and the displacement of local agricultural practices by large-scale, for-profit food corporations. These processes lead to **multispecies refugees** that must move to sustain their viability. Multispecies refugees refer to forced migration of human and nonhuman animals due to climate emergency threats to public health, such as extreme weather events, water scarcity, increasing rates of infectious diseases, and wildfires (Khazaal & Almiron, 2021). Since 2010, cross-border migration and mass movement of people displaced by climate change-related disasters has risen to 21.5 million (United Nations High Commission for Refugees, n.d.). As the planet warms, species are shifting where, when, and how they thrive: half of all Earth's species are on the move (Welch, 2017). "Human populations that rely on the animal world will similarly find subsistence increasingly difficult and so may exploit previously pristine areas or change farming practices, increasing the risk of exposure to animal pathogens" (p. 1). In turn, limiting these kinds of anthropogenic ecological damage requires addressing the structural DoH, including the root causes of climate emergency described in Chapter 4.

CAS, Determinants of Health, and Wicked Problems

A CAS approach involves examining and mapping wicked problems. Due to the dynamic nature of inequities and resulting injustices related to all three of the DoH and their synergies, they involve wicked problems—ones for which each endeavour to design a solution changes the understanding of the problem itself. Box 6.1 describes 10 main characteristics of wicked problems. Some of the wicked problems described in this book include

- designing targeted public policy to decrease health inequities;
- addressing health and social impacts of intersections of health care and 2SLGBTQIA+ identities;
- addressing the impacts of slow violence on Earth's life support systems;
- significantly decreasing childhood poverty;
- making public policy changes to halt and reverse rising infant mortality rates; and
- addressing the impacts of austerity measures after the 2008 financial crisis, ecosystem destruction, and global heating.

Wicked problems were first described by two faculty members at the University of California at Berkley: design science professor Horst Rittel and planning professor Melvin Webber (Rittel & Webber, 1973). Wicked problems refer to social, scientific, economic and political problems (to name a few) that are difficult or impossible to solve due to their complex and interconnected nature. "Wicked problems lack clarity in both their aims and solutions, and are subject to real-world constraints which hinder risk-free attempts to find a solution" (Wong, 2023).

Wicked problems cannot be solved in a traditional linear fashion, because the problem definition constantly changes and evolves as possible new solutions are considered and/or implemented (Rittel & Webber, 1973)—solutions to wicked problems are not right or wrong, simply "better," "worse," "good enough," or "not good enough." Every wicked problem is essentially unique and novel. There are so many factors and conditions, all embedded in dynamic social contexts, that no two wicked problems are alike, and the solutions to them will always be custom designed and fitted (Rittel & Webber, 1973). Ideas to consider for understanding "problem wickedness" include the following:

1) *You don't understand the problem until you have developed a solution.* Indeed, there is no definitive statement of "The Problem" since it is ill-structured, with an evolving set of interlocking issues and constraints (Rittel & Webber, 1973). For example, during the COVID-19 pandemic, social distancing, masking, and vaccination (the solutions) eventually led to a deeper understanding of determining virus transmission and designing effective preventive measures (the problems). In other words, these problems were not well understood until the solutions were implemented.

2) *Every solution to a wicked problem is a "one-shot operation"* and every attempt has consequences. As Rittel stated, "One cannot build a freeway to see how it works" (Rittel & Webber, 1973). This is the paradox of wicked problems: you cannot learn about the problem without trying solutions, but every solution you try is expensive and has lasting unintended consequences that are likely to create new wicked problems (Rittel & Webber, 1973). For example, a carbon tax is increasingly implemented in many jurisdictions as a public policy solution to curb atmospheric damage leading to global heating. Opposition to the carbon tax is largely rooted in neoliberal, market-driven ideologies. However, neoliberal public policies also come with other aspects of neoliberalism, such as austerity measures and retrenchment of social insurance programs in neoliberal welfare states. These harms to achieving equity across the social DoH are then likely to increase when political parties opposing the carbon tax are elected into power.

Box 6.1: Ten Main Characteristics of Wicked Problems

According to Rittel and Webber (1973), there are 10 important characteristics of wicked problems:

1. They do not have a definitive formulation or problem statement;
2. They do not have a "stopping rule." In other words, these problems lack an inherent logic that signals when they are solved;

3. Their solutions are not true or false, only good or bad;
4. Due to the countless inter-webbed, tangled components of a wicked problem, there is no way to test the solution to a wicked problem;
5. They cannot be studied through trial and error. Their solutions are irreversible so, as Rittel and Webber (1973) put it, "every trial counts";
6. There is no end to the number of solutions or approaches to a wicked problem;
7. All wicked problems are essentially unique;
8. Wicked problems can always be described as the symptom of other problems;
9. The way a wicked problem is described or formulated determines (confines) its possible solutions.

Source: Johnson-Woods, 2023.

THE CAS OF ALBERTA TAR SANDS: "A SLOW INDUSTRIAL GENOCIDE"

The Alberta Tar Sands are a crucial instance of long-term synergies among planet health and environmental public policy in Canada, corporate profit, and human ecosystems. They systematically illustrate the technical aspects of oil extraction and processing and how mega-corporations, rather than Canadian climate change mitigation policy initiatives, have directed the longitudinal impacts of the tar sands.

Overview of the Alberta Tar Sands

Tar sands are found in about 70 countries and they create significant wicked problems for humans and planet health. Alberta, Canada, is home to the largest industrial project on the globe. Table 6.2 ranks the top eight Alberta Oil Sands companies according to their oil reserves, which refer to the estimate of the amount of crude oil located in a particular economic region with the potential of being extracted (Society of

Table 6.2: Top Eight Alberta Oil Sands Companies: Oil Reserves

Rank	Company	Reserves (in millions of barrels)
1	Suncor Energy	10,935.35
2	Canadian Natural Resources (CNRL)	6.867.53
3	Cenovus Energy	5,613.97
4	ConocoPhillips	5,520.38
5	ExxonMobil	4,844.35
6	Shell	3,670.18
7	PetroChina	3,225.71
8	Athabasca Oil Corporation	3,162.50

Source: Rainforest Action Network, n.d.

Petroleum Engineers, 2019). These numbers demonstrate the enormity of corporate control, not only of current operations in the Alberta Tar Sands, but the reach of these corporations into future profits based on the planned extraction of millions of barrels of oil. Venezuela, Saudi Arabia, and Canada are the three leading countries with the most oil reserves. Tailings ponds from the Alberta Tar Sands contain a "toxic slurry" of heavy metals and hydrocarbons from the bitumen separation process (Leahy, 2019). When oil is processed, the remaining water and solids are discharged into vast tailings ponds that have now surpassed 1.9 trillion litres in Alberta. Their volumes continue to grow each year, with a cumulative clean-up cost of 66.5 billion (CAD) as of 2024. Currently, taxpayers are at risk of paying to cover the costs of cleaning up toxic tailing ponds, which continue to grow (Parkland Institute, 2023). The oil company Syncrude's tailings ponds, at 540 million cubic metres in volume, form one of the world's largest dams, second only to China's Three Gorges Dam. Statistically significant increases in cancers of the blood and lymphatic system, biliary tract, and soft tissue were found in individuals, including many First Nations families living in Fort Chipewyan, which lies in a depositional basin of tar ponds byproducts. Women in the area were found to have a 3.5 times higher risk of lung cancer (Timoney, 2007) when compared to the general population of women. The incidence of a rare form of biliary duct cancer has steadily increased over the past 30 years in Alberta, and rates are two to three times higher in First Nations communities when compared with non-First Nations populations (Tenenbaum, 2009).

In Alberta, "the feverish expansion of oil sands development is based on the untested assumption that mined landscapes can be recovered to something close to the pre-development ecosystem after mining is complete. Reclamation is the final step that mining companies are required to complete before mine closure" (Grant et al., 2008, p. 1). As of 2008, the Government of Alberta certified only 0.2% of the total land base disturbed by fossil fuel extraction as reclaimed. This percentage did not include tailings that companies propose to incorporate into the reclaimed landscape—a remarkably erroneous proposition, given that the toxic tailing lakes are the largest human-made structure in the world and can be seen from space (Hatch & Price, 2008). These 2008 findings have endured over time. In 2019, the largest Big Oil corporations, by far, were Syncrude, Suncor, and National Resources Ltd. Profits are remarkable: Suncor Energy's annual net income for 2022 was 6.98 billion (USD), a 112.44% increase from 2021 (Kirsch, 2021). The total reclaimed land by these three corporations was 14,614 hectares (1,461 square kilometers) (Canada Action, 2019). In 2019, the tar sands covered a total of 22,000 square kilometers in Alberta. Therefore, as of 2019, the total land reclaimed was just over 1,461 square kilometers, or 0.6%. If the land reclamation by these Big Oil corporations and the Canadian government continues at its current pace (from 0.2% in 2008 to 0.6% in 2023), it will take approximately 825,000 years to reclaim the land in Alberta that is damaged by the tar sands. These land reclamation claims are arguably disingenuous, if not unethical.

A development with significant human, environmental, social, and economic costs, the tar sands provide a disturbing modern instance of the ways that the fluidity of financial capital within global capitalism and the pursuit of profit can trigger direct and indirect health impacts that are wide-ranging and distributed unequally across populations. Policy intervention to mitigate harm is correspondingly complex:

> Canada does have some claim to credibility on the climate action front. As early as 2007, Alberta's provincial government instituted a carbon tax on large industrial emitters, which has raised US $350 million (CAD $463 million) for energy research. At the Paris climate summit in 2015, Canada pushed for the ambitious 2.7 degrees Fahrenheit (1.5 degrees Celsius) global warming target. A national carbon tax went into effect April 1, 2019. (Leahy, 2019)

Yet, during the same year that the national carbon tax went into effect in 2019, the Texas-based Kinder Morgan corporation, owners of the 65-year-old Trans Mountain oil pipeline, announced that they would not expand the pipeline—rather, it would build much larger twin pipelines along most of the same 715-mile (1,150-km) route from Alberta to British Columbia on unceded Indigenous Secwepemc territory. In the face of what appeared to be responsible climate policy, under pressure from Big Oil's plans of "unlocking" new Pacific markets for the Alberta Tar Sands, the Canadian government spent CAD $4.5 billion to buy the project (Leahy, 2019). The expanded pipeline deal was undertaken despite organized and prominent opposition from Indigenous and environmental groups (Leahy, 2019).

Due to persistent lack of effective public policy responsibility to decrease fatal harms (mortality) and intergenerational health damage (morbidity), the tar sands are a contemporary example of social murder (MacNeil, 2019). Huseman and Short (2012) refer to the tar sands as a "slow industrial genocide" of the Indigenous Peoples of the Treaty 8 region in northern Alberta. **Slow industrial genocide** refers to the gradual, historical, and deadly health threats of industrial activities such as resource extraction (e.g., Alberta Tar Sands) and chemical processing (e.g., Chemical Valley in Sarnia, Ontario, and Cancer Alley in Louisiana, United States). These industry activities are referred to as industrial genocide because they fit the United Nations (UN) Convention on the Prevention and Punishment of the Crime of Genocide (UN, 1948), which states that genocide means acts committed with intent to destroy, in whole or in part, a national, ethnical, racial, or religious group. More specifically, the term *industrial genocide* is used in cases such as environmental racism, where racialized fatality is well known, yet these industrial activities continue unabated.

In 1899, when Treaty 8 was signed, the Cree and Anthapaskans (or Dene) peoples (including Beavers, Chipewyans, Dogribs, Slaveys, and Yellowknives) were the two major language groups in the region (Huseman & Short, 2012). Treaty negotiations were viewed differently by the First Nations and the settler government—the former having the primary concern of continuation of their traditional way of life, hunting, fishing and being free to roam their territories and the latter having the primary interest of opening up the area to settler populations and industrial exploitation (Huseman & Short, 2012). The slow industrial genocide of the tar sands unfolded within a CAS involving colonialism, genocide, and serious, persistent intergenerational health damage.

The Alberta Tar Sands as a CAS

In the following discussion, evidence regarding the Alberta Tar Sands is applied to describe three central CAS characteristics: 1) *have interconnected relationships and parts that are not possible to disentangle*, 2) *have feedback loops*, and 3) *are self-organizing into system-wide coherent patterns*, demonstrating the emergence of control.

1. *Have interconnected relationships and parts that are not possible to disentangle.* Already-existing intergenerational health damage due to colonialist and misogynist policy (e.g., Indigenous land dispossession, disruption of lifeways, and targeted genocide) are *not possible to separate or disentangle* from toxic human and land-health impacts of the tar sands since their inception in 1967. For example, there is robust evidence of the impacts of the colonial governance strategies of cultural genocide (Battiste & Henderson, 2021; Henderson, 2021; Huseman & Short, 2012), as well as genocide as stated in criteria of the UN Convention on the Prevention and Punishment of the Crime of Genocide (UN, 1948; see Chapter 5). The intergenerational impacts of centuries-old settler assaults on Indigenous Peoples were already fortified by Canadian policy and governance since first contact in the

early 1600s. The Alberta Tar Sands then interacted with, and amplified, these centuries-old colonial assaults. The historical injustices of colonial land dispossession, genocide, and profound disruption of Indigenous lifeways cannot be disentangled from current injustices perpetrated on First Nations Peoples in Treaty 8 territory where the tar sands proliferate.

2. *Have feedback loops.* The tar sands are a pressing example of a CAS feedback loop. Figure 6.2 illustrates such a feedback loop across the social, ecological, and structural DoH. Although the figure depicts three interconnected and moving gears, the edges of the gears are intentionally uneven and do not depict a smoothly moving, mechanistic, and predictable

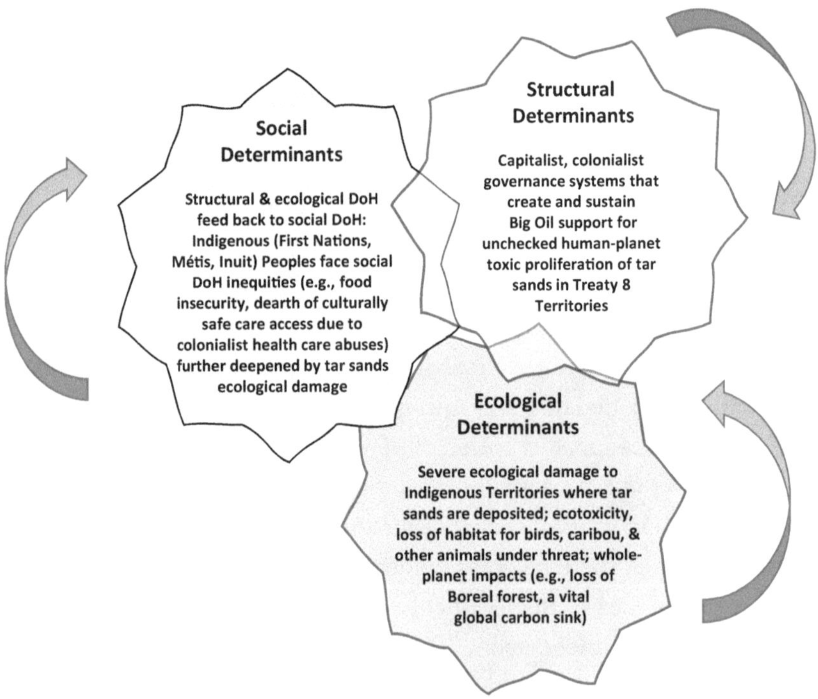

Figure 6.2: CAS Feedback Loop: Snapshot of Social, Ecological, and Structural DoH of the Alberta Tar Sands

Source: Created by author.

system. Consistent with complexity science and wicked problems, the DoH are moving within a CAS and the outcomes are neither smooth nor mechanically predictable. We can only ever describe a system snapshot at any given moment in time. A tar sands feedback loop may be described with the following phases. First, starting with the structural DoH, there is a lack of systematic government monitoring of Alberta Tar Sands clean-up legislation (MacNeil, 2019). This process is rooted in capitalist, colonialist governance systems that create and sustain Big Oil contributions to unchecked human-planet related toxin proliferation in Treaty 8 Territory.

Second, this process leads directly to severe impacts for the ecological DoH, producing ecological damage over time in the geographic area where the tar sands are deposited, as well as whole-planet impacts involving greenhouse gas emissions: industrial development and wildfires in the tar sands region have cleared or degraded nearly 2 million acres of boreal forest since the turn of the millennium, putting a vital habitat for birds, caribou, and other animals at risk—consequently, the tar sands are an urgent climate issue because the boreal forest is a vital global carbon sink, absorbing much more carbon from the atmosphere than it releases (Greenpeace Canada, 2021). The ongoing outcome is that significant increases in tar sands profits (mainly Syncrude, Suncor, and Canadian Natural Resources Ltd.) are supported by government policy inaction over time (MacNeil, 2019).

Third, since the social DoH form a CAS with the structural and ecological DoH, there are direct consequences for human and ecological health. These consequences feedback into the structural determinants that created them. For example, it is well known that the health of Indigenous Peoples is disproportionately damaged by the tar sands because they are located in Indigenous Territory: about 23,000 Indigenous Peoples from 18 First Nations and 6 Métis settlements live in the Alberta Tar Sands region (Natural Resources Canada, 2016). Inequities in the social DoH, such as food insecurity and the dearth of culturally safe access to health services created by colonialist health care abuses (Amster, 2022), are further deepened by tar sands health damage to Treaty 8 Indigenous Peoples. The result is creation of a direct feedback loop to the structural DoH, such as the capitalist, colonialist governance policies that initiated tar sands destruction that continues to perpetuate wicked problems that are the result of the tar sands. The three main tar sands producers are supported by decades-old resistance of public policy and governance decision makers to protect the lands and livelihoods of First Nations People in Treaty 8 Territory (Huseman & Short, 2012).

3. *Are self-organizing into system-wide coherent patterns.* The tar sands also illustrate the CAS characteristic of emergence of control. Processes occurring at the fine scale bring about emergent higher-level regimes (ways of organizing a system, creating prevailing patterns over time) that in turn feed back to control or regulate what occurs at the fine scale, leading to the emergence of control—interactions in the system create and maintain a regime that reinforces the system state, a phenomenon known as lock-in (Vergragt et al., 2011). For example, within social systems, institutions emerge to control the interactions among individuals in society (Centre for Complex Systems Studies, n.d.). In the case of the tar sands, institutional control has emerged with governmental and industry lock-in to fossil fuel extraction. Over the past 30 years, despite government attempts to move towards weaning Canada off fossil fuel extraction, Canada's climate policy has thus far been largely ineffective (MacNeil, 2019). Tar sands expansion plans demonstrate industry lock-in due to increasing government support of the tar sands (Janzwood, 2020). Importantly, in some jurisdictions such as Alberta, social system and public lock-in is demonstrated by increasing pro-Big Oil sentiments of the public, such as Alberta's election in 2023 of The United Conservative Party, whose main election policy platform was supporting and increasing fossil fuel extraction in the province (Lawson, 2022).

THE CAS OF THE COVID-19 PANDEMIC

The COVID-19 pandemic is another pressing case example of a CAS wicked problem. This discussion explores three important characteristics of CAS: they 1) *are dynamic, unpredictable, and multidimensional*, 2) *have feedback loops*, and 3) are self-organizing into *system-wide coherent patterns*, demonstrating the emergence of control. Structural DoH (e.g., climate emergency, social murder, necropolitics), ecological DoH (e.g., ecosystem changes leading to the proliferation of planetary zoonoses), and social DoH (e.g., housing and food insecurity, barriers in access to health care) are each dynamic, unpredictable, and multidimensional systems in and of themselves. Nonetheless, all three of these broad DoH areas operate together and cannot be broken down into their constituent parts. For example, structural DoH, such as public policy–induced inequities in the social DoH, were well in place before the pandemic. They provided the substrate for who became ill, who died, and who bore the burden of care, thus imperiling themselves in the workplace, where the "who" was/is predominately racialized and marginalized people and communities.

1. *Are dynamic, unpredictable, and multidimensional.* Harms in the area of the ecological DoH were demonstrably evident before the pandemic, thus deepening the unpredictable and multidimensional nature of the pandemic. For example, as described in Chapter 4, inequitable DoH exposure to watershed and air pollution, ozone layer depletion, exposure to workplace chemicals, and exposure to psychological stress, produced measurable harms to health across the lifecourse. As a result, harms and deaths associated with the virus itself were magnified by already impaired immune systems caused by inequitable exposure to environmental health hazards. Eventually, evidence showed that the dynamics of COVID-19 deaths were unequally distributed across marginalized and racialized peoples in Canada and globally. These processes are gendered and racialized because the pandemic rests on historical and current structures

of misogyny and racism (McGibbon, 2021). Structural DoH, such as pre-existing systemic oppressions, dictated the colour and social class of COVID-19 social murder in a dynamic and unpredictable way. "The local everyday experience of dying from COVID-19 [was/]is coordinated within ruling relations that are extralocal or external to the experience, where deaths are gendered, racialized, and class-based" (McGibbon, 2021, p. 36). As evidenced in Box 6.2, the pandemic is a living social experiment that is also a clear barometer of synergies with existing inequities in the social DoH, including systemic oppressions related to intersections of the isms (McGibbon, 2021).

Box 6.2: Social Murder and Necropolitics of COVID-19: Illness and Death by Income Quintile

- Absolute inequalities in age-standardized COVID-19 mortality were largest (differences of 24 to 46 deaths per 100,000) for
  - residents of lowest-income areas (compared to highest-income areas)
  - residents of apartments (compared to those in single-detached homes)
  - residents in areas with the highest concentration of individuals who are visible minorities, recently immigrated to Canada, or were born outside of Canada and those who have no knowledge of either official language (compared to areas with lowest concentration of this composite measure).
- These findings are aligned with public health's understanding of the role of systemic issues, such as racism, economic inequality, and other social determinants of health, in shaping inequitable distributions of health risk.
- Men experienced higher rates of COVID-19 mortality than women. However, the magnitude of this sex/gender gap was even larger in areas with lower income and greater concentration of individuals who recently immigrated or were born outside of Canada, who

were designated as visible minorities and were not proficient in either official language.

- In the lowest income and highest ethnocultural areas respectively, there were more deaths among men (31 deaths) than women (29 deaths) per 100,000 population. Although the trend of more men dying than women persisted, in the highest-income and lowest ethnocultural areas, there were significantly less deaths: men (8 deaths) and women (9 deaths) per 100,000 population respectively.

Source: Statistics Canada, 2022.

These inequities, determined by multidimensional structural DoH, created the substrate for the social murder and necropolitics of COVID-19. For example, the elderly, immunocompromised, and those with conditions such as asthma, cardiovascular disease, hypertension, chronic kidney disease, or obesity experienced higher risk of becoming severely ill if infected with the COVID-19 virus (Singu et al., 2020). Although it was known that these conditions already fell along social class and racialized lines, introducing a new system component, the COVID-19 pandemic, meant that impacts across the isms were even more dynamic and unpredictable. As detailed in Chapter 1, eventually, research demonstrated the racialization of pandemic impacts, where there was a strong association between high coronavirus death rates and low income, conditions of work and visible minority status (Etowa et al., 2020), and low levels of education and recent immigrant status (Wherry, 2020).

2. *Have feedback loops*. Lawler et al. (2021) described a COVID-19 ecosystem feedback loop. First, anthropogenic changes created increased likelihood of zoonotic disease emergence such as the COVID-19 virus, further described in Chapter 4. These changes included land-use alterations, wildlife trade, intensive livestock production, and climate emergency. Second, the

biodiversity and ecosystem effects of the COVID-19 pandemic were diverse and interconnected. For example, government responses to the pandemic were necessarily directed to goods and services that were considered to be more essential (Lawler et al., 2021). This process resulted in significantly decreased funding for ecosystem conservation in many areas, ultimately hampering effective global biodiversity conservation, including achieving UN Convention on Biological Diversity's Aichi targets (20 specific targets to address and mitigate biodiversity loss across the globe) (Lawler et al., 2021; Tsioumani, 2020).

Another biodiversity and ecosystem impact of COVID-19 is related to Indigenous Peoples' ownership or stewardship of approximately 40 percent of the global terrestrial protected areas (Garnett et al., 2018; Lawler et al., 2021). Indigenous Peoples' engagement in biodiversity conservation also results in improved conservation for many of the world's most biodiverse regions, along with more innovative and cost-effective conservation and management (Trewin et al., 2021). The central role of Indigenous Peoples in biodiversity and ecosystem protection was obstructed due to inadequate efforts to protect Indigenous communities from COVID-19 in Canada, where conflicts between the interests of Indigenous Peoples and extractive industries intensified during the pandemic (Bernauer & Slowey, 2020; Lawler et al., 2021).

Third, these COVID-19 biodiversity and ecosystem impacts can consequently exacerbate existing anthropogenic drivers (e.g., land use involving the encroachment of human activity on wildlife habitats). These impacts can then lead to further incidence of zoonosis and potential future health crises with unpredictable outcomes—the continuation of this cycle would reinforce a feedback loop with substantial implications for human health, economies, society, and the environment (Lawler et al., 2021).

3. *Are self-organizing into system-wide coherent patterns.* During the pandemic, Big Pharma (e.g., Pfizer and Moderna)

created system-wide, globally coherent patterns that shaped the COVID-19 pandemic survival and death rates by virtue of "capitalizing" on the selective manufacture and distribution of not only the COVID-19 vaccine itself, but financial and geographic access to immunization (Lexchin, 2021). Moderna was expected to earn US $18–20 billion from its COVID-19 vaccine in 2021, while receiving $5.75 billion in public funding to produce the vaccine; the corporation circulated the vaccine to 97% rich, 3% middle-income, and 0% low-income countries (Chow, 2021). Overall, Big Pharma profits were predicted to be in the trillion-dollar range, leading to a globe-wide pattern of vaccine nationalism—an economic strategy undertaken by some countries to hoard increasingly expensive vaccination supplies to increase availability in their own country. The aim was to stock up and vaccinate the nation as soon as possible, regardless of limited vaccine manufacturers' distribution for the rest of the world (Riaz et al. 2021). The stronghold of Big Pharma on vaccine supply had a feedback effect across the planet as rich countries such as Canada, the United States, and the United Kingdom refused to adjust their intellectual property laws to boost the production of vaccines globally (Meredith, 2021). The result was skyrocketing COVID-19 deaths in countries with limited vaccine access. These deaths fell along income and racialized lines because classism and racism were already significant predictors of morbidity and mortality before the pandemic.

Ultimately, these system-wide, coherent patterns of vaccine nationalism and legal measures to introduce stricter intellectual property controls are likely to continue, with rich countries scrambling to get ahead of each other in vaccine procurement and poor countries left with the crumb fest—a situation that will harm everyone on the planet because COVID-19 will continue to flourish in Global South countries, thus prolonging pandemic recovery and preventing global herd immunity (Tansey, 2020). In these ways, transnational profit had a ripple effect that cut across transnational Big Pharma profit, public policymaking in individual nations, and on-the-ground death in marginalized and racialized communities due to COVID-19.

The three COVID-19 CAS characteristics described above have an ongoing synergy with the other CAS characteristics, such as their interconnected and inseparable relationships and parts and multitudes of feedback loops. Similarly, the Alberta Tar Sands CAS demonstrates identifiable CAS characteristics, at least in the sense of useful snapshots at any given point in time. The innovative power of a CAS approach in comprehending these two wicked problems is that it frees us to move beyond attempting to grasp and rein in the millions of minute moving pieces of an enormous puzzle that can never be disentangled. Instead, a CAS application works towards producing clear (and sometimes fuzzy) maps of the messiness and overwhelming nature of problems such as those caused by the tar sands and the globe-wide public health crisis of the pandemic. Another interesting and vital aspect of CAS approaches is that they can provide solution-focused pathways to process the disturbing moral distress that accompanies wicked problems that cause extensive harm across the social, ecological, and structural DoH.

CONCLUSION

The ways that the social, ecological, and structural DoH interact are very difficult to pin down—their nature resists any kind of logical, predictable plan. One of the core reasons why it has taken so long to accept the fact that these problems are wicked and messy is that there is an embedded positivist notion that if we can just make enough lists, definitions, and linear diagrams, we can all agree what the issues are and hence arrive at the solutions. This, of course, is magical thinking. Instead, it is imperative that we find new ways to wean ourselves off the reductionist, Eurocentric thinking that makes us assume that solving problems is a finite process with a beginning and an end. This will not be easy to achieve, especially since we are also talking about "health," which is so heavily rooted in positivist approaches. This is why complexity science is becoming normalized as a way of thinking about and tackling inequities in the DoH—problems are much easier to "see" when we have numerous people within widely varying fields of knowledge, including first-voice and community-based knowledge, working together on solutions.

FURTHER READINGS

Begun, J. W., Zimmerman, B., & Dooley, K. (2003). Health care organizations as complex adaptive systems. In S. S. Mick & M. E. Wyttenbach (Eds.), *Advances in health care organization theory* (pp. 253–288). Jossey-Bass.

Huseman, J., & Short, D. (2012). "A slow industrial genocide": Tar sands and the Indigenous peoples of northern Alberta. *The International Journal of Human Rights, 16*(1), 216–237. https://doi.org/10.1080/13642987.2011.649593

McPhearson, T., Raymond, C. M., Gulsrud, N., Albert, C., Coles, N., Fagerholm, N., Nagatsu, M., Olafsson, A. S., Soininen, N., & Vierikko, K. (2021). Radical changes are needed for transformations to a good Anthropocene. *npj Urban Sustainability, 1*(1), 5. https://doi.org/10.1038/s42949-021-00017-x

Nayak, R., & Waterson, P. (2019). Global food safety as a complex adaptive system: Key concepts and future prospects. *Trends in Food Science & Technology, 91*, 409–425. https://doi.org/10.1016/j.tifs.2019.07.040

Naylor, A., Ford, J., Pearce, T., & Van Alstine, J. (2020). Conceptualizing climate vulnerability in complex adaptive systems. *One Earth, 2*(5), 444–454. https://doi.org/10.1016/j.oneear.2020.04.011

WEBSITES OF INTEREST

#ComplexityExplained—https://complexityexplained.github.io/

This website provides core explanations of complex adaptive system concepts, such as interactions, emergence, self-organization, and adaptation. The explanations are interactive, including depictions of herd immunity and vaccination rates, emergence of community structures and social networks, and many more.

Complexity Explorables—https://www.complexity-explorables.org/about/

This site is designed for people interested in hands on playing with interactive complex systems and complex dynamical processes. *Complexity Explorables* hosts different collections of interactive illustrations of models for complex systems in physics, mathematics, biology, chemistry, social sciences, neuroscience, epidemiology, network science, and ecology. You may want to start with social sciences (e.g., collective behaviour in schools of fish and flocking birds, classic complexity science examples) and ecology (e.g., forest fire dynamics).

Enid Lee Consultants—https://www.enidlee.com/

Enid Lee is an award-winning "anti-racist professional development specialist, leadership coach, and writer. She consults internationally on equitable education and supports educators in preparing all students to create and experience a world with greater justice, joy, and generosity." This website includes numerous tools for change, including Dr. Lee's equity tools, videos, articles, and books, as well as onsite and online anti-racist professional development sessions.

The Nobel Prize in Physics (2021)—https://www.nobelprize.org/prizes/physics/2021/popular-information/

This webpage details the 2021 Nobel Prize in Physics, shared by three Laureates (Syukuro Manabe, Klaus Hasselmann, and Giorgio Parisi) for their contributions to complex science related to humanity's impact on Earth's climate, offering critical insights into studying Earth's climate as a complex system.

Waterloo Institute for Complexity and Innovation—https://uwaterloo.ca/complexity-innovation/about/what-are-complex-systems

What are complex systems? This webpage delves deeper into complex systems, featuring brief interviews with interdisciplinary scholars that provide diverse examples of complex systems.

GLOSSARY

Complexity Science: Refers to the methodical investigation of emergent phenomena within systems. Complexity science stretches across disciplines, from physics and mathematics to biological and social sciences. Examples of these emergent phenomena include ecosystems, the human brain, ant colonies, and economic networks, which are all complex systems displaying collective behaviour, or emergence, beyond the sum of their parts (Jensen, 2022).

Emergence of Control: Refers to processes occurring at the fine scale that bring about emergent higher-level regimes (ways of organizing a system, prevailing patterns over time) that in turn feed back to regulate what occurs at the fine scale, leading to the emergence of control—interactions in the system create and maintain a regime that reinforces the system state (a phenomenon known as lock-in; Centre for Complex Systems Studies, n.d.).

Feedback Loops: Refer to a process that explains how the actions in one part of the system impact the other parts of the system, forming a feedback loop that can either enhance solutions to complex problems or worsen these problems (also see emergence of control).

Multispecies Refugees: Refer to forced migration of human and non-human animals due to climate emergency threats to public health, such as extreme weather events, water scarcity, increasing rates of infectious diseases, and wildfires (Khazaal & Almiron, 2021). Examples include cross-border migration and mass movement of people—for example people displaced by climate change-related disasters since 2010 has risen to 21.5 million (United Nations Commission for Refugees, 2023). As the planet warms, species are shifting where, when, and how they thrive: half of all Earth's species are on the move (Welch, 2017).

Permeable Boundaries: Refers to processes whereby the boundaries or limits of CAS, such as the social, ecological, and structural DoH, also have common building blocks or ideas that they share across these boundaries. For example, although each of the DoH areas have distinct definitions and properties (boundaries) in and of themselves, ideas such as the DoH impacts of neoliberal public policy cut across all three areas.

Slow Industrial Genocide: Refers to the gradual, historical, and deadly health threats of industrial activities such as resource extraction (e.g., the Alberta Tar Sands in Alberta, Canada) and chemical processing (e.g., Cancer Alley in Louisiana, United States). These industry activities are referred to industrial genocide because they fit the UN Convention on the Prevention and Punishment of the Crime of Genocide (UN, 1948) definition, which states that genocide means acts committed with intent to destroy, in whole or in part, a national, ethnical, racial, or religious group. Industrial genocide is used in cases such as environmental racism, where racialized fatality is well known, yet these industrial activities continue.

System-wide Coherent Patterns: Refer to the fact that there is no individual leader, no overall plan or collective intention devised together among the players. Nevertheless, the rules, operating individually and at a local level, broadly defined (e.g., community, individual, nation), are sufficient to produce globally coherent patterns that look as if someone, or at any rate something, is directing them (Paley, 2007).

Wicked Problems: Refer to social, scientific, economic, and political problems (to name a few) that are difficult or impossible to solve due to their complex and interconnected nature. "Wicked problems lack clarity in both their aims and solutions, and are subject to real-world constraints which hinder risk-free attempts to find a solution" (Wong, 2023).

REFERENCES

Amster, E. J. (2022). The past, present and future of race and colonialism in medicine. *Canadian Medical Association Journal, 194*(20), E708–E710. https://doi.org/10.1503/cmaj.212103

Azuma, K., Yanagi, U., Kagi, N., Kim, H., Ogata, M., & Hayashi, M. (2020). Environmental factors involved in SARS-CoV-2 transmission: Effect and role of indoor environmental quality in the strategy for COVID-19 infection control. *Environmental Health and Preventive Medicine, 25*(1), 1-16. https://doi.org/10.1186/s12199-020-00904-2

Battiste, M., & Henderson, S. (2021). Oppression and the health of Indigenous peoples. In E. McGibbon (Ed.), *Oppression: A social determinant of health* (pp. 85–99). Fernwood Publishing.

Begun, J. W., Zimmerman, B., & Dooley, K. (2003). Health care organizations as complex adaptive systems. In S. S. Mick & M. E. Wyttenbach (Eds.), *Advances in health care organization theory* (pp. 253–288). Jossey-Bass.

Bernauer, W., & Slowey, G. (2020). COVID-19, extractive industries, and Indigenous communities in Canada: Notes towards a political economy research agenda. *The Extractive Industries and Society, 7*(3), 844–846. https://doi.org/10.1016/j.exis.2020.05.012

Cabrera, D., & Cabrera, L. (2019). Complexity and systems thinking models in education: Applications for leaders. In J. M. Spector, B. C. Lockee, & M. C. Childress (Eds.), *Learning, design, and technology: An international compendium of theory, research, practice, and policy* (pp. 1727–1756). Springer Nature.

Canada Action. (2019, August 20). *How much of the oilsands has been reclaimed?* https://www.canadaaction.ca/how_much_of_the_oilsands_has_been_reclaimed

Capra, F. (1996). *The web of life: A new scientific understanding of living systems.* Anchor Books.

Capra, F. (2005). Complexity and life. *Theory, Culture & Society, 22*(5), 33–44. https://doi.org/10.1177/0263276405057046

Capra, F., & Luisi, P. L. (2014). *The systems view of life: A unifying vision.* Cambridge University Press.

Centre for Complex Systems Studies. (n.d.). Emergence of control in complex adaptive systems. Utrecht University. https://www.uu.nl/en/research/centre-for-complex-systems-studies-ccss/research/working-groups/emergence-of-control-in-complex-adaptive-systems

Chow, H. (2021). The Moderna vaccine should be a people's vaccine. *Global Justice Now.* https://mailchi.mp/globaljustice/lets-force-big-pharma-to-co-operate-608592?e=18d7ca0c9d

Etowa, J., Kohoun, B., Etowa, E. B., Kiros, G., Mbagwu, I., Muray, M., Dabone, C., Ubangha, L., & Nare, H. (2020). "Leaving no one behind": COVID-19 response in Black Canadian communities. *Witness: The Canadian Journal of Critical Nursing Discourse, 2*(2), 124–130. https://doi.org/10.25071/2291-5796.84

Garnett, S. T., Burgess, N. D., Fa, J. E., Fernández-Llamazares, Á., Molnár, Z., Robinson, C. J., Watson, J. E. M., Zander, K. K., Austin, B., Brondizio, E. S.,

French Collier, N., Duncan, T., Ellis, E., Geyle, H., Jackson, M. V., Jonas, H., Malmer, P., McGowan, B., Sivongxay, A., & Leiper, I. (2018). A spatial overview of the global importance of Indigenous lands for conservation. *Nature Sustainability, 1*(7), 369–374. https://doi.org/10.1038/s41893-018-0100-6

Grant, J., Dyer, S., & Woynillowicz, D. (2008). *Fact or fiction? Oil sands reclamation.* The Pembina Institute.

Greenpeace Canada. (2021, May 17). *Everything you need to know about the tar sands and how they impact you.* https://www.greenpeace.org/canada/en/story/3138/everything-you-need-to-know-about-the-tar-sands-and-how-they-impact-you/

Hatch, C., & Price, M. (2008). *Canada's toxic tar sands: The most destructive project on earth.* Environmental Defence.

Henderson, S. (2021). Aboriginal Peoples constitutional right to health. In E. McGibbon (Ed.), *Oppression: A social determinant of health.* Fernwood Publishing.

Holmes, E. C. (2022). *COVID-19—Lessons for zoonotic disease. Science, 375*(6585), 1114–1115. https://doi.org/10.1126/science.abn2222

Huseman, J., & Short, D. (2012). "A slow industrial genocide": Tar sands and the Indigenous peoples of northern Alberta. *The International Journal of Human Rights, 16*(1), 216–237. https://doi.org/10.1080/13642987.2011.649593

Janzwood, A. (2020). Explaining variation in oil sands pipeline projects. *Canadian Journal of Political Science, 53*(3), 540–559. https://doi.org/10.1017/S0008423920000190

Jensen, H. J. (2022). *Complexity science: The study of emergence.* Cambridge University Press.

Johnson-Woods, C. (2023, March 17). *The 10 characteristics of "wicked problems."* Resonance. https://www.resonanceglobal.com/blog/the-characteristics-of-wicked-problems

Khazaal, N., & Almiron, N. (Eds.). (2021). *Like an animal: Critical animal studies approaches to borders, displacement, and othering* (Vol. 5). Brill.

Kirsch, A. (2021). *Banking on climate chaos: Fossil fuel finance report, 2021.* Rainforest Action Network (RAN), BankTrack, Indigenous Environmental Network (IEN), Oil Change International (OCI), Reclaim Finance, & the Sierra Club. https://www.bankingonclimatechaos.org/bankingonclimatechaos2021/

Lawler, O. K., Allan, H. L., Baxter, P. W. J., Castagnino, R., Tor, M. C., Dann, L. E., Hungerford, J., Karmacharya, D., Lloyd, T. J., López-Jara, M. J., Massie, G. N., Novera, J., Rogers, A. M., & Kark, S. (2021). The COVID-19 pandemic is intricately linked to biodiversity loss and ecosystem health. *The Lancet Planetary Health, 5*(11), e840–e850. https://doi.org/10.1016/S2542-5196(21)00258-8

Lawson, J. (2022). Mounting turbulence in neoliberal globalization: Political economy, populist discourse, and policy in Alberta, Canada. *Social Sciences, 11*(5), 221–251. https://doi.org/10.3390/socsci11050221

Leahy, S. (2019, April 11). This is the world's most destructive oil operation—and it's growing. *National Geographic*. https://www.nationalgeographic.com/environment/article/alberta-canadas-tar-sands-is-growing-but-indigenous-people-fight-back

Lexchin, J. (2021). Obsessed by profits: Big Pharma and the corruption of health. In E. McGibbon (Ed.), *Oppression: A social determinant of health*. Fernwood Publishing.

MacNeil, R. (2019). *Thirty years of failure: Understanding Canadian climate policy*. Fernwood Publishing.

McGibbon, E. (2021). The COVID-19 pandemic: On the mechanisms of social murder. *Critical Studies: An International and Interdisciplinary Journal, 16*(1), 35–42. https://doi.org/10.51357/cs.v16i1.148

McGibbon, E., & McPherson, C. (2011). Applying intersectionality theory and complexity theory to address the social determinants of women's health. *Women's Health and Urban Life: An International Journal, 10*(1), 59–86.

Meredith, S. (2021, April 22). *Rich countries are refusing to waive the rights on COVID vaccines as global cases hit record levels*. CNBC News. https://www.cnbc.com/2021/04/22/covid-rich-countries-are-refusing-to-waive-ip-rights-on-vaccines.html

Morgan, G. (1998). *Images of organization: The executive edition*. Berrett-Koehler Publishers.

Natural Resources Canada. (2016). *Oil sands: A strategic resource for Canada and the global market: Indigenous Peoples*. https://natural-resources.canada.ca/sites/nrcan/files/energy/pdf/oilsands-sablesbitumineux/14-0696%20Oil%20Sands%20-%20Indigenous%20Peoples_e.pdf

Nayak, R., & Waterson, P. (2019). Global food safety as a complex adaptive system: Key concepts and future prospects. *Trends in Food Science & Technology, 91*, 409–425. https://doi.org/10.1016/j.tifs.2019.07.040

Naylor, A., Ford, J., Pearce, T., & Van Alstine, J. (2020). Conceptualizing climate vulnerability in complex adaptive systems. *One Earth, 2*(5), 444–454. https://doi.org/10.1016/j.oneear.2020.04.011

Okello, A. (2020). One Health: A cross-sectoral, holistic approach to reduce disease risk and build resilience. In *Development Co-operation Report 2020: Learning from crises, building resilience* (pp. 175–182). OECD. https://www.oecd-ilibrary.org/sites/8913694e-en/index.html?itemId=/content/component/8913694e-en

Paley, J. (2007). Complex adaptive systems and nursing. *Nursing Inquiry, 14*(3), 233–242. https://doi.org/10.1111/j.1440-1800.2007.00359.x

Parkland Institute. (2023). *Canada's balance sheet*. Environmental Defence Canada. https://environmentaldefence.ca/wp-content/uploads/2023/07/Canadas-balance-sheet_final-PDF.pdf

Phillipps, B., Skinner, K., Parker, B., & Neufeld, H. T. (2022). An intersectionality-based policy analysis examining the complexities of access to wild game and fish for urban Indigenous women in Northwestern Ontario. *Frontiers in Communication, 6*, 256. https://doi.org/10.3389/fcomm.2021.762083

Phillips, M. A., & Ritala, P. (2019). A complex adaptive systems agenda for ecosystem research methodology. *Technological Forecasting and Social Change, 148*(1), 119739. https://doi.org/10.1016/j.techfore.2019.119739

Rainforest Action Network. (n.d.). *List of tar sands companies*. https://www.ran.org/list-tar-sands-companies/

Reed, P. M., Hadjimichael, A., Moss, R. H., Brelsford, C., Burleyson, C. D., Cohen, S., Dyreson, A., Gold, D. F., Gupta, R. S., Keller, K., Konar, M., Monier, E., Morris, J., Srikrishnan, V., Voisin, N., & Yoon, J. (2022). Multisector dynamics: Advancing the science of complex adaptive human-Earth systems. *Earth's Future, 10*(3), e2021EF002621. https://doi.org/10.1029/2021EF002621

Riaz, M. M. A., Ahmad, U., Mohan, A., dos Santos Costa, A. C., Khan, H., Babar, M. S., Hasan, M. M., Essar, M. Y., & Zil-E-Ali, A. (2021). Global impact of vaccine nationalism during COVID-19 pandemic. *Tropical Medicine and Health, 49*(1), 101. https://doi.org/10.1186/s41182-021-00394-0

Rittel, H. W., & Webber, M. M. (1973). Wicked problems. *Man-made Futures, 26*(1), 272–280.

Rouse, W. B. (2008). Health care as a complex adaptive system: Implications for design and management. *The Bridge, 38*(1), 17–25. https://www.nae.edu/7704/HealthCareasaComplexAdaptiveSystemImplicationsforDesignandManagement

Sanger, T. (2019, November 1). *Time to step up for tax justice: Important international reforms to end tax-dodging and tax havens are on the horizon. Why isn't Canada doing more?* Canadian Centre for Policy Alternatives.

Singu, S., Acharya, A., Challagundla, K., & Byrareddy, S. N. (2020). Impact of social determinants of health on the emerging COVID-19 pandemic in the United States. *Frontiers in Public Health, 8*, 406. https://doi.org/10.3389/fpubh.2020.00406

Society of Petroleum Engineers. (2019). *Standards pertaining to the estimating and auditing of oil and gas reserves information* (rev. ed.). https://www.spe.org/industry/docs/Reserves_Audit_Standards_June%202019_Final.pdf

Statistics Canada. (2022, August 26). *Social inequalities in COVID-19 deaths in Canada*. Government of Canada. https://health-infobase.canada.ca/covid-19/inequalities-deaths/technical-report.html

Sturmberg, J. P., O'Halloran, D. M., & Martin, C. M. (2012). Understanding health system reform—A complex adaptive systems perspective.

Journal of Evaluation in Clinical Practice, 18(1), 202–208. https://doi.org/10.1111/j.1365-2753.2011.01792.x

Tansey, R. (2020, September 21). *Power and profit during a pandemic: Why the pharmaceutical industry needs more scrutiny not less* (K. Ainger, Ed.). Corporate Europe Observatory. https://corporateeurope.org/en/2020/09/power-and-profit-during-pandemic

Tenenbaum, D. J. (2009). Oil sands development: A risk worth taking? *Environmental Health Perspectives, 117*(4), A150–A156. https://doi.org/10.1289%2Fehp.117-a150

Timoney, K. P. (2007). *A study of water and sediment quality as related to public health issues, Fort Chipewyan, Alberta.* Nunee Health Board Society.

Trewin, D., Morgan-Bulled, D., & Cooper, S. (2021). *Australia state of the environment report.* Commonwealth of Australia. https://soe.dcceew.gov.au/climate/introduction

Tsioumani, E. (2020). Convention on biological diversity: A review of the post-2020 global biodiversity framework working group negotiations. *Environmental Policy & Law, 50*(1–2), 55–59. https://doi.org/10.3233/EPL-200207

United Nations (UN). (1948, December 9). *UN Treaty Collection: Convention on the prevention and punishment of the crime of genocide.* https://treaties.un.org/pages/ViewDetails.aspx?src=IND&mtdsg_no=IV-1&chapter=4&clang=_en#1

United Nations High Commission for Refugees. (n.d.). *Climate change and disaster displacement.* https://www.unhcr.org/what-we-do/build-better-futures/climate-change-and-displacement

Vergragt, P. J., Markusson, N., & Karlsson, H. (2011). Carbon capture and storage, bio-energy with carbon capture and storage, and the escape from the fossil-fuel lock-in. *Global Environmental Change, 21*(2), 282–292. https://doi.org/10.1016/j.gloenvcha.2011.01.020

Welch, C. (2017, April 27). Half of all species are on the move—And we're feeling it. *National Geographic.* https://www.nationalgeographic.com/science/article/climate-change-species-migration-disease

Wherry, A. (2020, June 13). *One country, two pandemics: What COVID-19 reveals about inequality in Canada.* CBC News. https://www.cbc.ca/news/politics/pandemic-covid-coronavirus-cerb-unemployment-1.5610404

Wong, E. (2023, October 16). *What are wicked problems and how might we solve them?* Interaction Design Foundation. https://www.interaction-design.org/literature/article/wicked-problems-5-steps-to-help-you-tackle-wicked-problems-by-combining-systems-thinking-with-agile-methodology

CHAPTER 7

Mobilizing for Democracy

CHAPTER OBJECTIVES

Using as many examples as possible:

1. Describe key features of the alternative political economy movement.
2. Discuss at least five current catalysts for mobilization towards an alternative political economy.
3. Describe and apply Gaventa's (2017) power cube in terms of entry points for action.
4. List and apply Emejulu's (2008) pathways for transformative action.
5. Discuss and apply Gene Sharpe's (1973) six overall areas for engaging in nonviolent action.

CRITICAL THINKING QUESTIONS

1. What are some of the main ways that an Earth-centred political economy differs from a neoliberal political economy?
2. What are some of the ways that Canada can start to move away from capitalist growth models?
3. What are some examples of catalysts for mobilization in your region? How would you apply the power cube to become involved?
4. What are some examples of alternative political economy initiatives already in place in your region? How would you apply Emejulu's (2008) methods of transformative action to become involved?
5. What might Vandana Shiva (2013) mean by "making peace with the Earth"?

INTRODUCTION

> Making peace with the Earth bears witness to the wars taking place in our times against the Earth and people. It also tells the stories of struggles to defend the Earth and people's rights to land and water, forests, seeds and biodiversity. It outlines how a paradigm shift to Earth-centered economics, politics and culture is our only chance of survival. (Shiva, 2013, p. 7)

The aim of Chapter 7 is to demonstrate entry points to take action and mobilize for participatory democracy to address inequities across the social, ecological, and structural DoH. Each of these areas are complex processes in and of themselves, and core foundations for mobilizing for change apply across all the DoH. The descriptions and word choices in this book reflect Raphael et al.'s (2022) exploration of the potential of using high valence terms (mobilizing high intellectual emotional responses such as anger) that make explicit the adverse outcomes of health-threatening public policy: structural violence, social murder, necropolitics, and slow violence, to name a few. Raphael et al. (2022) make the case that low valence and neutral approaches are not appreciably impacting the reduction of health inequities in Canada. This chapter builds on the high valence terms applied in the book, beginning with a brief description of the alternative political economy movement.

This renewal is based in the dismantling of existing ruling relations, such as the colonial and capitalist structures that have led us to the polycrisis of this point in history. Working knowledge of policy processes and political economies of health, discussed in Chapter 2, are an essential tool for citizen mobilization, because lack of basic political and policymaking knowledge makes it more difficult to successfully navigate the change processes. Current and well-developed inspirations for mobilization are then detailed, including the People's Health Movement (n.d.) and the Club of Rome's Earth4All mandate (Dixson-Declève et al., 2022). Engaging in decolonial futures is explored as a necessary process for the success of moving forward. John Gaventa's (2017) power cube is explained as a foundational way to map the various spaces, places, and forms of power when navigating entry points for action. The last two sections of the chapter take up some of the "nuts and bolts" of mobilization. Political sociologist Akwugo Emejulu's (2008) pathways for action ("learning for democracy") are listed and explored with practical applications. Gene Sharpe's (1973) germinal work about citizen mobilization, *198 Methods for Nonviolent Action* is then summarized, with specific attention to his six overall areas of engagement strategies. The chapter concludes with a living example of ongoing mobilization for change: the climate emergency.

TOWARDS AN ALTERNATIVE POLITICAL ECONOMY

> "If you want to act for solutions, then you need to actually take action—do something." (Anonymous)

The Alternative Political Economy Movement

There is increasing critique of public engagement that emerges within the confines of ruling relations (e.g., government surveys, invited consultations) that almost exclusively captures the ideas, opinions, and recommendations of the enfranchised—approaches that are most likely to reach white and middle-class people. These appraisals have led to a broad coalescence of Earth-centred, emancipatory governance approaches and corresponding critiques of neoliberal capitalist regimes that have piloted us to the current tipping point of survival, not only as communities but also in nation-state and planetary contexts. Human-induced, Western, Eurocentric views have dominated the political economies of global capitalism to the point where there is an embedded Western separation between humans, other-than-humans, and the land and air on which we rely (Ratima et al., 2019). In previous chapters, perspectives on the political economy of health were explained with numerous examples, emphasizing the imperative of disrupting neoliberal governance structures and fully integrating alternative political economies and ways of thinking. This section builds on these discussions to emphasize the imperative for **alternative political economies** that are health equity– and Earth-centred, that can engage in policy design to significantly decrease health and social inequities. Alternative political economy refers to a new paradigm for relations among governments, market forces, and civil society, which provides a pathway out of toxic neoliberal policies that are the root causes of inequitable sickness across the lifecourse, early death, and threats to Earth's life support systems. These economies aim to tackle unfettered capitalism, emphasizing the urgency of thinking and acting beyond the dominant neoliberal imperatives of profit that are leading to globe-wide destruction of ecospheres in the name of massive wealth accumulation for the very few. The alternative approaches discussed in this chapter are foundations in mobilizing for participatory democracy.

> Overcoming the limitations of the neoliberal discourse on the role of the state cannot be done by looking for more interventionist models within the neoliberal mould, but only by breaking this mould and developing an alternative framework that brings institutions and polices to its analytical core. (Chang, 2002, p. 557)

These ideas, once the stuff of "radical left-wing rhetoric" are entering mainstream public consciousness amid capitalism's end game of putting Earth's life support systems in peril and placing billions of people, worldwide, into grinding poverty. Across many Indigenous (First Nations, Inuit, Métis), Afrocentric, academic, and civil society movements (to name a few), a broad consensus is emerging that the machineries of current dominant political systems are the root causes of human and planet health destruction (Chang, 2002; Maloney, 2020; Schrecker, 2016; Thapliyal, 2022). It is these structures that must be dismantled. Social democratic political economies are based in the political philosophy of mass-scale wealth redistribution, which is surely a necessary ingredient for mobilization across class, gender, racialization, and marginalization in any alternative political economy. However, the field of political economy, itself crafted within Eurocentric patriarchy and colonialism, must find new ways to evolve within the contexts of increasing social murder, necropolitics, and anthropogenic Earth damage. Prominent strategies and inspirations for an alternative political economy, described further in this chapter, include the resurgence of Indigenous voices and knowledge systems, such as the Idle No More movement (n.d.); the People's Health Movement (PHM, n.d.); the participatory crafting of Global Health Watch, now in its 6th edition (Bloomsbury Publishing, 2022); the South American concept of Buen Viver, or "good living" (Everingham & Chassagne, 2020); and Club of Rome's Earth4All mandate (Dixson-Declève et al., 2022).

From "Winner-Take-All" Capitalism to Earth4All

> We know the pain points. Everyone knows we must end extreme poverty for billions. Everyone knows we must fix the inequality crisis. Everyone knows we need an energy revolution. Everyone knows our industrial diets are killing us, and the way we farm food is ripping through nature, driving a sixth mass extinction of species. We know human populations cannot increase endlessly. And we know our material footprint cannot expand infinitely on our finite, blue and green Earth. (Dixson-Declève et al., 2022, p. 1)

What, then, is the alternative to the Capitalocene (described in Chapter 5)? According to Moore (2017), our understandings of how capitalism is situated in the web of life is at the core of developing emancipatory strategies that tackle the urgent crises perpetrated by the Capitalocene. Given the inseparable synergies that make non-human life one-in-the-same with human life, any efforts towards human emancipation are not separate from emancipation of all life on Earth (Moore, 2017). Based on copious evidence, it is clear that any alternative economic systems cannot be credibly enacted without an emersed synergy with Earth systems and the inequitable distribution of anthropogenic damage that vastly accelerates inequities across the social DoH. There is now a coalescing globe-wide movement towards dismantling dominant neoliberal capitalist economies and creating Earth-centred alternative political economies that uproot the persistence of political choices that feed mass poverty, disenfranchisement, and social murder. Although we may not need to "reinvent the wheel," if the goal is achieving a just society, it is necessary to embark on a stark and definitive departure from current and dominant economic structures.

Confronting capitalism is no longer a fringe idea. Across the advanced capitalist world, a very recent and significant change is unfolding: "the ideological legitimacy of the neoliberal model of capitalism has collapsed" (Chibber, 2022, p. 1). This does not mean that capitalism is not currently the domineering global governance structure. Rather, there is a nascent expansion of an already-existing resurgence in left politics, a pathway that does not rely on cultivating a renewed left politics from within existing democratic political structures, where "the sense that we can really change anything through elections continues to wane" (Workman, 2011, p. 173). The ultimate failure of historical attempts at building an attractive alternative to capitalism in the Soviet Union, China, and elsewhere have discredited the idea of socialist, central planning due to the highly repressive character and the pervasive irrationalities of these economies (Wright, 2021). Yet, "for a growing and increasingly vocal minority, of mostly young activists, the concept of "communism" is beginning to lose a taint that has, for so long, been taken for granted" (Miéville, 2022, p. 2).

Immense inequalities and climate emergency offer material proof that these structures have not served us. What we need is a tangible process to achieve an alternative economic system based in explicit and verifiable principles of economic, fiscal, and environmental justice (Piketty, 2021) if we are to shock ourselves into tacking the enormous impacts of the Anthropocenes on the DoH across the globe. The Occupy Movement in 2011 and the popularity of Bernie Sanders' participatory socialist run for the US presidency are cited as concrete, recent examples of this political turn away from capitalism (Chibber, 2022; McBride, 2022). In synergy with these movements, and ignited by the slow, public murder of George Floyd by the Minneapolis police, thousands of citizens have confronted brutal and militarized police actions in protest of systemic practices of racist carceral oppression—inspiring massive solidarity protests and political conversations internationally (Miéville, 2021).

These mass movements of solidarity illustrate the crucial need for collectives of actors, emphasizing participation of the youngest and the poorest in political processes as a path to transform and even eliminate capitalism (Piketty, 2021). Piketty argues for **participatory socialism**, including the permanent recirculation of power and prosperity, social federalism, sustainable and fair globalization, and the solidarity of trade unions with participatory democracy, all of which are related to key social DoH. Over the last four decades, the negotiating strength of workers has been systematically weakened to the point that even in the richest nations on Earth, zero-hour contracts are now normal; these are contracts between an employer and a worker where the employer is not obliged to provide any minimum working hours (Dixson-Declève et al., 2022). "The common argument for the erosion of the power of trade unions and workers more generally has been to improve competitiveness in an increasingly globalized cut-throat economic world" (p. 108).

Club of Rome authors Dixson-Declève et al. (2022) argue that a Great Leap is now crucial for the deep-seated transformations (along with policy roadmaps) we need to make peace with ourselves and the Earth. The Club of Rome is a diverse international collective of leaders who identify broad-based and comprehensive solutions to complex global issues. The goal is to promote policy initiatives and action to support enacting solutions to multiple planetary emergencies (Club of Rome, n.d.). This **Earth4All mandate** involves five strands: ending poverty; addressing gross inequality, where income redistribution is non-negotiable; empowering women; making our food system healthy for people; and ecosystems stewardship (Dixson-Declève et al., 2022). These turnarounds are not an attempt to create an impossible-to-reach utopia because sufficient knowledge, funds, and technologies already exist in the world to implement them (Dixson-Declève et al., 2022). Specific strategies include concrete and measurable processes to implement proven life-saving measures as antidotes to structural pathogens, all of which reflect a direct focus on the social DoH. These strategies are reflected in the conclusions of many advocates of dismantling existing capitalist economic models. They include an unconditional basic income (Wright, 2021), gender parity, universal education, and fiscal justice (Piketty, 2021). The current polycrisis requires a precise focus on core principles of rethinking growth, rethinking efficiency, rethinking the state, rethinking the commons, and rethinking justice (McPhearson et al., 2021). The building of a socialist-oriented future increasingly stands out as a prominent, and in the case of the social DoH, a proven intervention for more rapidly building an alternative political economy for a livable and just future.

AN ALTERNATIVE POLITICAL ECONOMY: CATALYSTS FOR MOBILIZATION

Several significant social and civil society movements demonstrate a global cohesion in tackling the root causes of injustices that cause the growing wealth divide within nations and across Global North-South regions. These movements deeply inform alternatives to neoliberal capitalism within and across nations. The ideological underpinnings of these movements are reflected throughout this book, and they apply to Canadian as well as global collective action for political and social change to tackle the root causes of neoliberal epidemics, where health damage on a massive scale may be empirically traced to market-driven neoliberal political economies. In the following sections, an overview of some of these movements is discussed. The descriptions are not meant to be exhaustive. Rather, they provide an introduction to the existing foundations of solution-focused and collective actions to tackle neoliberal political, cultural, and economic dominance.

The People's Health Movement

The **People's Health Movement** (PHM, n.d.) is a global network that includes about 70 countries. It brings together grassroots health activists, civil society organizations, and academic institutions from around the world, particularly from low- and middle-income countries. Its vision focuses on equity, ecologically sustainable development, and peace. In 2000, concerned activists, academics, and health workers got together for the first People's Health Assembly. The founding document, The People's Charter for Health (PHM Global Secretariat, n.d.), was developed and the PHM was born. Guided by the charter, PHM works on various programs and activities and is committed to comprehensive primary health care and addressing the social, environmental, and economic DoH. "The world is facing a global health crisis characterized by growing inequities within and among nations and millions of preventable deaths, especially among the poor. These are in large degree due to unfair economic structures which lock people into poverty and poor health" (PHM, n.d.). The charter is both a tool for advocacy and a framework for action, endorsing the Declaration of Alma Ata (World Health Organization [WHO], 1978), which focused world attention on primary health care as the key to achieving an acceptable level of health throughout the world. The PHM affirms that health is a social, economic, and political issue, but above all, a fundamental human right.

One of the main projects of the PHM is Global Health Watch, further described below. PHM is also active in monitoring international legal and other governance changes to keep partners and friends updated on international pandemic governance negotiations and to facilitate progressive advocacy in this new era of global health governance. Some examples of PHM monitoring and reporting involve the reform of international systems of global health emergency response and pandemic preparedness, as well as discussions of a new international pandemic treaty that is reforming the legally binding instrument that defines rights and obligations of countries during global pandemic emergencies (PHM, n.d.).

Radical Transformation: Global Health Watch, the Alternative World Health Report

The launch of the sixth edition of the World Health Report "brought together voices from all over the world to reimagine health within a global ecosystem of justice, integrating social, economic, political, and environmental determinants of health, with stories of struggle and hope for a radical transformation" (Bloomsbury Publishing, 2022). The origins of the Alternative World Health Report began in 2003 at the World Health Assembly. The PHM, together with the Global Equity

Gauge Alliance and Medact, discussed the need for civil society to produce its own alternative World Health Report, due to 1) the inadequacy of the World Health Organization's reports, 2) the absence of a report that monitored the performance of global health institutions, and 3) the need to challenge the dominant neoliberal discourse in public-health policy with a more people-centred approach that highlights social justice (Global Health Watch, 2009). Ongoing development of the Alternative World Health Report promotes involvement of as many individuals and civil society organizations as possible. The Global Health Watch reports are increasingly catalyzing independent networks and initiatives to develop alternative regional and national health watches to accompany the Global Health Watch. The aims of The Watch are to

1. Promote human rights as the basis for health policy;
2. Counter-balance liberal and market-driven perspectives;
3. Shift the health policy agenda to recognize the political, social, and economic barriers to better health;
4. Improve civil society's capacity to hold national and international governments, global international financial institutions and corporations to account (including WHO and the World Bank);
5. Strengthen the links among civil society organizations around the world;
6. Provide a forum for magnifying the voice of the poor and vulnerable (Global Health Watch, 2009).

The Alternative World Health Reports emerged from a recognition that advocacy initiatives to address health inequities, including on the global stage, are fragmented and have a disease and issue-specific approach to health, as well as being guided (or distorted) by research and governance agendas (Bloomsbury Publishing, 2022). "The world experienced three years of the worst pandemic in a century. The misery and devastation caused during this period rattled most of us, although the virus is not solely to blame. Drug companies' greed, health system privatization, weakened global governance, and the inadequacy of public health systems" all contributed to the severity of pandemic outcomes (Bloomsbury Publishing, 2022). Using a political-economic lens, *Global Health Watch 6* (Bloomsbury Publishing, 2022) analyzes these issues and demonstrates connections between the social, economic, political, commercial, and environmental DoH and the structures of global power relations and underlying economic governance.

Global Health Watch acknowledged that the values underpinning the goal of health equity are often undermined by development policies emphasizing efficiency at the expense of fairness. In addition, market forces (neoliberalism) prevail at the expense of planning based on population needs. The diminished capacity and role of national governments and the public sector, particularly in poor countries, has further undermined the notion of social solidarity and democratic governance. The 2022 edition of Global Health Watch situates the elimination of neoliberalism as the main target for achieving justice in global health (Bloomsbury Publishing, 2022). Since 2005, a transnational network of researchers and campaigners broadly sharing this view, and operating on a shoestring budget, have periodically produced Global Health Watch as an alternative to the better known (and better funded) annual outputs of the World Health Organization and the World Bank (Kapilashrami & Schrecker, 2018). In 2014, the fourth report began with an overview of how four decades of neoliberal globalization increased inequality and undermined access to health care and opportunities for healthy life for many of the world's people, in countries rich and poor.

Buen Vivir: "Transformative Change within Earth's Physical Limits"

In the development of non-Western alternatives to neocolonial and neoliberal capitalism, the South American concept of **Buen Vivir** ("good living") supports the shifting of priorities away from capitalist growth models towards greater social and environmental well-being and meaningful human connections (Everingham & Chassange, 2020). Taking a Buen Vivir approach continues the degrowth momentum for transformative change in society within the Earth's physical limits, and counteracts the pursuit of limitless economic growth.

Buen Vivir dovetails with the degrowth movement, where human–nature relations are imagined in light of a radical reduction of matter–energy throughput in over-producing and over-consuming cultures (Heikkurinen, 2021). Redefining the parameters of how we understand "limits," Buen Vivir creates an ecosocial reset. In limiting unsustainable practices in development and tourism, a focus on Buen Vivir creates growth in other areas, such as social and environmental well-being and meaningful human connection. Buen Vivir can reorient the tourism industry towards localized tourism, and slow tourism because the principles of Buen Vivir require these alternatives to be small-scale, local, and benefiting host communities as well as tourists to increase the well-being for all. Although the movement emerged with the goal of reorienting away from capitalist growth models towards tourism as Buen Vivir, its principles and practices have gained broader uptake in the global movement towards an Earth future not grounded in capitalism.

Rethinking and Re-establishing the Public Commons

An integral aspect of the complex process of building solidarity within a growing participatory socialist political economy is the rethinking and re-establishing of the **public commons**, often referred to as the global commons (Dixson-Declève et al., 2022). It includes resources that are, once were, or need to be re-established as belonging in the public domain. The public commons includes land, natural resources, social media, personal data, the genetic commons, the global atmospheric commons, and all the natural resources that are at risk of destabilizing as a result of human pressures (Dixson-Declève et al, 2022; McPhearson et al., 2021). Rethinking and re-establishing the public commons refers to changes in the way we comprehend, govern, and exercise physical, cultural, and intellectual commons to safeguard their long-term availability and sustainability in service to all members of a society (Dixson-Declève et al., 2022). Emphasis is placed on building trust in local government and the experimentation process when working for change, as well as learning from social innovation (McPhearson et al., 2021).

Land was the first target of an assault on common inheritance across the globe, where confiscation, colonialism, and slavery replaced a degree of self-reliance. Over time, property rights became protected ahead of human rights, a conflict that is omnipresent across all times, including the current era (Dixson-Declève et al., 2022). Enclosure (privately owned for the sole benefit of the owner) of the commons was, and still is, a central driver of inequities in the social DoH.

> Even knowledge was enclosed, through the expansion of copyright and patents—in other words, intellectual property rights. Increasingly, by the late twentieth century, this appropriation of the commons was extended into the digital arena—capturing the value from personal data, for example—as well as into the biological world. Private claims were made on seeds and organisms all over the world, abusing the genetic commons that are necessary for long-term environmental integrity. (Dixson-Declève et al., 2022, p. 172)

The knowledge commons also remains a significant aspect of contemporary capitalist production, where the use of patents has secured vast public exclusion via restricted access to innovation, a process that secures profits (Wright, 2021). In contrast, in a democratic socialist economy, although there may be a remaining role for private intellectual property rights and limited patents, scientific and technical knowledge and information would be a part of a knowledge commons (Wright, 2021). "We know that the rich consume most of everything. Charging a fee for carbon emissions and then distributing all fees back to every citizen equally is fair and reflects the principle that we are all stewards of the atmospheric global commons" (Dixson-Declève et al., 2022. p. 162). Re-establishing the public commons is widely recognized as a central process for creating transformative political economies.

Idle No More

The Idle No More movement began when four women from Saskatchewan—Sylvia McAdam, Jessica Gordon, Nina Wilson and

Sheelah McLean—and Treaty People in Manitoba, Saskatchewan, and Alberta began a protest against the federal government's Bill C-45 (Beaulne-Stuebing, 2022). The bill, over 400 pages, proposed changes to the Indian Act, the Navigable Waters Protection Act, and the Environmental Protections Act, both of which proposed to dismantle environmental protection laws (Beaulne-Stuebing, 2022). The movement spread across the country with teach-ins, public forums, drumming, singing, and round dances in public spaces such as malls and provincial legislatures and Parliament Hill (Beaulne-Stuebing, 2022; Idle No More, n.d). Round dances are Indigenous social gatherings that extend a welcoming invitation to everyone in a celebration of friendship, diversity, and inclusivity (Miskanawah, n.d.).

Idle No More did not prevent the passage of Bill C-45 in December 2012; however, the Idle No More movement changed the social and political climate in Canada and helped lay foundations for the pivotal work of the Truth and Reconciliation Commission and the Missing and Murdered Indigenous Women and Girls Inquiry. Idle No More founders called for a refounded nation-to-nation relationship based on mutual respect:

> Born out of face-to-face organizing and popular education, but fluent in social media and new technologies, Idle No More has connected the most remote reserves to each other, to urbanized Indigenous Peoples, and to the non-Indigenous population... the movement grew rapidly into an inclusive, continent-wide network of urban and rural Indigenous Peoples working hand in hand with non-Indigenous allies to build a movement for Indigenous rights and the protection of land, water, and sky. (Idle No More, n.d.)

Idle No More, a grassroots, volunteer-led movement, became a pivotal foundation in pan-Canadian aspirations for sustainable development and the halting of natural resource extraction and destruction of habitats that are literally vital to all Canadians and the planet. An important example is clear-cut logging in old growth rainforests in Haida Gwaii Territory in British Columbia, described more fully in Chapter 4.

Indigenous Peoples have also led consciousness raising across Canada regarding the harms of vast pipeline construction and related environmental damage caused by vast oil extraction in Indigenous territories. As such, Indigenous Peoples continue to provide significant and inclusive leadership (everyone welcome, including settler Canadians) in the environmental justice movement, a key aspect of developing alternative, justice-based economies in Canada and globally.

Engaging in Decolonial Futures

The strategies and globe-wide impacts of historical and current colonialism mean that it is a pivotal substrate of the current polycrisis. As evidenced in the chapters of this book, the colonialist priority of capital accumulation has resulted in (and is resulting in) mass-scale ecosystem destruction, along with its exceptionally damaging impacts across the social DoH. The process of engaging in **decolonial futures** is intensely coupled with the success of the alternative political economy movement.

The Decolonial Turn

In a discussion about research methodologies to tackle inequities in the social DoH, Schrecker (2023), quoting Audre Lorde, calls for "downing of the master's tools," since positivist, Eurocentric, and colonialist research systems offer no effective template for accomplishing this process. Grosfoguel (2007) argues for a decolonial turn in the field of political economy itself, which "would require us to take seriously the epistemic perspective/cosmologies/insights of critical thinkers from and with subalternized racial/ethnic/sexual spaces and bodies" (p. 212). The term *subaltern* originated in the work of Antonio Gramsci (1971), referring to class, caste, gender, race, language, and cultural relegation to a servile, lower ranking. Subaltern continues to designate the importance of ongoing historical power/power over relationships (Prakash, 1994): "This postcolonial critique seeks to undo the Eurocentrism produced by the institution of the West's trajectory, its appropriation of the other in history" (p. 1475).

These unbalanced relations of power are grounded in a colonial past and a neocolonial present, including the pathways for dominant groups to reconfigure and reshape local meanings and sociopolitical structures (Anderson & McCann, 2002; Browne et al., 2005). In their analysis of a distinct Indigenous environmental justice, McGregor et al. (2020) question the legitimacy and applicability of political and legal mechanisms of nation states and international governing bodies because they continue to fail Indigenous Peoples globally and "they fail all life" (p. 35). The term *Anthropocene* itself is primarily driven by the ongoing dominance of Western, reductionist science and its subordination to market expansion imperatives that have little regard for limited planetary resources (Williams, 2017). In her work "Economic Literacy Otherwise: A Critical Reflection on Educating for Earth-Centred, Caring Economies in a Migrant-Settler Colony," Thapliyal (2022) calls for transformative development of "economic literacy otherwise," one that supports unlearning dominant economic logics of migrant settler colonialism and neoliberal development, and cultivating "alternative relational rather than exploitative, economic imaginaries and practices" (p. 14). Thapliyal draws her framing of economic literacy from the Decolonial Futures Collective, based in Indigenous conceptions of care, Earth-centredness, social justice, and solidarity:

> The Collective consists of researchers, artists, educators, students, and activists concerned with colonialism, racism, climate change, unsustainability, economic instability, mental health crises and the intensification of economic, social and ecological violence. Their work (including research, art and pedagogical experiments) aims to "enable healthier possibilities of (co)existence that are viable, but are unthinkable/unimaginable within dominant cognitive and affective frames of reference." (Decolonial Futures Network, 2022, p. 3, as cited in Thapiyal, 2022, p. 15)

Indigenous knowledges, described more fully in Chapter 4, grounded in decolonial praxis and centuries-old, already-Earth-centred ways of knowing and living on the land, are central beacons in any movement for developing an alternative Earth-centred political economy. In his work *For Our Nations to Live, Capitalism Must Die*, Glen

Coulthard (2013), a Yellowknives Dene and political scientist, asks: "how might we move beyond a resurgent Indigenous politic that seeks to inhibit the destructive effects of capital to one that strives to create Indigenous alternatives to it?" Coulthard problematizes the very notion of Indigenous resistance and protest within discourses of the Crown and dominant settler media, where Indigenous actions of mobilization and protest are labelled as reactionary, threatening, and disruptive. In the growing global movement to develop an alternative, Earth-centred economy, it is crucial to note that there must also be active settler participation and support of decolonizing the very instruments and governance systems that led to the current crises. Otherwise, settlers, including settler Canadians, will continue to buttress the Earth-damaging political economies of neoliberalism and capitalism.

Decolonizing

Decolonizing is a contested term, due to the deep embeddedness of colonialism over time, and the nature of structural participation in ongoing colonization. Decolonization is an iterative process, rather than an outcome. Postcolonial scholars emphasize that colonial oppression reaches backward and forward as a persistent influence on subjugated peoples (Paul, 2006). Decolonizing is ultimately an embodied process for settler colonizers—embodied in the sense of movement, action, thinking, feeling, and understanding. As such, decolonizing is about everyday performing of commitments, ethical decision making, and solidarities with Black, Indigenous and People of Colour (BIPOC), and their communities (McGibbon, 2019). It involves ongoing reflection about the truths of colonial damage, white privilege, and white supremacy, and implementing methodical, organized, targeted actions in the structural realm—requiring a seismic wake-up call to engage in serious and measurable commitments for institutional and public-policy change.

Over two decades ago, Dr. Cornell West, an African American philosopher, political activist, social critic, author, and public intellectual, presented at a Canadian conference about race and the academy. He analyzed historical progress in anti-racism work and the impacts of the civil rights movements in the United States. He clearly detailed how forward steps in the fight for equality of African-American people were systematically undone by white people over time. Dr. West's analysis was historically correct—white people, intentionally and unintentionally, at times create a veneer of complicity in the fight for racial equality, then, just as deftly, craft a countermove that undoes or obfuscates progress (McGibbon, 2019).

Decolonizing involves actively seeking knowledge about postcolonial histories and their ongoing impacts. Postcolonial theory has many origins across first-voice experience, oral histories, civil society organizations, and academic disciplines, to name a few. It provides a vocabulary for understanding the burden of history and how this history shapes present-day experiences and new forms of injustice (Browne et al., 2005)—"the unequal relations of power that are the legacy of a colonial past and neocolonial present, and the ways in which the cultures of dominant groups have redefined local meanings, and dictated social structures, including health care delivery systems" (Anderson et al., 2003, p. 197). Actions for decolonizing involve vocabularies and analytical lenses that critique the historical origins of colonization, neocolonialism, and their imperialist underpinnings. The concept of decolonization requires the postcolonial imperative to expose, resist, and transform the continuing presence and influence of colonial processes (McGibbon et al., 2013).

Developing and enacting an alternative Earth-centred political economy rests on many foundations. A key element of success is grappling with decolonizing the policy and governance structures that underpin existing political economies, ones that led to the present crisis. Without an embedded decolonization process, it will not be possible to fully achieve an Earth-centred alternative political economy. Lila Watson, Murri Indigenous Elder, activist, and visual artist in Australia underscored this solidarity: "If you have come here to help me, you are wasting your time, but if you have come because your liberation is bound up with mine, then let us work together" (Evans et al., 2024, para. 1). Engaging in decolonial futures means acting for mobilization with an embedded knowledge and understanding of the vast and ongoing impacts of the ongoing colonial project, whether it concerns areas such as the Alberta Tar Sands or the embedded racism in so many things associated with "health." Along with the centrality of learning for democracy and transformation described in this chapter, engaging in decolonial futures involves continuously questioning taken-for-granted, hidden ways of enacting policy and governance. These too are often "sly and treacherous." Learning about decolonization processes does not mean going to a two-day workshop, although this may be an important beginning step. As Dr. West explained during his conference keynote address described above, the problem often lies in naming this learning as an action in and of itself, providing the veneer of participation—although self-education is important, it is not a replacement for action to change oppressive circumstances.

NAVIGATING POWER FOR CHANGE: THE POWER CUBE

The urgency of increasing health and social inequities, and the climate emergency have dovetailed with collective mobilization movements such as the ones described above. Each of these areas can be understood as complex adaptive systems (CAS). As described in Chapter 6, they are dynamic, unpredictable, and multidimensional, with interconnected relationships and parts that are not possible to disentangle. When combined with the urgency of mobilization processes, which are also CAS, embracing this complexity is a prerequisite for navigating change processes, rather than reducing mobilization methods and practices into a series of concrete steps. The **power cube** (Figure 7.1) is a three-dimensional depiction of areas of power that are foundational to initiating and sustaining change for justice in complex systems-within-systems (Gaventa, 2017). The power cube is map of entry points—places, spaces, and forms of power—for citizen mobilization.

The power cube was first applied by John Gaventa at a meeting of the Development Research Centre on Citizenship, Participation and Accountability (Citizenship DRC) in 2002 (Gaventa, 2017). Citizenship DRC is a participatory research organization that has worked with universities, research institutes, and non-governmental organizations in more than 25 countries to explore the new ways that citizens are shaping

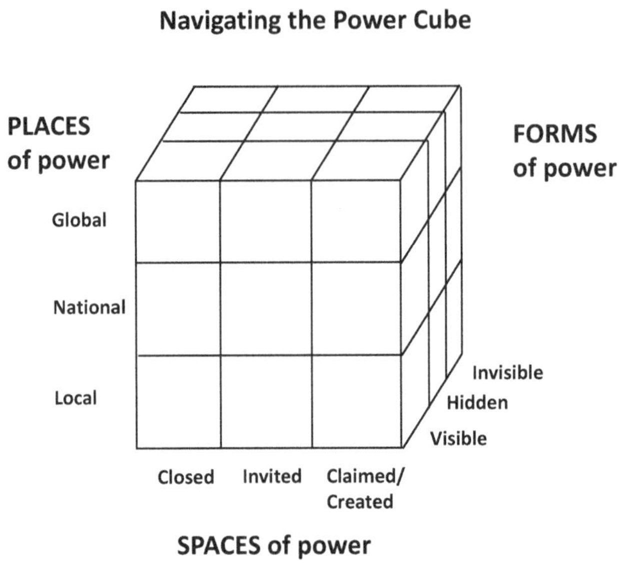

Figure 7.1: Navigating the Power Cube

Source: Adapted from Gaventa, 2007, 2021.

states and societies, and as a training tool with donors on rights-based approaches to international development (Citizenship DRC, n.d.). Gaventa (2006) described how conventional views of democracy and power failed to explain the realities of democratic rights violations in contexts of "enormous inequalities in wealth and appalling environmental living conditions [where] there was little visible conflict or action for change" (p. 24). Along with his colleagues, he sought approaches that could make implicit power perspectives more explicit, specifically for examining the forms of power in different political places and spaces. The power cube has therefore been widely applied within the international development sector as well as in organizations and projects focusing on justice, women's empowerment, climate change, resource development, environment, policy making, poverty reduction, and civic participation (Gaventa, 2017). It has also been used in the context of health care and mental health, agriculture, activism, arts, teaching, political ecology, housing, and water management (Gaventa, 2017).

Application of the power cube provides an accessible way to explain how power operates when aiming to change complex inequitable systems. In order to act for change at the micro, meso, and macro levels of power, it is important to know how power is embedded throughout a chosen issue. In Chapter 5, visible, hidden, and invisible forms of power were discussed and applied in contexts of the DoH. Power cube applications involve a multifaceted approach for exploring the visible, hidden, and invisible dimensions of power. This process is accomplished through mapping the various spaces and levels where stakeholders, including those with power to change public policy, experience and exercise these forms of power (Mozumder et al., 2020). The focus is on processes of governance and citizen participation within organizations and social relationships (Gaventa, 2017).

Places, Spaces, and Forms of Power

Places (or levels) of power refer to the places where participatory action takes place (Mozumder et al., 2020). These may be at the local level (e.g., community organizations, municipal governance), the national level (e.g., national networks or national assemblies), or the global level (e.g., regional organizations or systems).

Spaces of power refer to the potential arenas for participation and action (Institute of Development Studies [IDS], 2009). The notion of space is extensively used across literatures about power, policy, democracy, and citizen action (Gaventa, 2006). *Closed* spaces are decision-making spaces where only influential stakeholders (politicians, experts, managers, etc.), in closed-door meetings, can participate in decision making. These spaces are controlled by an elite group, such as bureaucrats, experts, and elected representatives who make decisions with minimal broad consultation or involvement. *Invited* spaces refer to instances where people with power make efforts to widen participation, moving from closed spaces to more "open" ones, and creating new spaces for more participation in decision making (Mozumder et al., 2020). With external pressure, or in an attempt to increase legitimacy, some policymakers may create invited spaces for outsiders to share their opinions. Here, a wider variety of stakeholders (users, citizens, or beneficiaries) may be invited to participate by various authorities (government or non-governmental organizations, agencies with power or influence that transcends national boundaries or governments). *Claimed* spaces are created spaces that are co-opted by less powerful stakeholders, from, or against, the power holders. Claimed space may also be created more autonomously at the grass-roots level. Claimed spaces can provide the less powerful with a chance to develop their agendas and create solidarity without control from power holders (IDS, 2009).

Forms of power refer to how power manifests in visible, hidden, and invisible ways (IDS, 2009). Chapter 5 (Table 5.1) provides case examples of how each form of power operates in sexualized violence on university campuses. *Visible* power includes the definable aspects of political power: formal rules, structures, authorities, institutions, and decision-making procedures (Nash et al., 2006). It refers to the conventional understanding of power that is negotiated through formal rules and structures, institutions, and procedures (e.g. governing boards, elected officials). Visible power is understood by the axiom: A has power over B to the extent that it can get B to do something that B would not otherwise do (Mozumder et al., 2020). In contrast, *hidden* power involves certain influential people and institutions maintaining their influence by controlling who gets to sit at the decision-making table and what gets put on the discussion and decision list. These dynamics may operate simultaneously at many levels to exclude and devalue the concerns and representation of less powerful groups (Mozumder et al., 2020). Hidden power focuses on the actual controls over decision making and the way certain powerful people and institutions maintain their influence over the process and often exclude and devalue concerns and agendas of less powerful groups (IDS, 2009). *Invisible power* refers to social and cultural norms, perceptions, and beliefs that condition or influence people's individual or collective views (Mozumder et al., 2020). This power operates by influencing how individuals think of their place in society and explains why some are prevented from questioning existing power relations (IDS, 2009). Visible conflict is hidden through internalization of powerlessness or lack of awareness (IDS, 2009). Direct application of the power cube to an urgent social, ecological, or structural DoH issue can uncover specific strategies and targets for action. Table 7.1 provides a template that can be copied and applied to analyze a specific DoH activism issue.

Table 7.1: Applying the Power Cube to a Specific DoH Action Issue

Chosen DoH Action Issue:	
Places of Power	
Places	**Application Examples of Chosen DoH Action Issue**
Global	
National	
Local	
Spaces	**Application Examples of Chosen DoH Action Issue**
Closed	
Invited	
Claimed/Created	
Forms	**Application Examples of Chosen DoH Action Issue**
Visible	
Hidden	
Invisible	
Analyzing Combined Places, Spaces, and Forms of Power: Some Possibilities	
Global, Closed, Visible	
National, Invited, Hidden	
Local, Claimed, Visible	

Source: Adapted from Gaventa, 2007.

LEARNING FOR DEMOCRACY

> In Germany, they first came for the Communists, and I didn't speak up because I wasn't a Communist. Then they came for the Jews, and I didn't speak up because I wasn't a Jew. Then they came for the trade unionists, and I didn't speak up because I wasn't a trade unionist. Then they came for the Catholics, and I didn't speak up because I was a Protestant. Then they came for me and by that time, no one was left to speak up. (Reverend Martin Niemoller, United States Holocaust Memorial Museum, 2023)

Gaventa's (2017) power cube demonstrates concrete entry points for mobilization, mapping the places, spaces, and forms of power that are central in developing and enacting alternatives to neoliberal capitalism, rapidly increasing inequities across the DoH, and rapid climate destruction. This section builds on this mapping of power by describing overarching pathways for **transformative action**. The work of political sociologist Akwugo Emejulu (2008) is applied to describe pathways for action in what Emejulu calls "learning for democracy." Emejulu provides a recipe for the actual "doing" of transformative change.

Explore alternatives: "Seeing that the status quo is not inevitable—that another world is possible" (Emejulu, 2008, p. 32)—questioning "the way things are", as described in this chapter and throughout the book. Examples of alternatives include social democratic political economy, the People's Health Movement, Global Health Watch and the Alternative World Health Report, Idle No More, the Club of Rome's Earth4All mandate, and social democracy.

Take sides: Developing alternate ways of thinking about current and dominant political approaches is about taking sides. This process involves taking the time to learn about political economies, especially neoliberalism, because it has been demonstrated to be the most lethal for humans, all living things, and the planet. Neutrality is situated in the perilous territory of agreeing with oppression. If we do not speak up, we are silently agreeing. In reference to South African Apartheid atrocities, Bishop Desmond Tutu famously stated: "If you are neutral in situations of injustice, then you have chosen the side of the oppressor. If an elephant has its foot on the tail of a mouse, and you say that you are neutral, the mouse will not appreciate your neutrality" (Ratcliffe, 2017).

The violent subtext of "neutrality" is that it creates and supports a stance of bystanding in the face of need—looking the other way when silence will support physical, spiritual, and psychological damage for humans, ecosystems, and all living creatures (McGibbon & Lukeman, 2019). Voting is an interesting example of being involved on one hand or perhaps bystanding on the other. If we say that "there is no point in voting because all the political parties are the same," then we are also saying that there is no alternative to the political economy of neoliberalism.

If we are completely discouraged by our options for voting, which is understandable in some instances, then we either seek out alternative ways to make political change or develop new options for the voting public (e.g., new framings of conventional political processes).

Neutrality is grounded in its close neighbour, "objectivity," both rooted in positivism as discussed in Chapter 2. It results in the violence of moral bystanding, where injustices are seen to be somebody else's problem/issue, both in terms of those experiencing the problem (e.g., people who live in poverty) as well as any felt responsibility to do something about it. Although moral bystanding is cloaked in ostensible objectivity and neutrality, it often involves decisions to actively engage in bystanding. If anyone else speaks up, they may be accused of a number of infractions, such as "being too negative," "taking things too seriously," "being biased," "being too political," and ironically, "not wanting to support change" (McGibbon & Lukeman, 2019). Taking sides is closely connected to developing political and policy literacy. Engaging in formal election processes—locally, regionally, nationally, and globally—is a formal way to take action. In Canada, this can involve finding and supporting a justice-minded member of provincial parliament (MPPs) or member of parliament (MPs, nationally) who is working publicly for action on pressing DoH issues such as climate emergency, the crisis of the unhoused, rising student debt, and health care privatization's damaging impacts on health care access for the disenfranchised and those living in poverty.

Develop political, political economy, and policy change literacy: Knowing and understanding how politics and policy are connected, and therefore, how to navigate power (such as within the power cube) (Gaventa, 2017) are foundational tools and skills for mobilization. This process can be supported by knowing your political compass and the political compasses of the major political parties (see Box 7.1 and Figure 7.2). Learn about the purpose of a policy brief (briefing note) and how to write them (see Chapter 2). Another way to increase political literacy, participate in mobilization, and "see" what alternatives look like is to follow alternative press and alternative information sources, such as The Breach, Aboriginal Peoples Television Network (APTN), Canadaland, Counterpunch, and The Conversation.

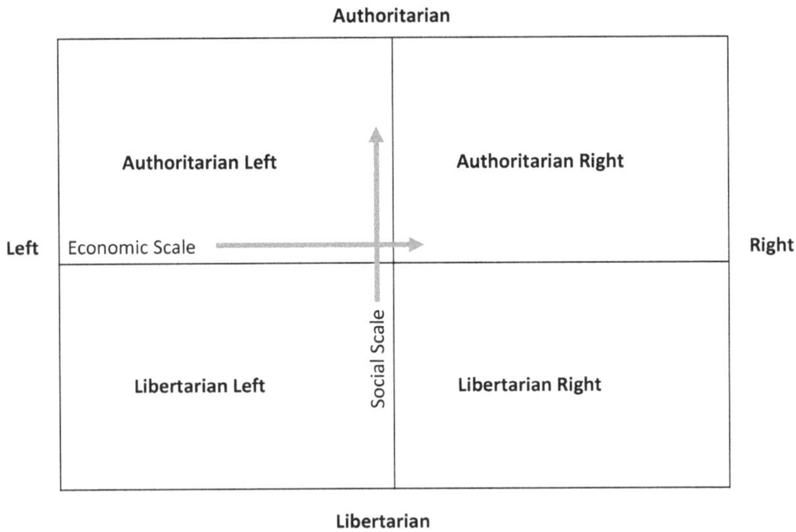

Figure 7.2: The Political Compass

Source: Pace News, n.d.

Box 7.1: What is Your Political Compass?

The Political Compass (Pace News, n.d.), designed by Wayne Brittenden, includes an online website that comprehensively examines political parties across the globe in terms of their Left, Right, Authoritarian, and Libertarian leanings. It also profiles political personalities applicable to all democracies and places them on a quadrant according to their political leanings. Website features enable comparison of the "politics of different countries and political figures past and present," depicting the political compasses of elections across nine countries, including Canada from 2005 to 2021.

You can therefore observe left to right and authoritarian to libertarian shifts at the country scale across time, and hence the overall political compass of the global countries analyzed in the Political Compass. Perhaps best of all, you can go online and "take the test," determining your own political compass. You can then compare your compass to the prevailing political compass of your country or the political compasses of prominent political global figures (and your friends and families if they'll take the test as well). The essential idea underlying the Political Compass is that Left and Right, although far from obsolete, are essentially a measure of economics:

> As political establishments adopt either enthusiastically or reluctantly the prevailing economic orthodoxy—the neo-liberal strain of capitalism—the Left-Right division between mainstream parties becomes increasingly blurred. Instead, party differences tend to be more about identity issues and in the narrowing debate, our social scale is more crucial than ever... We believe that, in an age of diminishing ideology, The Political Compass helps a new generation in particular to get a better idea of where they stand politically—and the sort of political company they keep. (Pace News, n.d.)

The website includes readings about the authoritarian left, the authoritarian right, the libertarian left, and the libertarian right, podcasts, and numerous other resources to increase political literacy.

Source: Pace News, n.d.

Expose the power of language: Learning for democracy means taking great care to name and analyze taken-for-granted ways that language dictates beliefs and values, and thus our action or lack of action. If the discourse (texts and talk) of alternative thinking and theorizing is not front and centre, then we are most likely sidestepping critical perspectives and hence opportunities for collective moral engagement and social change (McGibbon & Lukeman, 2019). This process is challenging because knowledge production is created within the language of the dominant, the peoples and governance systems who "won." For example, deeply embedded and centuries-old epistemic (related to knowledge or knowing) violence continues to privilege Eurocentric colonialist and patriarchal language and knowledge production, silencing the voices of the subaltern (Dotson, 2011). Resistance and transformation must be grounded in knowledge about how "the cat," described in

Chapter 1, operates in stealth ("in a sly and treacherous manner"), and increasingly through the language of digital communications, such as social media. Here, the mechanisms of corporate influence, operating at organizational and individual levels, are an example of hidden power (subtle and deliberately concealed), "as actors in the neoliberal knowledge economy struggle to meet market imperatives while ensuring that their products appear value-free" (Greenhalgh, 2016, p. 486). Raphael's (2021) eight social DoH discourses, described in detail in Chapter 3, are a clear example of how knowledge about patterns in DoH language can be translated into successfully changing public and policymaker perceptions about how to tackle inequities in the social DoH.

Act in solidarity: Supporting transformation and democracy means acting with unanimity, cooperation, mutual support, and cohesion—"engaging in a critical and committed way with communities and social movements for progressive social change" (Emejulu, 2008, p. 32). For examples of acting in solidarity with climate justice, see Climate Emergency Activism in a subsequent section of this chapter.

Work at the grassroots: Working for democracy also involves "being in everyday contact with people on their own ground and on their own terms" (Emejulu, 2008, p. 32), building on participatory action that is already strong or in urgent need of initiation or active support. Box 7.2 details possibilities of participatory action.

Box 7.2: Building on Participatory Activism

The following is a beginning list of suggestions about classic ways to get involved and continue to be involved. Reflecting Sharpe's (1973) 198 methods for nonviolent action, they have all stood the test of time as classic grassroots methods and strategies to "do something."

- Follow local, provincial, national, and international labour unions and protest initiatives (on social and other media). Union movements are among the oldest and most developed activism collectives.

- Find justice-minded websites that are interesting to you. These websites will have links to additional resources that can further your knowledge about justice issues that are important to you. They cross the full spectrum of increasing your knowledge and signing up for newsletters and calls for activism supports, joining an online community of people who are passionate about specific social justice-oriented issues, all the way to taking collective public action.
- Curate your social media so that it is community and activism-oriented. Be intentional about who you are following on social media—activists will have public calls to action (e.g., protests, petitions, blockades).
- Identify your skill sets and resources so that you can offer your supports and services to participate in activism issues that you are passionate about. Remember that not all activism needs to involve the front lines of activities such as protests. Your involvement can be engaging in crucial supportive activities such as assisting with transportation and/or babysitting, writing briefing notes, IT contributions such as website management, and trade skills such as carpentry.
- It is important to note that following and volunteerism is not necessarily activism; however, you will likely meet likeminded people who are activists in areas that you feel passionate about. Then you may step towards activism, which can involve activities such as joint lobbying of local governments on housing policy. Remember that social justice activist communities tend to be welcoming.
- When engaging in activism of any kind, a core responsibility is self-education to understand your positionality (social location) in the broader context of the issue you are engaging with and its root causes. This knowledge informs your entry points and how much space you will take up, including physical, cultural, verbal, intellectual, philosophical, and ideological space (to name a few). Also see the following section on allyship.

Allyship

Allyship is central in moving forward for collective development and/or support of an alternative political economy. Allyship is when those who experience privilege consistently work to recognize these privileges, and to actively work within an anti-oppressive, anti-colonial stance (McGibbon & Mbugua, 2018). Being an ally has a longstanding history in anti-racist literatures and activism (Bishop, 2015).

> [Allyship] is a lifelong process of building relationships based on trust, consistency, and accountability with marginalized and racialized individuals and/or groups of people... it is an active, consistent, and arduous practice of unlearning and re-evaluating, in which a person of privilege seeks to operate in solidarity with a marginalized group of people. (The Anti-Oppression Network, n.d.)

According to Utt (2013), we cannot simply decide we are allies. Being in solidarity is an important process to which we can aspire. However, it is ultimately the choice of those with whom we wish to develop allyship regarding whether they trust us enough to call us an ally (Utt, 2013).

Voice is one of the foundations of allyship—being constantly mindful of whose voices are considered important, or even listened to, in efforts towards collective action (McGibbon & Mbugua, 2018). Since we are already immersed in Eurocentric, biomedical, colonialist meanings of health, including planet health, attending to silenced voices is a core requisite for mobilization. Those who act in allyship recognize that people who experience oppression can never take a break—the isms never go away, and they are experienced relentlessly (The Anti-Oppression Network, n.d.). Those of us with privileges also have the privilege of looking the other way. For example, "People of color have no choice but to weather the storm of racism every single day of their lives. Women have no choice but to weather the storm of misogyny every day of their lives. Differently abled people have no choice but to deal with and respond to ableism every day of their lives" (Utt, 2013). Allyship is about consistently and mindfully not taking breaks, not looking the other way in the face of human and Earth impacts across the DoH, and for those with the various kinds of privilege, openly talking about our own privileged positions. We build our capacity to receive criticism, to be accountable for our mistakes, and to recognize that mistakes are a turning point for us to move forward, to grow, and to do things differently (Bishop, 2015; Utt, 2020).

Performative or performance activism is when individuals engage in advocating solely for the purpose of maintaining a progressive social image regarding a particular issue, problem, or trend, rather than providing meaningful and progressive support for a social cause (Lucie, 2021). Examples include Blackout Tuesday, a social media–promoted event originally organized within the music industry in response to the murder of George Floyd, the murder of Ahmaud Arbery, and the killing of Breonna Taylor (Abdalla et al., 2022). Supporters of the Black Lives Matter movement were encouraged to not spend any money or only spend money at Black-owned businesses for 24 hours. Many thousands of people changed their profile pictures and posted black squares on their social media in the absence of any reference to action that they could take to stop racism. These posts effectively obscured and appropriated space and attention on social media platforms from actually informative posts related to the Black Lives Matter movement and anti-racism protests. As a result, critical, collective organizing was seriously hampered by performative social media postings on Blackout Tuesday (Abdulla et al., 2022).

Acknowledgement of Indigenous territories is a complex example of performative activism. On the one hand, land acknowledgement facilitates questioning and advocacy that is vital for anti-oppression and anti-Indigenous racism (Gerson, 2023). For example, universities and health care institutions (to a lesser extent) may have policies of acknowledgement of Indigenous territories at the beginnings of meetings, and university academic staff may add a geographically specific land acknowledgement as part of their email signature. If nothing else, in some circles these actions reinforce a "coming to know" among settler Canadians of the names and locations of Indigenous Treaty Territories across the country, signifying that these treaties are still legal, nation-to-nation agreements. However, land acknowledgement is also a form of performance activism if there is no systematic, measurable integration of Indigenous-led knowledges and anti-Indigenous racism initiatives in the teaching and administrative structures of these institutions.

198 METHODS OF NONVIOLENT ACTION

Gene Sharpe, an American political scientist and the founder of the Albert Einstein Institution, a non-profit organization dedicated to advancing the study of nonviolent action, researched and catalogued 198 methods for nonviolent action in his germinal work, *The Politics of Nonviolent Action* (1973). Nonviolent action methods have been implemented (some of them for centuries) to catalyze mobilization for justice. "Wise strategy, attention to the dynamics of nonviolent struggle, and careful selection of methods can increase a group's chances of success" (The Albert Einstein Institution, n.d.). Box 7.3 is a summary of Sharpe's (1973) six overall areas for enacting his 198 methods for nonviolent action. Building on each of the urgent areas of DoH action discussed throughout the book, these examples provide another clear roadmap for mobilization across places, spaces, and forms of power.

Box 7.3: 198 Methods of Nonviolent Action

Gene Sharpe's six overall areas for enacting his 198 methods for nonviolent action:

The Methods of Nonviolent Protest and Persuasion

Formal Statements (e.g., public speeches, letters of support or opposition, group or mass petitions, slogans, caricatures, and symbols); *Group Representations* (e.g., mock awards, group lobbying, picketing); *Symbolic Public Acts* (e.g., wearing of symbols, paint as protest, symbolic reclamations, new signs and names); *Pressures on Individuals* (e.g., vigils, sit-ins, protests outside or inside public offices); *Drama and Music* (e.g., humorous skits, pranks, performances of plays and music, singing); *Processions* (e.g., marches, parades, pilgrimages, motorcades); *Honouring the Dead* (e.g., political mourning, mock funerals, demonstrative funerals, homage at burial); *Public Assemblies* (e.g., assemblies of protest or support, protest meetings, teach-ins); *Withdrawal and Renunciation* (e.g., walk-outs, silence, renouncing honours).

The Methods of Social Noncooperation

Ostracism of Persons (e.g., selective social boycott); *Noncooperation with Social Events, Customs, and Institutions* (e.g., suspension of social and sports activities, student strike, social disobedience, stay-at-home); *Withdrawal from the Social System* (e.g., stay-at-home, total personal noncooperation, collective disappearance, protest emigration—hijrat).

The Methods of Economic Noncooperation: Economic Boycotts

Actions by Consumers (e.g., consumers' boycott, nonconsumption of boycotted goods, rent withholding, international consumers' boycott); *Action by Workers, Producers, Owners, and Management* (e.g., boycotts: workers, producers, suppliers, handlers; refusal to let or sell property, merchants' "general strike"); *Action by Holders of Financial Resources* (e.g., withdrawal of bank deposits; refusal to pay fees, dues, debts, interest); *Actions by Governments* (e.g., domestic embargo, international sellers' embargo, international buyers' embargo, international trade embargo).

The Methods of Economic Noncooperation: The Strike

Symbolic Strikes (e.g., protest strike, quickie walkout [lightning strike]); *Agricultural Farm Workers' Strikes*; *Strikes by Special Groups* (e.g., prisoners' strike, craft strike, professional strike); *Ordinary Industrial Strikes* (e.g., industry strike); *Restricted Strikes* (e.g., slowdown strike, working-to-rule strike, reporting "sick" [sick-in], strike by resignation); *Multi-industry Strikes* (e.g., general strike).

The Methods of Political Noncooperation

Rejection of Authority (e.g., withholding/withdrawal of allegiance; refusal of public support; literature and speeches, advocating resistance); *Citizens'*

(*continued*)

Noncooperation with Government (e.g., boycott of legislative bodies, government depts., agencies, and other bodies; refusal of assistance to enforcement agents; removal of own signs and placemarks); *Citizens' Alternatives to Obedience* (e.g., reluctant and slow compliance; refusal of an assemblage or meeting to disperse; noncooperation with conscription and deportation; civil disobedience of "illegitimate" laws); *Action by Government Personnel* (e.g., selective refusal of assistance by government aides; general administrative noncooperation); *International Governmental Action* (e.g., delay and cancellation of diplomatic events; withdrawal from international organizations, refusal of membership in international bodies; expulsion from international organizations).

The Methods of Nonviolent Intervention

Psychological Intervention (e.g., the fast, hunger strike); *Physical Intervention* (e.g., sit-ins, nonviolent raids, nonviolent occupation); *Social Intervention* (e.g., overloading of facilities, social media, alternative social institutions, alternative communication systems); *Economic Intervention* (e.g., defiance of blockades, alternative markets, alternative economic institutions); *Political Intervention* (e.g., overloading of administrative systems; civil disobedience of "neutral" laws; dual sovereignty and parallel government).

Source: Albert Einstein Institution, n.d.; Sharpe, 1973.

ANOTHER LIVING APPLICATION: CLIMATE EMERGENCY ACTIVISM

> Global environmental justice activism and research, in fact, is moving beyond demanding equity in the distribution of environmental harms and benefits to a call for the structural transformation of the economy and our relationship with nature as a means to address social, political, economic and environmental crises. (Pintauro, 2017)

Climate emergency activism is a globe-wide case study in how to apply the principles and practices of mobilization discussed in this chapter. Despite disturbing predictions regarding the immediacy of action that is necessary to curtail irreversible damage and the numerous indicators of increasing climate destruction, climate activist initiatives and interventions prevail. The Intergovernmental Panel on Climate Change's (IPCC) Sixth Assessment Report, released in March 2023, paints a bleak picture of the climate emergency. As detailed in this book, the report highlights the increasingly devastating consequences of rising greenhouse gas emissions, resulting in large-scale environmental and infrastructural destruction, loss of livelihoods, food insecurity, extreme weather events, and loss of biodiversity. In lieu of many countries' failures to respond proportionately to the climate emergency, activists across the globe have intervened across all of the spaces, places, and forms of power, at on-the-ground levels as well as in the structural policy and governance realm. In a departure from green economy initiatives, which incentivize individual consumers to solve the climate emergency through responsible forms of consumption and self-regulation, climate activism evokes collective solidarity and demands action by public policymakers and industry in global, national, and local spheres of power and influence.

The Carnegie Endowment for International Peace's (n.d.) Climate Protest Tracker has followed and recorded global trends in climate policy protests since 2022. Thirty-three climate policy protests, each with greater than 500 participants, have been recorded. Of these, 10 included over 10,000 participants. Climate policy protests in France in October 2022 saw over 100,000 people join in solidarity against the French government's climate emergency inaction and rising prices in the energy sector (Carnegie Endowment for International Peace, n.d.). The Global Climate Strike protests of 2023 saw over 300,000 people call for drastic action on climate change and divestment from fossil fuel industries. Young people made up a significant proportion of those in attendance. These numbers represent a 10-fold increase from the previous years' Global Climate Strike protests in March 2022 and September 2022, which saw a peak of over 30,000 participants globally (Carnegie Endowment for International Peace, n.d.).

Mass climate protests have provoked significant policy change at the nation state level. The "Fight for Our Future" protests in the United States in April of 2022—which demanded that the Biden administration fulfill their campaign promise of enacting comprehensive climate legislation—saw Congress pass the Inflation Reduction Act, which featured over $300 billion in climate-response spending for the following August. President Biden signed the act into law shortly thereafter (Malus et al., 2022). The "Last Generation" highway protest in Germany in April 2023 demanded that the German government enact more stringent climate policies in light of hosting the 2023 annual Petersburg Climate Dialogue. In response, German Chancellor Olaf Scholz proposed the tripling of solar and wind power by 2030, in accordance with a target proposed by the International Renewable Energy Agency (Wehrmann, 2023).

Across the globe, climate activism has extended into legal action against governments, with the intent of provoking government action to protect the well-being of current and future generations (David Suzuki Foundation, n.d.). In October 2019, 15 Canadian young people filed a pre-trial motion to strike, declaring that the Canadian government was in violation of their rights by failing to act sufficiently on climate change. The plaintiffs are pursuing an Order that would require the Canadian government to implement a Climate Recovery Plan (*La Rose et al. v. His Majesty the King; formerly Her Majesty the Queen*) (Climate Change Litigation Databases, 2019a). Remarkably, the lawsuit was dismissed in Federal Court in October 2020 for failure to state a reasonable cause of action. The plaintiffs appealed the decision in November 2020 and as of February 2023, the plaintiffs' lawyers have appeared before a panel of Federal Court of Appeal judges. The plaintiffs are continuing to push to have their case proceed to trial pending the ruling of the appeal (David Suzuki Foundation, n.d.). These young people represent a larger movement of young activists holding their governments accountable for the climate emergency. Similar youth-led cases are pending in other countries, such as *Juliana v. United States* (Climate Change Litigation Databases, 2015), where the principal laws being challenged are the Public Trust Doctrine of the Ninth Amendment, the Fifth Amendment (entitlement to due process) and the Fifth Amendment (equal protection). The action by these plaintiffs asserted that the federal government violated their constitutional rights by causing dangerous carbon dioxide concentration emissions. Results in this case are still pending as of spring 2024.

Climate activists have pursued legal action not only against complacent governments but also against environmentally destructive conglomerate corporations. In a 2019 precedent-setting case brought before the Netherlands government by MilieuDefensie (MilieuDefensie, n.d.) alongside co-plaintiffs and over 17,000 Dutch citizens, it was ruled that oil giant Shell would reduce its 2010-level emissions by 45 percent by 2030 and achieve zero emissions by 2050 (*MilieuDefensie et al. v. Royal Dutch Shell plc*) (Climate Change Litigation Databases, 2019b). This verdict represents a very significant achievement for climate activists and serves as a warning to other industrial giants that "business as usual" is now subject to contestation (BBC News, 2021).

Indigenous land defenders play a pivotal global role in activism against the climate emergency. Between 2020 and 2022 in Fairy Creek, British Columbia, fierce opposition by protestors to old-growth logging became the largest act of civil disobedience in Canadian history (McSheffrey, 2023). The protestors, consisting of climate activists and Indigenous land defenders known as the "Rainforest Flying Squad," worked strategically to defend what is believed to be the last unprotected (from logging corporations) old-growth watershed on southern Vancouver Island (Moye, 2021). Over the two-year period, more than 1,000 peaceful protestors were arrested and physically removed from the land and trees they occupied in Fairy Creek (McSheffrey, 2023). As of June 2023, the British Colombia (BC) government has extended a legal order deferring logging in Fairy Creek until February 1, 2025. This extension came at the request of leadership from Pacheedaht First Nation (McSheffrey, 2023). The June 2023 statement from the Ministry of Forests reads, "The Province and First Nations will continue collaborating on long-term forest ecosystem management of the Fairy Creek watershed, including the management of old-growth forests" (McSheffrey, 2023). While the fate of old-growth in Fairy Creek remains uncertain, Indigenous land defenders and their allies achieved the postponement of old-growth logging and provoked further deliberation by government officials. Member of Parliament (MP) Patrick Weiler introduced a motion in Parliament in May 2023 that would prevent logging on federal land and halt exports of old growth logs and products from Canada by 2030.

The 2022 United Nations Environment Programme's (UNEP, 2022) Emissions Gap Report concluded that the current state of the climate emergency will require a rapid transformation of society, and that the international community falls far from meeting the Paris Agreement goals. The report warns of "no credible pathway" to limiting warming to 1.5 degrees Celsius (UN News, 2022). In scenarios where emissions are not rapidly reduced, global temperature increase will likely exceed 1.5°C between 2026 and 2042 (central estimate of between 2030 and 2032). In the highest emissions scenario, the 2°C threshold will likely be exceeded between 2034 and 2052. In a scenario of modest mitigation, where emissions remain close to current levels, the 2°C threshold would be exceeded between 2038 and 2072 (Hausfather, 2020). These predictions are substantiated by data-driven approaches for quantifying the signal of climate change in historical observations and for constraining the uncertainty in climate model projections (Diffenbaugh & Barnes, 2023). In 2023, using seven different predictive models, these researchers found that the 1.5°C threshold would be reached in 2025. The 2°C threshold was predicted to occur in approximately 20–24 years. Although these predictions may be contested on their scientific merit, the results are sufficient to warrant an abundance of caution in accepting the potential results of stalling in any way in terms of climate emergency mitigation responsibility and accountability. The efforts of climate activists demonstrate that mobilizing for democracy is a viable alternative to the age of extinction.

CONCLUSION

Mobilization is an age-old tool for collectively lifting ourselves up. In Chapter 2, the centrality of policy and political knowledge was discussed, including political literacy, and how it must become part of teaching and mentoring processes across as many forms of education as possible. The same can be said for mobilization and mobilization literacy. If we are not simultaneously learning about how to change injustices that we are enraged about, then we may be left with a deep sense of futility and moral distress—a sense that there is no point in acting. Moral distress is when we know the right course of action, but institutional and other constraints prevent us from acting. The perpetrators of structural inequities and structural violence are counting on both a lack of policy literacy and a lack of mobilization literacy among the populace. However, as this book and many other works like it demonstrate, it is entirely possible to "bell the cat" so that we will know when it is about and thus prevent its "sly and treacherous" advance.

FURTHER READINGS

Densu, K. (2018). Omenala: Toward an African-centered ecophilosophy and political ecology. *Journal of Black Studies, 49*(1), 29–52. https://doi.org/10.1177/0021934717729503

Emejulu, A. (2008). Learning for democracy: Ten propositions and ten proposals. In *Reclaiming social purpose in community education: The Edinburgh Papers 2008*. University of Edinburgh.

Maloney, M. (2020). Practical pathways to ecological law: Greenprints and a bioregional, regenerative governance approach for Australia. In K. Anker, P. D. Burdon, G. Garver, M. Maloney, & C. Sbert (Eds.), *From environmental to ecological law* (pp. 237–251). Routledge.

McGibbon, E., & Lukeman, S. (2019). Critical social justice: The moral imperative for critical perspectives. *Witness: The Canadian Journal of Critical Nursing Discourse, 1*(1), 3–12. https://doi.org/10.25071/2291-5796.21

Ratima, M., Martin, D., Castleden, H., & Delormier, T. (2019). Indigenous voices and knowledge systems—Promoting planetary health, health equity, and sustainable development now and for future generations. *Global Health Promotion, 26*(Suppl. 3), 3–5. https://doi.org/10.1177/1757975919838487

WEBSITES OF INTEREST

The Degrowth Movement—https://degrowth.info/degrowth

In response to capitalism's imperative of unfettered growth at the expense of planetary health, the Degrowth Movement advances "degrowth" as an economic alternative and philosophy towards transforming society to ensure environmental justice and a good life for all within planetary boundaries.

Gaventa's Power Cube: Understanding Power for Social Change—https://www.powercube.net/analyse-power/what-is-the-powercube/background-to-the-powercube/

This interactive website facilitates the investigation of different forms, spaces, and levels of power. The power cube analysis facilitates a heightened understanding of how these different forms of power interact to produce distinct expressions of power and oppression.

Global Nonviolent Database—https://nvdatabase.swarthmore.edu/

The aims of this website include provision of free access to information about hundreds of cases of nonviolent action for learning and for citizen action, researching campaigns that have reached a point of completion. Cases are drawn from all continents and most countries. People are shown struggling for human rights, economic justice, democracy, national and ethnic identity, environmental sustainability, and peace. This site seeks to make available comparative information that will support researchers and writers to develop strategic knowledge and theory about nonviolent action for justice.

Greenprints—https://www.greenprints.org.au/

Greenprints "provides a practical, step-by-step approach to help people understand both the big picture and the small details, of how to create systems change, transform our societies, and thrive within our ecological limits... It demystifies and connects the many existing concepts, models, and methods that can be used to create sustainable and regenerative communities and organizations."

Organizing for Power, Organizing for Change—https://www.organizingforpower.org/

This website offers what activist Lisa Fithian calls "building blocks" for change which facilitate our ability to think critically about our work. Click "Resources" to access exercises on healing from internalized oppression, challenging oppressive moments, and understanding and recognizing white privilege.

Radical Citizen Media (RCM)—https://radicalcitizenmedia.com/

RCM is an "independent media outlet that visually documents the peace movement, activist community, and contemporary issues from a progressive perspective in Edmonton, Alberta. The site operates with the philosophy that the best way to report on an event or issue is to present it as it happens, so that viewers can draw meanings for themselves."

GLOSSARY

Alternative Political Economy: Refers to a new paradigm for relations among governments, market forces, and civil society, which provides a pathway out of toxic neoliberal policies that are the root causes of inequitable sickness across the lifecourse as well as and early death. Current and well-developed inspirations for mobilization include the People's Health Movement (PHM, n.d.); the participatory crafting of Global Health Watch, now in its 6th edition (Bloomsbury Publishing, 2022); the South American concept of Buen Viver ("good living") (Everingham & Chassagne, 2020); and Club of Rome's Earth4All mandate (Dixson-Declève et al., 2022).

Buen Vivir: Refers to the South American concept of "good living," a movement that focuses on the development of non-Western alternatives to neocolonial and neoliberal capitalism. Buen Vivir supports the shifting of priorities away from capitalist growth models towards greater social and environmental well-being and meaningful human connections (Everingham & Chassange, 2020).

Decolonial Futures: Refer to systematically addressing unbalanced relations of local, regional, and global power that are grounded in a colonial past and a neocolonial present, including the pathways for dominant groups to reconfigure and reshape local meanings and sociopolitical structures (Anderson & McCann, 2002; Browne et al., 2005). Decolonial futures involve decolonizing processes, such as commitments, ethical decision making, and solidarities with Black, Indigenous and People of Colour and their communities (McGibbon, 2019).

Earth4All Mandate: Refers to the Club of Rome's five strands for achieving planet and human sustainability: ending poverty; addressing gross inequality, where income redistribution is non-negotiable; empowering women; making our food system healthy for people; and ecosystems (Dixson-Declève et al., 2022). The Club of Rome is a "platform of diverse thought leaders who identify holistic solutions to complex global issues and promote policy initiatives and action to enable humanity to emerge from multiple planetary emergencies" (Club of Rome, n.d.).

Participatory Socialism: Refers to the collective and permanent re-distribution and re-circulation of power and prosperity. social federalism, sustainable and fair globalization, and the solidarity of trade unions with participatory democracy (Piketty, 2021). Social federalism involves addressing unusually decentralized federalism in countries such as Canada, where the delivery of services crucial to social democracy, such as health care, education, social assistance, are for the great majority of recipients, an exclusively provincial jurisdiction.

People's Health Movement: Refers to a global network that includes about 70 countries and brings together grassroots health activists, civil society organizations, and academic institutions from around the world, particularly from low- and middle-income countries. Its vision focuses on equity, ecologically-sustainable development, and peace (People's Health Movement, n.d.).

Power Cube: Refers to a three-dimensional depiction of areas of power that are foundational to initiating and sustaining change for justice in complex systems-within-systems (Gaventa, 2017). The cube is map of entry points—places, spaces, and forms of power—for citizen mobilization.

Public Commons: Often known as the global commons, the public commons refers to resources that are, once were, or need to be re-established as in the public domain. These resources include land, natural resources, social media, personal data, the genetic commons, the global atmospheric commons, and all the natural resources that are at risk of destabilizing as a result of human pressures (Dixson-Declève et al., 2022; McPhearson et al., 2021).

Transformative Action: Refers to specific kinds of action that create and sustain collective work for social justice, referred to as "learning for democracy" by political sociologist Akwugo Emejulu (2008). Transformative action involves exploring alternatives, taking sides, exposing the power of language, acting in solidarity, and working at the grassroots.

REFERENCES

Abdalla, A., D'Souza, N., Gill, R., Jadavji, R., & Meneguzzi, C. (2022). Social media as a stage: A behind the scenes analysis of performative activism, "cancel culture," and effective allyship. *McMaster Undergraduate Journal of Social Psychology, 3*(1), 83–122. https://journals.mcmaster.ca/mujsp/article/view/3139

Albert Einstein Institution. (n.d.). *198 methods of non-violence action.* https://www.aeinstein.org/198-methods-of-nonviolent-action

Anderson, J. M., & McCann, E. K. (2002). Toward a post-colonial feminist methodology in nursing research: Exploring the convergence of post-colonial and Black feminist scholarship. *Nurse Researcher, 9*(3), 7–27. https://doi.org/10.7748/nr2002.04.9.3.7.c6186

Anderson, J., Perry, J., Blue, C., Browne, A., Henderson, A., Khan, K. B., Reimer-Kirkham, S., Lynam, M. J., Semeniuk, P., & Smye, V. (2003). "Rewriting" cultural safety within the postcolonial and postnational feminist project: Toward new epistemologies of healing. *Advances in Nursing Science, 26*(3), 196–214.

Anti-Oppression Network. (n.d.). *Allyship.* https://theantioppressionnetwork.com/allyship/

BBC News. (2021, May 26). *Shell: Netherlands court orders oil giant to cut emissions.* https://www.bbc.com/news/world-europe-57257982

Beaulne-Stuebing, L. (2022, November 26). *How Idle No More transformed Canada.* CBC Radio. https://www.cbc.ca/radio/unreserved/idle-no-more-reconciliation-1.6663310

Bishop, A. (2015). *Becoming an ally: Breaking the cycle of oppression in people* (3rd ed.). Fernwood Publishing.

Bloomsbury Publishing. (2022). *Global Health Watch 6: In the shadow of the pandemic.*

Browne A. J., Smye, V. L., & Varcoe, C. (2005). The relevance of postcolonial theoretical perspectives to research in Aboriginal health. *Canadian Journal of Nursing Research, 37*(4), 16–37. https://cjnr.archive.mcgill.ca/article/view/1969

Carnegie Endowment for International Peace. (n.d.). *Climate protest tracker.* https://carnegieendowment.org/features/climate-protest-tracker

Chang, H. J. (2002). Breaking the mould: An institutionalist political economy alternative to the neo-liberal theory of the market and the state. *Cambridge Journal of Economics, 26*(5), 539–559. https://www.jstor.org/stable/23600312

Chibber, V. (2022). *The class matrix: Social theory after the cultural turn.* Harvard University Press.

Climate Change Litigation Databases. (2015). *Juliana v. United States.* Sabin Center for Climate Change Law. https://climatecasechart.com/case/juliana-v-united-states/

Climate Change Litigation Databases. (2019a). *La Rose et al. v. His Majesty the King; formerly Her Majesty the Queen.* Sabin Center for Climate Change Law. http://climatecasechart.com/non-us-case/la-rose-v-her-majesty-the-queen/

Climate Change Litigation Databases. (2019b). *MilieuDefensie et al. v. Royal Dutch Shell plc.* https://climatecasechart.com/non-us-case/milieudefensie-et-al-v-royal-dutch-shell-plc/

Club of Rome. (n.d.). *About us.* https://www.clubofrome.org/about-us/

Coulthard, G. (2013, November 5). *For our nations to live, capitalism must die.* Nations Rising. https://www.nationsrising.org/for-our-nations-to-live-capitalism-must-die/

David Suzuki Foundation (n.d.). *Youth climate lawsuit: Youth go to court for climate justice.* https://davidsuzuki.org/project/youth-climate-lawsuit/

Development Research Centre on Citizenship, Participation, and Accountability (Citizenship DRC). (n.d.). *What is Citizenship DRC?* http://archive.ids.ac.uk/drccitizen/pages/about.html

Diffenbaugh, N. S., & Barnes, E. A. (2023). Data-driven predictions of the time remaining until critical global warming thresholds are reached. *Proceedings of the National Academy of Sciences, 120*(6), e2207183120. https://doi.org/10.1073/pnas.2207183120

Dixson-Declève, S., Gaffney, O., Ghosh, J., Randers, J., Rockström, J., & Stoknes, P. E. (2022). *Earth for all: A survival guide for humanity.* New Society Publishers.

Dotson, K. (2011). Tracking epistemic violence, tracking practices of silencing. *Hypatia, 26*(2), 236–257. https://doi.org/10.1111/j.1527-2001.2011.01177.x

Emejulu, A. (2008). Learning for democracy: Ten propositions and ten proposals. In *Reclaiming social purpose in community education: The Edinburgh Papers 2008* (pp. 29–32). University of Edinburgh.

Evans, N., Hemphill, F., Han, D., & Kitchens, K. (2024). *Our liberation is bound together.* Embracing equity. https://www.embracingequity.org/post/our-liberation-is-bound-together

Everingham, P., & Chassagne, N. (2020). Post COVID-19 ecological and social reset: Moving away from capitalist growth models towards tourism as Buen Vivir. *Tourism Geographies, 22*(3), 555–566. https://doi.org/10.1080/14616688.2020.1762119

Gaventa, J. (2006). Finding the spaces for change: A power analysis. *Institute of Development Studies Bulletin, 37*(6), 23–33. https://doi.org/10.1111/j.1759-5436.2006.tb00320.x

Gaventa, J. (2007). Levels, spaces and forms of power: Analysing opportunities for change. In F. Berenskoetter & M. J. Williams (Eds.), *Power in World Politics.* Routledge.

Gaventa, J. (2017, December 18). *What have we learned from the powercube?* Institute of Development Studies. https://www.ids.ac.uk/news/what-have-we-learned-from-the-powercube/

Gaventa, J. (2021). Linking the prepositions: Using power analysis to inform strategies for social action. *Journal of Political Power,* 14(1), 109–130. https://doi.org/10.1080/2158379X.2021.1878409

Gerson, H. (2023). The land acknowledgement at Columbia University: Performance and/or activism? *The Morningside Review, 19.* https://journals.library.columbia.edu/index.php/TMR/article/view/9815

Global Health Watch. (2009). *About the GHW.* https://www.ghwatch.org/about.html

Gramsci, A. (1971). *Selections from the Prison Notebooks* (Q. Hoare & G. N. Smith, Eds. & Trans.). Lawrence and Wishart.

Greenhalgh, S. (2016). Neoliberal science, Chinese style: Making and managing the "obesity epidemic." *Social Studies of Science, 46*(4), 485–510. https://doi.org/10.1177/0306312716655501

Grosfoguel, R. (2007). The epistemic decolonial turn: Beyond political-economy paradigms. *Cultural Studies, 21*(2–3), 211–223. https://doi.org/10.1080/09502380601162514

Hausfather, Z. (2020, December 4). *Analysis: When might the world exceed 1.5C and 2C of global warming?* Carbon Brief. https://www.carbonbrief.org/analysis-when-might-the-world-exceed-1-5c-and-2c-of-global-warming/

Heikkurinen, P. (2021). The nature of degrowth: Theorising the core of nature for the degrowth movement. *Environmental Values, 30*(3), 367–385. https://doi.org/10.3197/096327120X15973379803681

Idle No More. (n.d.). *About the movement.* https://idlenomore.ca/about-the-movement/

Intergovernmental Panel on Climate Change (IPCC). (2023, March 20). *Sixth assessment report: Synthesis report.* https://www.ipcc.ch/assessment-report/ar6/

Institute of Development Studies (IDS). (2009). *Power pack: Understanding power for social change*. Powercube. https://www.powercube.net/wp-content/uploads/2010/01/PowerPack_web_version.pdf

Kapilashrami, A., & Schrecker, T. (2018). Global Health Watch: Challenging entrenched ideas in global health. *British Medical Journal, 360*, k956. https://doi.org/10.1136/bmj.k956

Lucie, S. (2021). A passive performative: Alternative models of human agency. *Journal of Dramatic Theory and Criticism, 35*(2), 113–116. https://doi.org/10.1353/dtc.2021.0008

Maloney, M. (2020). Practical pathways to ecological law: Greenprints and a bioregional, regenerative governance approach for Australia. In K. Anker, P. Burdon, G. Garver, M. Maloney, & C. Sbert (Eds.), *From environmental to ecological law* (pp. 237–251). Routledge.

Malus, H., Cooney, M., & Alt, C. (2022, April 27). *Fight for our future: Activists demand action on climate and justice*. Center for American Progress. https://www.americanprogress.org/article/fight-for-our-future-activists-demand-action-on-climate-and-justice/

McBride, S. (2022). *Escaping dystopia: Rebuilding a public domain*. Bristol University Press.

McGibbon, E. (2019). Truth and reconciliation: Health care organizational leadership. *Healthcare Management Forum, 32*(1), 20–24. https://doi.org/10.1177/0840470418803379

McGibbon, E., & Lukeman, S. (2019). Critical social justice: The moral imperative for critical perspectives in nursing. *Witness: The Canadian Journal of Critical Nursing Discourse, 1*(1), 3–12. https://doi.org/10.25071/2291-5796.21

McGibbon, E., & Mbugua, J. (2018). Race and racialization in health, health care, and nursing education. In M. McIntyre & C. McDonald (Eds.), *Realities of Canadian nursing* (5th ed.). Wolters Kluwer Health.

McGibbon, E., Mulaudzi, M., Didham, P., Barton, S., & Sochan, A. (2013). Towards decolonizing nursing: The colonization of nursing and strategies to increase the counter-narrative. *Nursing Inquiry, 21*(3), 179–191. https://doi.org/10.1111/nin.12042

McPhearson, T., Raymond, C. M., Gulsrud, N., Albert, C., Coles, N., Fagerholm, N., Nagatsu, M., Olafsson, A. S., Soininen, N., & Vierikko, K. (2021). Radical changes are needed for transformations to a good Anthropocene. *npj Urban Sustainability, 1*(1), 5. https://doi.org/10.1038/s42949-021-00017-x

McGregor, D., Whitaker, S., & Sritharan, M. (2020). Indigenous environmental justice and sustainability. *Current Opinion in Environmental Sustainability, 43*, 35–50. https://doi.org/10.1016/j.cosust.2020.01.007

McSheffrey, E. (2023, June 2). *B.C. extends order to stop old-growth logging in Fairy Creek watershed*. Global News. https://globalnews.ca/news/9742092/bc-extends-order-stop-old-growth-logging-fairy-creek/

Miéville, C. (2022). *A spectre, haunting: On the communist manifesto.* Haymarket Books.
MilieuDefensie. (n.d.). *We are suing ING in a ground breaking new climate case.* Friends of the Earth Netherlands. https://en.milieudefensie.nl/
Miskanawah. (n.d.). *Join for our 18th annual friendship round dance.* https://miskanawah.ca/annual-round-dance
Moore, J. W. (2017). The Capitalocene, Part I: On the nature and origins of our ecological crisis. *The Journal of Peasant Studies, 44*(3), 594–630. https://doi.org/10.1080/03066150.2016.1235036
Moye, J. (2021, August 28). *In British Columbia, the fight for old growth rages on.* Outside. https://www.outsideonline.com/outdoor-adventure/environment/old-growth-trees-british-columbia-rainforest-flying-squad/
Mozumder, M. M. H., Pyhälä, A., Wahab, M. A., Sarkki, S., Schneider, P., & Islam, M. M. (2020). Governance and power dynamics in a small-scale hilsa shad (*Tenualosa ilisha*) fishery: A case study from Bangladesh. *Sustainability, 12*(14), 5738. https://doi.org/10.3390/su12145738
Nash, R., Hudson, A., & Luttrell, C. (2006). *Mapping political context: A toolkit for civil society organisations.* Overseas Development Institute.
Pace News. (n.d.). *The political compass.* https://www.politicalcompass.org/
Paul, D. N. (2006). *We were not the savages: Collision between European and Native American civilizations.* Fernwood Publishing.
People's Health Movement (PHM). (n.d.). *About the People's Health Movement.* https://phmovement.org/about
PHM Global Secretariat. (n.d.). *The People's Charter for Health.* https://phmovement.org/the-peoples-charter-for-health
Piketty, T. (2021). *Time for socialism: Dispatches from a world on fire, 2016–2021.* Yale University Press.
Pintauro, K. (2017, March 16). Environmental justice in the Anthropocene symposium, April 24–25. *Colorado State University College News.* https://source.colostate.edu/soges-host-environmental-justice-anthropocene-symposium-april/
Prakash, G. (1994). Subaltern studies as postcolonial criticism. *The American Historical Review, 99*(5), 1475–1490.
Raphael, D. (2021). Raising the volume on the social determinants of health in Canada and elsewhere. In E. McGibbon (Ed.), *Oppression: A social determinant of health* (2nd ed.). Fernwood Publishing.
Raphael, D., Bryant, T., Govender, P., Medvedyuk, S., & Mendly-Zambo, Z. (2022). Desperately seeking reductions in health inequalities in Canada: Polemics and anger mobilization as the way forward? *Sociology of Health & Illness, 44*(1), 130–146. https://doi.org/10.1111/1467-9566.13399
Ratcliffe, S. (Ed.). (2017). *Oxford essential quotations* (5th ed.). Oxford University Press.

Ratima, M., Martin, D., Castleden, H., & Delormier, T. (2019). Indigenous voices and knowledge systems—Promoting planetary health, health equity, and sustainable development now and for future generations. *Global Health Promotion, 26*(Suppl. 3), 3–5. https://doi.org/10.1177/1757975919838487

Schrecker, T. (2016). Neoliberalism and health: The linkages and the dangers. *Sociology Compass, 10*(10), 952–971. https://doi.org/10.1111/soc4.12408

Schrecker, T. (2023). Downing the master's tools? New research strategies to address social determinants of health inequalities. *International Journal of Social Determinants of Health and Health Services, 53*(3), 253–265. https://doi.org/10.1177/27551938231161932

Sharpe, G. (1973). *The politics of nonviolent action*. Porter Sargent.

Shiva, V. (2013). *Making peace with the earth*. Pluto Press.

Thapliyal, N. (2022). Economic literacy otherwise: A critical reflection on educating for earth-centred, caring economies in a migrant-settler colony. *Policy & Practice: A Development Education Review,* (35), 14–33. https://www.developmenteducationreview.com/issue/issue-35/economic-literacy-otherwise-critical-reflection-educating-earth-centred-caring

United Nations Environment Programme (UNEP). (2022, October 27). *Emissions gap report 2022: The closing window—Climate crisis calls for rapid transformation of societies.* https://www.unep.org/emissions-gap-report-2022

United Nations News. (2022, October 27). *Climate change: No "credible pathway" to 1.5C limit, UNEP warns.* https://news.un.org/en/story/2022/10/1129912

United States Holocaust Memorial Museum. (2023, April 11). *Martin Niemöller: "First they came for..."* Holocaust Encyclopedia. https://encyclopedia.ushmm.org/content/en/article/martin-niemoeller-first-they-came-for-the-socialists

Utt, J. (2013, November 8). *So you call yourself an ally: 10 things all "allies" need to know*. Everyday Feminism. https://everydayfeminism.com/2013/11/things-allies-need-to-know/

Wehrmann, B. (2023, June 5). *German chancellor promises monitoring of renewables expansion to stay on track for 2030 target*. Journalism for the Energy Transition. https://www.cleanenergywire.org/news/german-chancellor-promises-monitoring-renewables-expansion-stay-track-2030-target

Williams, L. (2017). Empowerment and the ecological determinants of health: Three critical capacities for practitioners. *Health Promotion International, 32*(4), 711–722. https://doi.org/10.1093/heapro/daw011

Workman, T. (2011). The left after politics. *Studies in Political Economy, 87*(1), 173–183.

World Health Organization (WHO). (1978). *Declaration of Alma-Ata*.

Wright, E. O. (2021). *How to be an anti-capitalist in the twenty-first century*. Verso Books.

INDEX

MIX
Papier | Fördert gute Waldnutzung
FSC® C083411

Kolibri 360 GmbH
Ferdinand-Jühlke-Straße 7
99095 Erfurt, Deutschland
produktsicherheit@kolibri360.de